NOC and NIC Linkages

to NANDA-I and Clinical Conditions

Supporting Critical Reasoning and Quality Care

NOC and NIC Linkages
to NANDA-I and Clinical Conditions

Supporting Critical Reasoning and Quality Care

Marion Johnson, PhD, RN

Sue Moorhead, PhD, RN

Gloria Bulechek, PhD, RN, FAAN

Howard Butcher, PhD, RN, PMHCNS-BC

Meridean Maas, PhD, RN, FAAN

Elizabeth Swanson, PhD, RN

Center for Nursing Classification
& Clinical Effectiveness
Sharon Sweeney, BSB, Center Coordinator
The University of Iowa
College of Nursing

ELSEVIER
MOSBY

KH

ELSEVIER
MOSBY

3251 Riverport Lane
Maryland Heights, MO 63043

Notice

Knowledge and best practice in this field are constantly changing. As new research and experience broaden
our knowledge, changes in practice, treatment and drug therapy may become necessary or appropriate.
Readers are advised to check the most current information provided (i) on procedures featured or (ii) by
the manufacturer of each product to be administered, to verify the recommended dose or formula, the
method and duration of administration, and contraindications. It is the responsibility of the practitioner,
relying on their own experience and knowledge of the patient, to make diagnoses, to determine dosages and
the best treatment for each individual patient, and to take all appropriate safety precautions. To the fullest
extent of the law, neither the Publisher nor the [Editors/Authors] [delete as appropriate] assumes any liabil-
ity for any injury and/or damage to persons or property arising out of or related to any use of the material
contained in this book.

The Publisher

Senior Editor: Sandra Clark
Senior Developmental Editor: Charlene Ketchum
Publishing Services Manager: Jeffrey Patterson
Project Manager: Mary G. Stueck
Designer: Kimberly Denando

Printed in the United States of America

Last digit is the print number: 9 8 7 6 5 4 3 2 1

1/16/15

This edition of the book consists of four parts. Part I includes three chapters that describe the languages and their uses. Part II provides the linkages among NANDA-I diagnoses, NOC outcomes, and NIC interventions. Parts I and II were included in the previous editions of this text. Part III is new; it describes links between NOC and NIC and selected clinical conditions. Part IV, also included previously, includes appendixes listing NOC and NIC labels and definitions.

The title for the third edition of the book changed to reflect the addition of links to clinical conditions. The major portion of the book continues to contain the NOC and NIC linkages to NANDA-I diagnoses, but now with the addition of linkages for ten common clinical conditions that nurses see frequently in their practice. The conditions include Asthma, Chronic Obstructive Pulmonary Disease, Colon and Rectal Cancer, Diabetes Mellitus, Depression, Heart Failure, Hypertension, Pneumonia, Stroke, and Total Joint Replacement: Knee/Hip. These conditions are prevalent in the United States, are often chronic, and can carry considerable cost for the patient and for society.

The standardized nursing languages used in the book are 2009–2011 diagnoses of NANDA International, the Nursing Outcomes Classification (NOC) terms published in the 4th edition, and the Nursing Intervention Classification (NIC) terms published in the 5th edition. The illustration of how these three languages can be linked together shows the relationship among nursing diagnoses, outcomes, and interventions and can facilitate clinical reasoning. The book can assist nurses to develop plans of care for individual patients or for patient populations, and can be of use in electronic information systems. Providing linkages among a nursing diagnosis, an outcome, and the interventions selected to manage the diagnosis and meet the outcome allows for the evaluation of nursing care for patient populations and the determination of nursing effectiveness.

Part I of the book contains three chapters. The first two are similar to chapters in previous editions and the third chapter is completely new. Chapter 1 provides a brief overview of the three languages, a description of how the linkage work has progressed over time, and the changes found in the presentation of the linkages. Chapter 2 focuses on how the linkages can be used in designing nursing care, computer-based information systems, and in clinical reasoning and decision-making. It provides an overview of using the Outcome-Present State (OPT) Model as an example of clinical reasoning that can be particularly helpful when teaching students. Chapter 3 takes a different focus, discussing how the languages can be used in the design and application of electronic nursing information systems. This chapter will be useful to nurses who need to identify the information they want from an electronic system and how they can make use of it, as well as information technology nurses who assist in system design and implementation in their organization. The authors are interested in feedback on the usefulness of this chapter and whether it or a similar chapter should be included in future editions.

Part II consists of the linkages between NANDA-I diagnoses, NOC outcomes, and NIC interventions. The links are entered through the NANDA-I diagnosis. The diagnoses are listed alphabetically with two exceptions: (1) the "risk for" diagnoses are in one section following the diagnoses focused on actual problems and health promotion; and (2) the major concept is used for determining how the diagnosis is listed. For example, Impaired Swallowing will be found under Swallowing, Impaired, and Imbalanced Nutrition: Less than Body Requirements is under Nutrition, Imbalanced: Less than Body Requirements. Suggested NOC outcomes are linked to each of the diagnoses, and suggested NIC interventions are linked to each of the outcomes. Definitions for the diagnosis and outcomes are provided in the table, and Part IV: Appendixes provides definitions for both the outcomes and the interventions.

Changes have been made in the selection of the outcomes and the interventions. The outcomes selected reflect the measurement of: (1) the reversal of the problem identified in an actual diagnosis, (2) improvement of the patient state identified by the defining characteristics of the nursing diagnosis and (3) the actual problem to be prevented as well as outcomes that address the related factors in the "risk for" diagnoses. Interventions to consider choosing for the related factors precede each NANDA-I, NOC, NIC linkages. This assists in identifying those outcomes and interventions that directly address the current patient state as defined by the diagnosis and defining characteristics. Clinical reasoning notes were added to some of the diagnoses to clarify the reason for a selection or to identify why some outcomes/interventions were chosen or not chosen. These are major changes in the reasoning process used to identify outcomes and interventions; previously outcomes and interventions that addressed the diagnosis, defining characteristics, and related factors were included in the all linkages.

The "risk for" diagnoses linkages were revised to prevent repeating the same or similar outcomes and interventions used with an actual diagnosis when there is a corresponding "risk for" diagnosis; for example, Situational Low Self-Esteem and Risk for Situational Low Self-Esteem.

In previous editions, the outcomes for measuring prevention of the "risk for" state, in this case low self-esteem, were generally a modified repetition of the outcomes for measuring resolution of the actual state, chronic low self-esteem. In this edition, the outcome Self-Esteem that measures whether low self-esteem occurs when using the diagnosis Risk for Situational Low Self-Esteem is presented as the outcome to measure the occurrence of the "risk" problem. Interventions to achieve this outcome can be found with the actual diagnosis, Chronic Low Self-Esteem. Following this outcome are a list of NOC outcomes and a list of interventions associated with the risk factors for low self-esteem. The interventions are not linked to the outcomes because the list of outcomes can include only a few or many labels; if the list is over 20 labels, it becomes prohibitive to provide interventions for each of the outcomes, especially when an intervention can be applicable to more than one outcome. Again, these are major changes in the reasoning process behind the presentation of the "risk for" diagnoses, and feedback from users of this text on the usefulness, or not, of these changes would be appreciated.

Part III is a new section in this edition. It includes the ten clinical conditions identified previously. Each condition has a brief description that includes the prevalence, mortality, and cost as appropriate for each condition, as well as a concise overview of the course of the condition and/or the symptoms of the condition. This description is followed by a generic plan of care that illustrates the use of NOC outcomes and NIC interventions for the clinical condition. The care plans generally do not encompass the condition from diagnosis throughout the course of the illness because many of the conditions are chronic and will last for the remainder of the the patient's life. This section is a brief illustration of the use of NOC outcomes and NIC interventions if the clinical condition is described using a term that does not appear in NANDA-I. Possible outcomes are presented with a brief list of interventions appropriate for the clinical condition. In most instances the reader can readily identify the nursing diagnosis that might represent the patient state implied in the outcome.

As with previous editions, we appreciate all feedback; positive and negative, regarding what to change and what not to change and how to strengthen the book for the various users. This is of particular interest because of the changes made in this edition.

Marion Johnson

UNIFYING NURSING LANGUAGES

Consider the English language. There are as many variations as there are nationalities who claim it as their mother tongue. In the United Kingdom, for example, people put their shopping in the boot. In North America, people put boots on their feet and shopping purchases in the trunk. Even as I write this foreword, the differences in language are apparent. There is a squiggly red line underneath my UK English spelling of the word "center" and the only way to make it go away is to change my default language to US English.

Although amusing anecdotes illustrating how we are divided by our common language make wonderful dinner conversations, safe clinical practice and effective research and education rely on consistency within language, particularly in relation to nursing diagnoses, interventions, and outcomes.

The fact that you are holding a book that addresses this issue means that you are a person who recognises that you can be part of the solution.

NANDA International and the Center for Nursing Classification and Clinical Effectiveness at the University of Iowa's College of Nursing (the Center) continue to develop and promulgate the world's foremost evidence-based nursing classifications of nursing diagnoses, interventions, and outcomes. This book demonstrates the positive impact that a closer working relationship between NANDA International and the Center can have on patient safety.

As President of NANDA International, I am personally committed to further developing this relationship for the benefit of safer patient care and commend this work to you.

Professor Dickon Weir-Hughes
President, NANDA International

CONTRIBUTORS

Joanne Dochterman, PhD
Professor Emerita
The University of Iowa
College of Nursing
Iowa City, Iowa

Barbara J. Head, PhD, RN
Assistant Professor Emerita
University of Nebraska Medical
    Center
Omaha, Nebraska

Cindy A. Scherb, PhD, RN
Professor
Graduate Programs in Nursing
Winona State University
University Center Rochester
Rochester, Minnesota

REVIEWERS

Jane M. Brokel, RN, PhD
College of Nursing
The University of Iowa
Iowa City, Iowa

Jeanette M. Daly, RN, PhD
Department of Family Medicine
University of Iowa
Iowa City, Iowa

PRIOR CONTRIBUTORS

Joanne McCloskey Dochterman

CONTENTS

CHAPTER 1

Languages and Development of the Linkages

Sue Moorhead and Joanne McCloskey Dochterman

THE LANGUAGES

Nursing is striving to build a knowledge base that supports professional practice and improves the quality of care provided by nurses in a variety of settings across the health care continuum. This need for representation and classification of the knowledge base of nursing continues to be an issue for the profession (Kautz, Kuiper, Pesut, & Williams, 2006). Essential to this knowledge base is knowledge of nursing diagnoses, patient outcomes, and nursing interventions (Lavin, Meyers, & Ellis, 2007). Experience helps nurses gain expertise in nursing practice and clarify the relationships of problems, outcomes, and interventions in a specialty area or with a specific patient population. Today the Internet also serves as a resource for nurses seeking current professional practice information.

As early as 1969 Abdellah stated that nursing diagnoses were the foundation of nursing science (Abdellah, 1969). The need for uniform or standardized nursing languages (SNL) has been discussed in nursing literature for the past 35 years (Anderson, Keenan, & Jones, 2009; Bakken & Currie, 2011; Clancy, Delaney, Morrison, & Gunn, 2006; Dochterman & Jones, 2003; Fischetti, 2008; Gebbie & Lavin, 1975; Hunt, Sproat, & Kitzmiller, 2004; Jones, 1997; Keenan & Aquilino, 1998; Lunney, Delaney, Duffy, Moorhead, & Welton, 2005; Maas, 1985; McCloskey & Bulechek, 1994; McCormick, 1991; Muller-Staub, Needham, Odenbreit, Lavin, & Van Achterberg, 2007; Pesut, 2006; Zielstorff, 1994). A uniform nursing language serves several purposes, including the following:

- Provides a standard language to facilitate communication both among nurses and between nurses and other health care professionals, as well as the public

- Allows the collection and analysis of uniform information documenting nursing's contribution to patient care
- Facilitates the evaluation and improvement of nursing care through outcome evaluation
- Fosters the development of nursing knowledge to support the nursing process
- Supports the development of electronic clinical information systems and electronic health records
- Provides the concepts for electronic data warehouses for quality improvement initiatives and effectiveness research
- Provides information for the formulation of organizational and public policy concerning health and nursing care
- Facilitates teaching clinical reasoning skills to nursing students and novice nurses

The contribution of standardized languages to the practice and development of nursing is described in detail in the articles previously cited as well as in the books describing the Nursing Interventions Classification (Bulechek, Butcher, & Dochterman, 2008; Dochterman & Bulechek, 2004; McCloskey & Bulechek, 1992, 1996, 2000) and the Nursing Outcomes Classification (Johnson & Maas, 1997; Johnson, Maas, & Moorhead, 2000; Moorhead, Johnson, & Maas, 2004; Moorhead, Johnson, Maas, & Swanson, 2008).

This book illustrates linkages between three of the standardized languages recognized by the American Nurses Association (ANA): (1) the diagnoses developed by NANDA International (NANDA-I), (2) the interventions of the Nursing Interventions Classification (NIC), and (3) the outcomes of the Nursing Outcomes Classification (NOC). The provision of links between these classifications is a major advancement in facilitating the use of these standardized nursing languages in practice, education, and research. The implementation of NANDA-I, NOC, and NIC (NNN) has also increased the practicality and efficiency of managing nursing data (Lavin, Avant, Craft-Rosenberg, Herdman, & Gebbie, 2004). Nurses are faced with complicated clinical situations where the interpretation of patient data is complex and diverse (Lunney, 2003) and is driven by the context of care (Levin, Lunney, & Krainovich-Miller, 2004). These linkages support the critical thinking and reasoning skills needed by nurses to care for patients with multiple chronic conditions. The link between the use of standardized nursing languages and critical thinking is well documented in the nursing literature (Bartlett et al., 2008; Bland et al., 2009; Farren, 2010; Fesler-Birch, 2005; Kautz et al., 2006, Lunney, 2003, 2006, 2009; Pesut & Herman, 1998, 1999; Simmons, Lanuza, Fonteyn, Hicks, & Holm, 2003). A review of the literature by Anderson and colleagues (2009) identified that NANDA-I, NIC, and NOC demonstrated the "strongest and most noteworthy patterns of sustainability" (p. 89). For the first time this book provides linkages of NOC and NIC to some common clinical conditions that nurses treat with other disciplines. For those unfamiliar with the languages, a brief overview of each classification follows.

NANDA International

The use of standardized nursing language began in the 1970s with the development of NANDA's diagnostic classification. A nursing diagnosis is "a clinical judgment about individual, family, or community responses to actual or potential health problems/life processes. A nursing diagnosis provides the basis for selection of nursing interventions to achieve outcomes for which the nurse is accountable" (NANDA International, 2009, p. 419). Nursing diagnoses describe actual, potential (is at risk for development), and health promotion needs. The elements of an actual NANDA-I diagnosis are the label, the definition of the diagnosis, the defining characteristics (signs and symptoms), and the related factors (causative or associated factors), as illustrated in Table 1-1. The elements of a potential diagnosis as defined by NANDA-I are the label, the definition, and the associated risk factors. The elements of a health promotion diagnosis are the label, definition, and defining characteristics; an exception to this is the *Readiness for Enhanced Resilience* that also includes related factors.

NANDA was established in 1973 when a group of nurses met in St. Louis, Missouri, and organized the first National Conference Group for the Classification of Nursing Diagnoses (Gebbie & Lavin, 1975). In 2002 the name of the organization was changed to NANDA International to better reflect the membership from multiple countries. NANDA International is a membership organization directed by an elected president and board of directors. The Diagnosis Development Committee (DDC) reviews new and refined diagnoses submitted by members and a taxonomy committee adds diagnoses to the taxonomic structure and refines the taxonomy. In 2009 the NANDA-I classification included 202 diagnoses; *Taxonomy II* was first published in 2003 with 13 domains and 36 classes. NANDA-I representatives, along with representatives from NIC and NOC, participated in the development of the *Taxonomy of Nursing Practice*,

TABLE 1-1   One Example of a NANDA-I Diagnosis
Self-Esteem, Situational Low—00120
DEFINITION: Development of a negative perception of self-worth in response to a current situation (specify)
DEFINING CHARACTERISTICS: Evaluation of self as unable to deal with events; evaluation of self as unable to deal with situations; expressions of helplessness; expressions of uselessness; indecisive behavior; nonassertive behavior; self-negating verbalizations; verbally reports current situational challenge to self-worth
RELATED FACTORS: Behavior inconsistent with values; developmental changes; disturbed body image; failures; functional impairment; lack of recognition; loss; rejections; social role changes

From NANDA International. (2009). *Nursing diagnoses: Definitions and classification 2009-2011* (p. 193). West Sussex, United Kingdom: Wiley-Blackwell.

a unifying structure for the placement of diagnoses, interventions, and outcomes, published in 2003 (Dochterman & Jones, 2003). NANDA-I terminology has been translated into 15 languages and is used in 32 countries. The NANDA-I organization publishes a classification book every 3 years and sponsors the *International Journal of Nursing Terminologies and Classifications*, previously titled *Nursing Diagnosis: The Journal of Nursing Language and Classification*. More information about the organization and the classification can be found at *www.NANDA.org*.

NIC

Research to develop a vocabulary and classification of nursing interventions began in 1987 with the formation of a research team led by Joanne McCloskey (now Joanne Dochterman) and Gloria Bulechek at the University of Iowa. The team developed the Nursing Interventions Classification (NIC)—a comprehensive, standardized classification of nursing interventions, first published in 1992. Unlike a nursing diagnosis or patient outcome in which the focus of concern is the patient, the focus of concern with nursing interventions is nursing behavior—nursing actions that assist the patient to progress toward a desired outcome.

An intervention is defined as:

Any treatment, based upon clinical judgment and knowledge, that a nurse performs to enhance patient/client outcomes. Nursing interventions include both direct and indirect care; those aimed at individuals, families, and the community; and those for nurse-initiated, physician-initiated and other provider-initiated treatments (Bulechek, Butcher, & Dochterman, 2008, p. xxii).

Each NIC intervention consists of a label name, a definition, a set of activities that indicate the actions and principles constituting the delivery of the intervention, and a short list of background readings, as illustrated in Table 1-2. The intervention label name and the definition are the content of the intervention that is standardized and should not be changed when NIC is used to document care. Care can be individualized, however, through the choice of activities. From a list of approximately 10 to 30 activities per intervention, the nurse selects the activities most appropriate for the specific individual, family, or community. The nurse can add new

activities if needed; however, all modifications and additions should be congruent with the definition of the intervention.

The NIC is continually updated and has been published in five editions; the 2008 edition contains 542 interventions and more than 12,000 activities. The interventions are grouped for ease of use into 30 classes and 7 domains to create the taxonomy for the classification. NIC can be used in all settings (from intensive care units to home care, hospice care, and primary care settings) and in all specialties (from pediatrics and obstetrics to cardiology and gerontology). Although the entire classification describes the domain of nursing, some of the interventions can be provided by other disciplines. Health care providers other than nurses are welcome to use NIC to describe their treatments.

The classification book as well as multiple other publications cited in this book document the years of research required to develop and test the classification and its taxonomic structure. NIC interventions have been linked to NANDA-I diagnoses, to Omaha System problems, to the Resident Assessment Instrument used in long-term care facilities, to OASIS (Outcome and Assessment Information Set) categories for home health care, and to NOC outcomes. The NIC classification has been translated into nine languages. The classification is continually updated through an ongoing process of feedback and review from users. Review work is conducted between editions of the NIC book and new interventions are developed and added from those submitted. A list of publications are available from the Center for Nursing Classification and Clinical Effectiveness at The University of Iowa, College of Nursing, Iowa City, IA 52242. Current information is available at *www.nursing.uiowa.edu/cnc*.

NOC

In 1991 a research team, led by Marion and Meridean Maas, was formed at the University of Iowa to develop a classification of patient outcomes correlated with nursing care. The work of the research team resulted in the Nursing Outcomes Classification (NOC)—a comprehensive, standardized classification of patient outcomes that can be used to evaluate the results of nursing interventions, first published in 1997.

Patient outcomes serve as the criteria against which to judge the success of a nursing intervention.

TABLE 1-2	One Example of a NIC Intervention

Self-Esteem Enhancement—5400

DEFINITION: Assisting a patient to increase his/her personal judgment of self-worth

Activities

Monitor patient's statements of self-worth

Determine patient's locus of control

Determine patient's confidence in own judgment

Encourage patient to identify strengths

Encourage eye contact in communicating with others

Reinforce the personal strengths that patient identifies

Provide experiences that increase patient's autonomy, as appropriate

Assist patient to identify positive responses from others

Refrain from negatively criticizing

Refrain from teasing

Convey confidence in patient's ability to handle situation

Assist in setting realistic goals to achieve higher self-esteem

Assist patient to accept dependence on others, as appropriate

Assist patient to reexamine negative perceptions of self

Encourage increased responsibility for self, as appropriate

Assist patient to identify the impact of peer group on feelings of self-worth

Explore previous achievements of success

Explore reasons for self-criticism or guilt

Encourage the patient to evaluate own behavior

Encourage patient to accept new challenges

Reward or praise patient's progress toward reaching goals

Facilitate an environment and activities that will increase self-esteem

Assist patient to identify significance of culture, religion, race, gender, and age on self-esteem

Instruct parents on the importance of their interest and support in their children's development of a positive self-concept

Instruct parents to set clear expectations and to define limits with their children

Teach parents to recognize children's accomplishments

Monitor frequency of self-negating verbalizations

Monitor lack of follow-through in goal attainment

Monitor levels of self-esteem over time, as appropriate

Make positive statements about patient

From Bulechek, G., Butcher, H., & Dochterman, J. (Eds.). (2008). *Nursing interventions classification (NIC)* (5th ed., pp. 641–642). St. Louis: Mosby Elsevier.
1st edition 1992

BACKGROUND READINGS

Bunten, D. (2001). Normal changes with aging. In M. L. Maas, K. C. Buckwalter, M. D. Hardy, T. Tripp-Reimer, M. G. Titler, & J. P. Specht (Eds.), *Nursing care of older adults: Diagnoses, outcomes, & interventions* (p. 519). St. Louis: Mosby.

Byers, P. H. (1990). Enhancing the self-esteem of inpatient alcoholics. *Issues in Mental Health Nursing, 11*(4), 337–346.

Luckmann, J., & Sorensen, K. C. (1987). *Medical-surgical nursing* (3rd ed.). Philadelphia: W. B. Saunders.

Norris, J., & Kunes-Connell, M. (1985). Self-esteem disturbance. *Nursing Clinics of North America, 20*(4), 745–761.

Reasoner, R. W. (1983). Enhancement of self-esteem in children and adolescents. *Family and Community Health, 6*(2), 51–63.

Whall, A. L., & Parent, C. J. (1991). Self-esteem disturbance. In M. Maas, K. Buckwalter, & M. Hardy (Eds.), *Nursing diagnosis and interventions for the elderly* (pp. 480–488). Redwood City, CA: Addison-Wesley.

An outcome is defined as "an individual, family, or community state, behavior, or perception that is measured along a continuum in response to a nursing intervention(s)" (Moorhead et al., 2008, p. 30). It is recognized that a number of variables, in addition to the intervention, influence patient outcomes. These variables range from the process used in providing the care, including the actions of other health care providers; to organizational and environmental variables that influence how interventions are selected and provided; to patient characteristics, including the patient's physical and emotional health, as well as the life circumstances experienced by the patient. Because the outcomes describe the status of the patient, other disciplines may find them useful for the evaluation of their interventions.

Each NOC outcome has a label name, a definition, a list of indicators to evaluate patient status in relation to the outcome, a five-point Likert scale to measure patient status, and a short list of references used in the development of the outcome, as illustrated in Table 1-3. The scales allow measurement of the outcome status at any point on a continuum from most negative to most positive, as well as identification of changes in patient status at different points in time. In contrast to the information provided by a goal statement, that is, whether or not a goal is met, NOC outcomes can be used to monitor progress, or lack of progress, throughout an episode of care and across different care settings. The outcomes have been developed to be used in all settings, all specialties, and across the care continuum. The fourth edition of the classification published in 2008 contained 385 outcomes grouped into 33 classes and 7 domains for ease of use. The classification is continually updated to include new outcomes and to revise older outcomes based on new research or user feedback.

The NOC classification books and numerous other publications document the extensive research to develop and validate NOC. The outcomes have been linked to: NANDA-I diagnoses, Omaha System problems, Gordon's functional patterns, the Long-Term Care Minimum Data Set, the Resident Assessment Instrument used in long-term care facilities, and to NIC interventions. The NOC classification has been translated into 10 languages and is experiencing growing use across the United States and worldwide. Current information about NOC is available on the Center for Nursing Classification and Clinical Effectiveness web page: *www.nursing.uiowa.edu/cnc*.

DEVELOPMENT OF THE LINKAGES

Part II of the book links NANDA-I diagnoses, NOC outcomes, and NIC interventions. The work represents the judgment of selected members of the NIC and NOC research teams, including academicians, clinicians, and students. Data collected during the evaluation of NOC outcomes in clinical sites were used when available. The data showed aggregated links between NOC outcomes, NIC interventions, and NANDA-I diagnoses based on clinician's selections for individual patients. The aggregated data provided information about the outcomes and interventions clinicians select for nursing diagnoses that served as a resource to compare clinical decisions and expert opinion for some of the diagnoses. *However, it is important to recognize that the linkages in this book are not intended to be prescriptive and do not replace the clinical judgment of the nurse.* In addition to the linkages provided in this book, users may select other outcomes and interventions for a particular diagnosis for an individual patient. The linkages presented here illustrate how three distinct nursing languages can be connected and used together when planning care for an individual patient or a group of patients.

Description of the Linkages

The linkages in this book are between the NANDA-I diagnoses, the NIC interventions, and the NOC outcomes. A linkage can be defined as that which directs the relationship or association of concepts. The links between the NANDA-I diagnoses and the NOC outcomes suggest the relationships between the patient's problem or current status and those aspects of the problem or status that are expected to be resolved or improved by one or more interventions. The links between the NANDA-I diagnoses and the NIC interventions suggest the relationship between the patient's problem and the nursing actions that will resolve or diminish the problem. The links between the NOC outcomes and the NIC interventions suggest a similar relationship focused on the resolution of a problem and the nursing actions directed at problem resolution, that is, the outcome that the intervention(s) (are) expected to influence.

TABLE 1-3 One Example of a NOC Outcome

Self-Esteem—1205

DOMAIN: Psychosocial Health (III)

CLASS: Psychological Well-Being (M)

SCALE(S): Never positive to Consistently positive (k)

DEFINITION: Personal judgment of self-worth

OUTCOME TARGET RATING: Maintain at _____   Increase to _____

CARE RECIPIENT:

DATA SOURCE:

	Never Positive	Rarely Positive	Sometimes Positive	Often Positive	Consistently Positive	
Self-Esteem Overall Rating	1	2	3	4	5	
Indicators:						
120501 Verbalizations of self-acceptance	1	2	3	4	5	NA
120502 Acceptance of self-limitations	1	2	3	4	5	NA
120503 Maintenance of erect posture	1	2	3	4	5	NA
120504 Maintenance of eye contact	1	2	3	4	5	NA
120505 Description of self	1	2	3	4	5	NA
120506 Regard for others	1	2	3	4	5	NA
120507 Open communication	1	2	3	4	5	NA
120508 Fulfillment of personally significant roles	1	2	3	4	5	NA
120509 Maintenance of grooming and hygiene	1	2	3	4	5	NA
120510 Balance of participation and listening in groups	1	2	3	4	5	NA
120511 Confidence level	1	2	3	4	5	NA
120512 Acceptance of compliments from others	1	2	3	4	5	NA
120513 Expected response from others	1	2	3	4	5	NA
120514 Acceptance of constructive criticism	1	2	3	4	5	NA
120515 Willingness to confront others	1	2	3	4	5	NA
120521 Description of success in work	1	2	3	4	5	NA
120522 Description of success in school	1	2	3	4	5	NA
120517 Description of success in social groups	1	2	3	4	5	NA
120518 Description of pride in self	1	2	3	4	5	NA
120519 Feelings about self-worth	1	2	3	4	5	NA

From Moorhead, S., Johnson, M., Maas, M., & Swanson, E. (Eds.). (2008). *Nursing outcomes classification (NOC)* (4th ed., p. 638). St. Louis: Mosby Elsevier.

1st edition 1997; Revised 4th edition

OUTCOME CONTENT REFERENCES

Bonham, P., & Cheney, A. (1982). Concept of self: A framework for nursing assessment. In P. L. Chinn (Ed.), *Advances in nursing theory development* (pp. 173–189). Rockville, MD: Aspen.

Coopersmith, S. (1967). *The antecedents of self-esteem.* San Francisco: W. H. Freeman.

Crandall, R. (1973). The measurement of self-esteem and related constructs. In J. P. Robinson & P. R. Shaver (Eds.), *Measures of social psychological attitudes.* Ann Arbor, MI: Institute for Social Research, University of Michigan.

Fitts, W. (1965). *Manual for the Tennessee Self-Concept Scale.* Nashville: Counselor Recordings & Tests.

Groh, C. J., & Whall, A. L. (2001). Self-esteem disturbance. In M. Maas, K. Buckwalter, M. Hardy, T. Tripp-Reimer, M. Titler, & J. Specht (Eds.), *Nursing care of older adults: Diagnoses, outcomes & interventions* (pp. 593–600). St. Louis: Mosby.

Larson, J. (1989). Validation of the defining characteristics of disturbance in self-esteem in patients with anorexia nervosa. In R. Carroll-Johnson (Ed.), *Classification of nursing diagnoses: Proceedings of the eighth conference (North American Nursing Diagnosis Association)* (pp. 307–312). Philadelphia: J.B. Lippincott.

Nugent, W. R., & Thomas, J. W. (1993). Validation of a clinical measure of self-esteem. *Research on Social Work Practice, 3*(2), 191–207.

Roid, G., & Fitts, W. (1988). *Tennessee Self-Concept Scale: Revised manual.* Los Angeles: Western Psychological Services.

Rosenberg, M. (1965). *Society & adolescent self image.* Princeton, NJ: Princeton University Press.

Stanwyck, D. (1983). Self-esteem through the life span. *Family and Community Health, 6*(2), 11–28.

The concept names and definitions used in the linkages are those in the 2009-2011 edition of *NANDA International Nursing Diagnoses: Definitions & Classification* (2009), the fifth edition of *Nursing Interventions Classification (NIC)* (Bulechek et al., 2008), and the fourth edition of *Nursing Outcomes Classification (NOC)* (Moorhead et al., 2008). The NANDA-I diagnosis is the starting point for the linkages. The diagnoses are listed in alphabetical order except for the risk diagnoses, which are listed alphabetically following the other diagnoses. However, the NANDA-I diagnostic name has been reordered when the initial term does not specify the concept of concern in the diagnostic label; for example, *Ineffective Thermoregulation* is presented in these linkages as *Thermoregulation: Ineffective*. Listing the diagnostic concept before the modifier facilitates the ease with which a diagnosis can be located. Each diagnosis contains the diagnostic name and the definition. Suggested NOC outcomes with associated NIC interventions are provided for each diagnosis. The definition for each of the selected outcomes is provided in the linkage table and in Appendix A. The interventions are identified as major or suggested interventions for achieving each of the recommended outcomes for a particular diagnosis. The optional category of nursing inerventions, used in the previous two editions of this book, is not used in this edition of the linkages. Definitions of the NIC interventions used in the linkages are listed in Appendix B. The alphabetical ordering of the diagnoses does not reflect the taxonomic structure used by NANDA-I. Likewise, the taxonomic and coding structures of NIC and NOC are not reflected in these linkages. The current taxonomic structure for each of these languages can be found in the books describing each language.

Development of the Linkages to NANDA-I

Previous linkage work in the first edition, *Nursing Diagnoses, Outcomes, & Interventions: NANDA, NOC, and NIC Linkages* (Johnson, Bulechek, Dochterman, Maas, & Moorhead, 2001) and the second edition, *NANDA, NOC, and NIC Linkages: Nursing Diagnoses, Outcomes, and Interventions* (Johnson et al., 2006) provided the starting point for revising and updating the links in this third edition. Prior linkage work used for the first edition included the development of links between NANDA diagnoses and NIC interventions, NANDA diagnoses and NOC outcomes, and NIC

interventions and NOC outcomes. Linkage work used for the current edition included the suggested outcomes for each NANDA-I diagnosis from the fourth edition of the *Nursing Outcomes Classification (NOC)* (Moorhead et al., 2008) and suggested interventions for each NANDA-I diagnosis in the fifth edition of the *Nursing Interventions Classification (NIC)* available online (Bulechek et al., 2008).

Third Edition Revision and Update

Linkages and methods developed for the first and second editions served as the basis for linkage revision in the third edition. The following steps were used to develop the current linkages:

1. Outcomes used in the second linkage book were compared with outcomes suggested for a diagnosis in the fourth edition of the NOC book (Moorhead et al., 2008). In many instances the outcomes in the second linkage book and the suggested outcomes in the current NOC book were the same. In other instances additional outcomes had been added to the list of suggested outcomes in the NOC book and these were added to the diagnosis in the linkage book. In a few instances some of the outcomes in the second linkage book were no longer on the suggested list in the current NOC book. Before these were removed, they were reviewed by all of the authors and sometimes the decision was made to retain them in the linkage book.

2. Interventions selected for each outcome in the second linkage book were reviewed against the interventions selected for the diagnosis in the current NIC book (Bulechek et al., 2008). Again, deletion or addition of interventions was based on author review and published linkages from other authors. The general tendency was to retain interventions rather than eliminate them. This provides more realistic options for clinicians when selecting interventions for patients of various ages and with diverse medical diagnoses and related problems.

3. Terminology for all three languages was updated to reflect changes in the editions used for each of the languages.

4. Formatting and technical changes were made in the linkages. To understand these changes carefully read the introductions to each section in Part II.

The final phase in the development of the linkages was second-level refinement. Because one person completed the initial links, it was important that others reviewed the linkage work. Reviewers were the other authors of this book and, in some instances, clinicians and graduate students with clinical expertise. Suggested changes were made in the linkages if there was agreement among the reviewers. If reviewer agreement was not reached, the suggested changes were presented to the authors for discussion and final decision.

The revision of linkages for this book required close scrutiny by the authors of previous and current linkage books. As a result, the linkages in this book, although similar to previously published linkage data, are not identical to the linkages found in this book's first or second edition or in the current editions of NIC and NOC. The decision to include or eliminate a particular outcome for a diagnosis based on the interventions recommended for that diagnosis was another source of controversy. For example, there were a few times when an outcome used in the linkage book was not linked to the diagnosis in the NOC book. This occurred if the appropriateness of the outcome became apparent when considering the interventions recommended for the diagnosis. Although rare, another difference occurred when not all of the interventions selected for a specific diagnosis in the NIC book were found in the linkage table. This transpired because not all possible outcomes that might be selected for a diagnosis are included in the linkage and some of the interventions would be more appropriate for the missing outcomes. Considering the number of diagnostic, outcome, and intervention linkages in this edition, the number of times there are significant differences between these linkages and those in the NOC and NIC books is minimal.

Clinical evaluation and testing of the linkages found in this book are needed. Clinical sites that use the three languages can aggregate and analyze data collected at their site to determine the outcomes and interventions selected for both nursing and medical diagnoses. The data can also be analyzed to determine which diagnoses, outcomes, and interventions are selected for patient populations delineated by age, medical diagnosis, or other parameters of interest. The linkages can also be tested in research studies that focus on selected patient populations or selected practice sites. Feedback from clinicians and others using the work will assist the authors to refine the linkages

for future editions. Previous linkage books have been translated into five languages, increasing the opportunities for international reviews of the linkage work. This is important because there may be cultural differences in how these classifications are linked.

Development of the Linkages to Clinical Conditions

New to this edition is a section that focuses on linkages to common clinical conditions that are treated with other disciplines. We focused on high-frequency, high-cost conditions that can be identified either by medical diagnoses or by adverse events, which nurses attempt to prevent. Each condition has a short summary about the condition followed by NOC outcomes and NIC interventions commonly used when providing care for patients with these conditions. In this section NANDA International diagnoses are not used in the linkages because these interventions are closely related to the medical condition or serious complication. These linkages can be found in Part III.

CONCLUSION

NANDA-I, NIC, and NOC can be used together or separately. Together they represent the domain of nursing in all settings and specialties. They have been recognized by the American Nurses Association (ANA) and Health Level 7 (HL7, the electronic messaging standards' organization in the United States) and included in the National Library of Medicine's Metathesaurus for a Unified Medical Language System (UMLS), the Cumulative Index to Nursing Literature (CINAHL), and the Systematized Nomenclature of Medicine-Clinical Terms (SNOMED-CT). Representatives from the three developing groups created the *Taxonomy of Nursing Practice* published by the American Nurses Association in 2003 (Dochterman & Jones, 2003). This common organizing structure should facilitate the use of all three languages. Multiple clinical agencies and educational settings across the United States and worldwide are using one or more of these nursing languages for the documentation of patient care and for the education of nursing students. In this book, we provide linkages between NOC outcomes and NIC interventions for NANDA-I diagnoses. Linking the three languages assists clinicians and students to select the outcomes and interventions most appropriate for the nursing diagnoses of their clients.

REFERENCES

Abdellah, F. G. (1969). The nature of nursing science. *Nursing Research, 18,* 390–393.

Anderson, C. A., Keenan, G., & Jones, J. (2009). Using bibliometrics to support your selection of a nursing terminology set. *CIN, Computers, Informatics, Nursing, 27*(2), 82–98.

Bakken, S., & Currie, L. M. (2011). Standardized terminologies and integrated information systems: Building blocks for transforming data into nursing knowledge. In P. S. Cowen & S. Moorhead (Eds.), *Current issues in nursing* (8th ed., pp. 287–296). St. Louis: Mosby Elsevier.

Bartlett, R., Bland, A., Rossen, E., Kautz, D., Benfield, S., & Carnevale, T. (2008). Evaluation of the Outcome-Present State Test Model as a way to teach clinical reasoning. *Journal of Nursing Education, 47*(8), 337–344.

Bland, A., Rossen, E., Bartlett, R., Kautz, D., Carnevale, T., & Benfield, S. (2009). Implementation and testing of the OPT model as a teaching strategy in an undergraduate psychiatric nursing course. *Nursing Education Perspectives, 30*(1), 14–21.

Bulechek, G. M., Butcher, H., & Dochterman, J. M. (Eds.). (2008). *Nursing interventions classification (NIC)* (5th ed.). St. Louis: Mosby/Elsevier.

Clancy, T. R., Delaney, C. W., Morrison, B., & Gunn, J. K. (2006). The benefits of standardized nursing languages in complex adaptive systems such as hospitals. *Journal of Nursing Administration, 36*(9), 426–434.

Dochterman, J. M., & Bulechek, G. M. (Eds.). (2004). *Nursing interventions classification (NIC)* (4th ed.). St. Louis: Mosby.

Dochterman, J. M., & Jones, D. A. (Eds.). (2003). *Unifying nursing languages: The harmonization of NANDA, NIC, and NOC.* Washington, DC: American Nurses Association.

Farren, A. T. (2010). An educational strategy for teaching standardized nursing languages. *International Journal of Nursing Terminologies and Classifications, 21*(1), 3–10.

Fesler-Birch, D. (2005). Critical thinking and patient outcomes: A review. *Nursing Outlook, 53*(2), 59–65.

Fischetti, N. (2008). Using standardized nursing languages: A case study exemplar in management of diabetes mellitus. *International Journal of Nursing Terminologies & Classifications, 19*(4), 163–166.

Gebbie, K., & Lavin. M. A. (1975). *Proceedings of the first national conference on the classification of nursing diagnoses.* St. Louis: Mosby.

Hunt, E. C., Sproat, S. B., & Kitzmiller, R. R. (2004). *The nursing informatics implementation guide.* New York: Springer.

Johnson, M., Bulechek, G., Dochterman, J. M., Maas, M., & Moorhead, S. (2001). *Nursing diagnoses, outcomes, & interventions: NANDA, NOC, and NIC linkages.* St. Louis: Mosby.

Johnson, M., Bulechek, G., Butcher, H., Dochterman, J. M., Maas, M., Moorhead, S., & Swanson, E. (2006). *NANDA, NOC, and NIC linkages: Nursing diagnoses, outcomes, and interventions* (2nd ed.). St. Louis: Mosby.

Johnson, M., & Maas, M. (Eds.). (1997). *Nursing outcomes classification (NOC)* (1st ed.). St. Louis: Mosby.

Johnson, M., Maas, M., & Moorhead, S. (Eds.). (2000). *Nursing outcomes classification (NOC)* (2nd ed.). St. Louis: Mosby.

Jones, D. L. (1997). Building the information infrastructure required for managed care. *Image: Journal of Nursing Scholarship, 29*(4), 377–382.

Kautz, D. D., Kuiper, R., Pesut, D. J., & Williams, R. L. (2006). Using NANDA, NIC, and NOC (NNN) language for clinical reasoning with the Outcome-Present State Test (OPT) Model. *International Journal of Nursing Terminologies and Classifications, 17*(3), 129–138.

Keenan, G., & Aquilino, M. L. (1998). Standardized nomenclatures: Keys to continuity of care, nursing accountability, and nursing effectiveness. *Outcomes Management for Nursing Practice, 2*(2), 81–85.

Lavin, M. A., Avant, K., Craft-Rosenberg, M., Herdman, T. H., & Gebbie, K. (2004). Context for the study of the economic influence of nursing diagnoses on patient outcomes, *International Journal of Nursing Terminologies and Classifications, 15*(2), 39–47.

Lavin, M. A., Meyers, G. A., & Ellis, P. (2007). A dialogue on the future of nursing practice. *International Journal of Nursing Terminologies and Classifications, 18*(3), 74–83.

Levin, R. F., Lunney, M., & Krainovich-Miller, B. (2004). Improving diagnostic accuracy using an evidence-based nursing model. *International Journal of Nursing Terminologies and Classifications, 15*(4), 114–122.

Lunney, M. (2003). Critical thinking and accuracy of nursing diagnoses. *International Journal of Nursing Terminologies and Classifications, 14*(3), 96–107.

Lunney, M. (2006). Helping nurses use NANDA, NOC, and NIC: Novice to expert. *Nurse Educator, 31*(1), 40–46.

Lunney, M. (2009). *Critical thinking to achieve positive health outcomes: Nursing case studies and analyses.* Ames, IA: Wiley-Blackwell.

Lunney, M., Delaney, C., Duffy, M., Moorhead, S., & Welton, J. (2005). Advocating standardized nursing languages in electronic health records. *Journal of Nursing Administration, 35*(1), 1–3.

Maas, M. L. (1985). Nursing diagnosis: A leadership strategy for nursing administrators. *Journal of Nursing Administration, 1*(6), 39–42.

McCloskey, J. C., & Bulechek, G. M. (Eds.). (1992). *Nursing interventions classification (NIC)* (1st ed.). St. Louis: Mosby Year Book.

McCloskey, J. C., & Bulechek, G. M. (1994). Standardizing the language for nursing treatments: An overview of the issues. *Nursing Outlook, 42*(2), 56–63.

McCloskey, J. C., & Bulechek, G. M. (Eds.). (1996). *Nursing interventions classification (NIC)* (2nd ed.). St. Louis: Mosby Year Book.

McCloskey, J. C., & Bulechek, G. M. (Eds.). (2000). *Nursing interventions classification (NIC)* (3rd ed.). St. Louis: Mosby.

McCormick, K. A. (1991). Future data needs for quality of care monitoring, DRG considerations, reimbursement, and outcome measurement. *Image: Journal of Nursing Scholarship, 23*(1), 29–32.

Moorhead, S., Johnson, M., & Maas, M. (Eds.). (2004). *Nursing outcomes classification (NOC)* (3rd ed.). St. Louis: Mosby.

Moorhead, S., Johnson, M., Maas, M., & Swanson, E. (Eds.). (2008). *Nursing outcomes classification (NOC)* (4th ed.). St. Louis: Mosby Elsevier.

Muller-Staub, M., Needham, I., Odenbreit, M., Lavin, M. A., & Van Achterberg, T. (2007). Improved quality of nursing documentation: Results of nursing diagnoses, interventions, and outcomes implementation study. *International Journal of Nursing Terminologies & Classifications*, 18(1), 5–17.

NANDA International. (2009). *Nursing diagnoses: Definitions and classification 2009-2011*. West Sussex, United Kingdom: Wiley-Blackwell.

North American Nursing Diagnosis Association. (1999). *Nursing diagnoses: Definitions & classification 1999-2000*. Philadelphia: Author.

Pesut, D. J. (2006). 21st century nursing knowledge work: Reasoning into the future. In C. Weaver, C. W. Delaney, P. Weber, & R. Carr (Eds.), *Nursing and informatics for the 21st century: An international look at practice, trends and the future* (pp. 13–23). Chicago: Health Care Information and Management Systems Society.

Pesut, D., & Herman, J. (1998). OPT: Transformation of nursing process for contemporary practice. *Nursing Outlook*, 46(1), 29–36.

Pesut, D. J., & Herman, J. (1999). *Clinical reasoning: The art & science of critical & creative thinking*. Albany, NY: Delmar.

Simmons, B., Lanuza, D., Fonteyn, M., Hicks, F., & Holm, K. (2003). Clinical reasoning in experienced nurses. *Western Journal of Nursing Research*, 25(6), 701–719.

Zielstorff, R. D. (1994). National data bases: Nursing's challenge, classification of nursing diagnoses. In R. M. Carroll-Johnson & M. Paquette (Eds.), *Classification of nursing diagnoses: Proceedings of the Tenth Conference* (pp. 34–42). Philadelphia: J.B. Lippincott.

CHAPTER 2

Use of Linkages for Clinical Reasoning and Quality Improvement

Howard Butcher and Marion Johnson

Daniel Pink (2005) convincingly explains in *A Whole New Mind: Moving from the Information Age to the Conceptual Age* that we are entering a new age, an age that requires a new form of thinking. For nearly a century Western society in particular has been dominated by narrowly reductive and deeply analytical thinking, which has culminated in our current "information age." In the information age, it has been essential that nurses be what Peter Drucker (2001) named "knowledge workers," theoretical thinkers, as well as gleaners and managers of information. However, according to Pink (2005), the "conceptual age" is currently rising in place of the information age. The conceptual age requires "big picture thinkers" who are concept users, pattern recognizers, meaning makers, and relationship seers.

Similar to Pink, Howard Gardner (2006) in *Five Minds for the Future* asserts that in this age of accelerating globalization, mounting quantities of information, and the growing hegemony of science and technology, new ways of learning and thinking are required in education and the professions. In particular, Gardner (2006) identifies the "disciplined mind" as one of the five "new minds of the future." Disciplines represent a radically different view of phenomena and therefore constitute a distinctive way of thinking about the world. Gardner (2006) asserts that "it is essential for individuals in the future to think in ways that characterize the major disciplines" (p. 31). As a scientific, professional, and practice discipline, "nursing has a unique and distinctive content or knowledge base" (Butcher, 2004a, p. 73). Nursing classification systems not only identify the essential content of nursing but also provide a way of organizing and structuring nursing knowledge (Butcher, 2011). Nursing diagnoses, interventions, and outcomes—specifically *NANDA International Nursing Diagnoses: Definitions & Classification*

2009-2011 (2009), the fifth edition of *Nursing Interventions Classification* (Bulechek, Butcher, & Dochterman, 2008), and the fourth edition of *Nursing Outcomes Classification* (Moorhead, Johnson, Maas, & Swanson, 2008), together referred to as NNN—provide the blueprint for "big picture" disciplinary thinking, as well as the structure and content for nursing knowledge development, care planning, and clinical decision making.

In addition to disciplinary thinking, Gardner (2006) identifies the "synthesizing mind" as the second essential way of thinking required for the future. The synthesizing is the ability to "knit together information from disparate sources into a coherent whole" (Gardner, 2006, p. 46). Gardner specifically identifies taxonomies, such as the nursing classification systems in this text, as an illustration of disciplinary knowledge synthesis. *The linkages between nursing diagnoses and clinical conditions, with nursing interventions and outcomes, are in essence a "synthesis of synthesis" integrating nursing knowledge into a cohesive whole. The linkages in this text provide a discipline-specific "conceptual roadmap" or blueprint for linking diagnoses, interventions, and outcomes that prepare nurses for "big picture" thinking in the emerging conceptual age.* The linkages can be used for designing evidence-based care for patient populations or for individual patients. They provide a standardized language that can be used in software development for electronic nursing information systems. The linkages can assist educators to teach clinical decision making and develop curricula and can be used by researchers to test nursing interventions, to evaluate the connections suggested in the linkages, and to develop mid-range theories.

A series of high-profile reports—*To Err Is Human: Building a Safer Health System* (Kohn, Corrigan, & Donaldson, 2000), *Crossing the Quality Chasm: A New*

Health System for the 21st Century (Institute of Medicine [IOM], 2001), *Keeping Patients Safe: Transforming the Work Environment of Nurses* (Page, 2003), and *Health Professions Education: A Bridge to Quality* (Greiner & Knebel, 2003)—have drawn considerable attention to significant problems related to the quality of care in the health care system. Chassin, Galvin, and the National Roundtable on Health Care Quality (1988) characterized "the burden of harm conveyed by the collective impact of our quality problems is staggering" (p. 1004). Quality is lacking in terms of providing care that is safe, effective, patient-centered, timely, efficient, and equitable (IOM, 2001). As a means to begin to address the challenge of preparing nurses with the knowledge, skills, and attitudes needed to improve quality and safety, the *Quality and Safety Education for Nurses (QSEN)* funded by the Robert Wood Johnson Foundation identified six competencies that can be used as a framework for *reforming* nursing education (Cronenwett et al., 2007). While some progress has been made in bridging the "quality chasm," a report by the Agency for Healthcare Research and Quality (AHRQ) concluded that although "the safety of health care has improved since 2000, more needs to be done" (AHRQ, 2008, p. 1). A vast majority of surveyed health care leaders believe that health care quality and efficiency will improve only with fundamental change. Nearly 9 out of 10 respondents to the latest Commonwealth Fund/Modern Healthcare Opinion Leaders Survey indicated the health care system needs radical system reform, with only 8% claiming that modest changes are all that is necessary (Kirchheimer, 2008).

Among the recommendations to bridge the health care "quality gap," the IOM (2001) identified a number of critical strategies designed to improve patient outcomes including: (1) evidence-based planned care, (2) computer-aided evidence-based clinical decision making, and (3) use of outcome measurements for continuous quality improvement. The use of the nursing classification systems and their linkages presented in this text not only describes the essential content of nursing diagnoses, interventions, and outcomes but also provides the means for achieving quality improvement by providing nursing content for the following goals: (1) designing nursing care; (2) developing computer-based information systems; (3) teaching and practicing clinical decision making; and (4) testing the effectiveness of interventions designed to achieve desired patient outcomes.

DESIGNING NURSING CARE

Nurses use a decision-making process to determine a nursing diagnosis, project a desired outcome, and select interventions to achieve the outcome. The linkages in this book are designed to assist nurses in making decisions about selecting the most appropriate interventions and outcomes for specific NANDA-I diagnoses and selected clinical conditions when planning care. It is important to keep in mind that the linkages are only guides; the nurse must continually evaluate the situation and adjust the diagnoses, outcomes, and interventions to match each patient's or population's unique needs. Thus the use of nursing taxonomies and their linkages is not a prescriptive formula and does not replace clinical decision making. Rather, the linkages provide possible choices and thus facilitate nursing judgments for designing care based on knowledge and understanding of each patient's unique situation, accurate interpretation of assessment information and data, and validation of assessment data with supporting evidence. In other words, nurses must use the linkages within the context of critical reasoning to ensure care is individualized, evidence-based, safe, and therapeutic. The use of suggested linkages does not alter the skills that nurses need and use in making decisions about patient care. "The skills the nurse must have to use the nursing process are: intellectual, interpersonal, and technical. Intellectual skills entail problem solving, critical thinking, and making nursing judgments" (Yura & Walsh, 1973, p. 69). When using the linkages, these intellectual skills are directed toward evaluating and selecting or rejecting the outcomes and interventions provided for each nursing diagnosis. Accurate nursing judgments lead to the effective designing of patient care. When the linkages presented in this book are used in conjunction with current nursing protocols, care plans, care maps, and evidence-based practice guidelines, then not only will nursing care be discipline-specific but also the use of NNN linkages will promote consistent documentation, evaluation, and communication of nursing practice in multiple settings and across disciplines.

The first clinical decision the nurse must make when using the linkages is to determine the nursing diagnosis. There is general agreement that before a nursing diagnosis is determined, an assessment of the patient status must be done. Rubenfeld and Scheffer (1999) state that assessment includes both data collection and data analysis or, as they describe it, "finding clues" and "making sense of the clues" (p. 130). They detail a number of steps used in assessment that enable the nurse to draw conclusions about the patient's strengths and health concerns, that is, to make a diagnosis. They further suggest categorizing health concerns as (1) problems for referral (issues addressed by other health care providers), (2) interdisciplinary problems (issues addressed collaboratively with other providers), and (3) nursing diagnoses (issues addressed primarily by the nurse).

The diagnosis is used as the entry point for accessing the linkages. This is true when planning the care for one patient (an individual care plan) or for a group of patients (a critical path). However, identification of the nursing diagnosis for a group of patients requires an additional step: the collection and analysis of data to determine the diagnoses that occur most frequently and are important to address for the entire population. Once a nursing diagnosis is determined, the nurse can locate the diagnosis in the linkage tables and determine if any of the suggested outcomes are appropriate for the individual patient or patient group. When selecting the outcome, the nurse should consider the following factors: (1) the defining characteristics of the diagnosis, (2) the related factors of the diagnosis, (3) the patient characteristics that can affect outcome achievement, (4) the outcomes generally associated with the diagnosis, and (5) the preferences of the patient. It is important to note that the outcomes presented in the linkage work reflect a desired end-state outcome related to the patient state to be achieved. For example, the suggested outcomes for the diagnosis *Skin Integrity, Impaired,* include the following: *Allergic Response: Localized; Burn Healing; Tissue Integrity: Skin & Mucous Membranes; Wound Healing: Primary Intention;* and *Wound Healing: Secondary Intention.* These outcomes and their associated indictors can measure resolution of the defining characteristics and the overall diagnosis.

Outcomes that address the related factors, often etiological, antecedent, or associated factors in a NANDA-I diagnosis, must often be resolved before

the actual end-state outcome is achieved. If the related factor is impaired circulation, the outcome *Circulation Status* might be selected; if the related factor is imbalanced nutritional state, the outcome *Nutritional Status, Nutritional Status: Nutrient Intake,* or one of the other measures of nutritional status might be selected. In other situations, selecting interventions to influence the related factors may be appropriate. If the related factor is mechanical, such as pressure, *Pressure Management* could be the intervention of choice; if the related factor is radiation, *Radiation Therapy Management* could be selected. Examples of outcomes selected by clinicians for seven NANDA-I diagnoses are reported in the literature with a discussion of some of the factors that might impact selection (Moorhead & Johnson, 2004).

After the outcome is selected, the nurse can consider the interventions suggested in the linkage work to assist in the selection of intervention(s) for the individual or group. The major interventions are the most closely related to both the diagnosis and the outcome and should be considered first. If the major intervention is not selected, consideration should be given to the suggested interventions. Bulechek and colleagues (2008) identify six factors to consider when selecting a nursing intervention. They are (1) the desired patient outcome, (2) the characteristics of the nursing diagnosis, (3) the research base associated with the intervention, (4) the feasibility of implementing the intervention, (5) the acceptability of the intervention to the patient, and (6) the capability of the nurse. In addition, estimates of time and education necessary to perform each intervention are provided. This information will be helpful to the nurse when selecting interventions for a particular patient (Bulechek et al., 2008). All of these factors should be considered when using the linkage work; the linkages can assist the nurse by suggesting interventions associated with both the outcome and the diagnosis, but cannot replace the nurse's judgment when selecting an intervention.

HEALTH INFORMATION TECHNOLOGIES

Computerized clinical information systems will become even more prevalent in health care organizations as the need to capture clinical data useful for evaluation expands rapidly and plays an increasing role in achieving quality improvement. On February 17, 2009, President Barack Obama signed into law the American Recovery and Reinvestment Act of 2009 (ARRA), which contained provisions for stimulus expenditures related to health information technology, including more than $20 billion for the development and adoption of electronic record systems (Wilson, 2011). Nurses have a critical role in using information in a systematized, organized manner to increase the quality of care (Dickerson, 2011). Nurses have recognized the importance of computer information technology in collecting, documenting, and quantifying nursing's domain of care, and have accepted the significance of information technology (IT) in determining health outcomes impacted by nursing care (Wilson, 2011). McBride (2006) clearly described how information technology (IT) will assist in achieving the IOM's quality initiatives, including facilitating the ability of nurses to document and share information, to use online benchmarking and tracking of patient outcomes, and to employ IT to link nursing processes (such as interventions to outcomes). Computer information systems are being used to reduce errors by standardizing and automating decisions, and identifying errors. Online databases that include evidence-based practice protocols, care plans, and critical paths provide nurses and health care professionals quick access to a mass of knowledge designed to enhance clinical decision making. Electronic records have the potential to make a significant contribution to patient safety and to the quality, effectiveness, and efficiency of health care (Lee, 2011). Electronic health records allow health care providers to quickly access the latest patient information digitally across settings, providing for a more complete documentation of the patient's health information and potentially limiting the duplication of services. Computerized decision support systems aid in clinical decision making by providing access to best evidence-based guidelines at the point of care (Wilson, 2011). Health care purchasers and managed care entities rely on statistical information derived from these systems to determine how health care dollars will be allocated. As health care information systems expand, each discipline must identify the data elements required to evaluate the processes and outcomes of care.

Although the development of nursing information systems was identified as a high priority as early as 1988 (National Center for Nursing Research, 1988), the construction of systems that use standardized data elements remains in the early stages of development. "If nurses do not develop and adopt the tools needed to participate in this information-driven environment, opportunities to provide nursing services may significantly diminish in the future" (Jones, 1997, p. 377). Database development requires a common language and a standard way to organize data. Standardized nursing languages or terminologies are vital to the discipline of nurses because they provide consistent terms to communicate nursing knowledge. This minimizes the bias created when nurses use terminology based on their own mental models of care (Clancy, Delaney, Morrison, & Gunn, 2006). Furthermore, standardized nursing languages allow for the coding of nursing diagnoses, interventions, and outcomes to enable the capture, storage, retrieval, and transformation of nursing care information (Bakken & Currie, 2011). In an effort to advance nursing in preparation for the electronic patient record, the American Nurses Association (ANA) developed a set of standards for nursing data sets in information systems. Standards include those related to nomenclatures, clinical content linkages, the data repository, and general system requirements (American Nurses Association, 1997). The ANA recognizes the NANDA-I, NOC, and NIC vocabularies as approved nomenclatures. By organizing nursing information into meaningful categories of data for analysis, the NANDA-I/NOC/NIC linkages are the "building blocks" for electronic clinical information systems (Lang, 2008, p. 233). All three languages have been registered in HL7 (Health Level 7), the U.S. standards' organization for health care. They are all licensed for inclusion in SNOMED-CT (Systematized Nomenclature of Medicine-Clinical Terms), a comprehensive reference terminology that is poised to become the recognized reference terminology for health information exchanges of important sections of the electronic health record.

Nurses' documentation of the diagnoses they treat, the interventions used to treat the diagnoses, and the resulting outcome responses to interventions in computerized information systems is necessary for the development of large local, regional, national, and international nursing databases (Iowa Intervention Project, 1997; Keenan & Aquilino, 1998). Large clinical databases are needed to assess nursing effectiveness, generate hypotheses for testing with controlled research designs, and refine the linkages among diagnoses, interventions, and outcomes based on clinical and research evidence. These database uses are essential for nursing knowledge development, for research-based practice, and to influence health policy. Busy clinicians, however, cannot afford the time to repeatedly sort through each standardized language in alphabetical form in a computerized system.

Five nursing-developed terminological sets that integrate nursing diagnoses, interventions, and outcomes are recognized by the American Nurses Association. The five nursing terminologies are Clinical Care Classification (CCC), International Classification on Nursing Practice (ICNP), Omaha System, Perioperative Nursing Data Set (PNDS), and NANDA-I/NIC/NOC (NNN). A systematic study of these five terminological sets indicates that because the Omaha System, PNDS, and the CCC systems are narrow in scope and non-comprehensive systems, they have significantly fewer publications and much smaller co-author publishing networks (Anderson, Keenan, & Jones, 2009). For example, articles focusing on the research, application, and implementation of NNN are found in 21 countries and 28 states while Omaha System classification is used in 5 countries and 16 states. The authors found NNN has more publications (journal articles, abstracts, books, book chapters, dissertations); in fact, NNN was used in 879 publications, as compared to a total of 261 publications for the other four terminology sets combined. Thus it is not surprising that NNN is the most common standardized terminology set used in health care information systems. The NANDA-I/NOC/NIC linkages presented in this book assist with the organization and structuring of nursing clinical information systems that are the most efficient for nurses' documentation of their practice. The taxonomies provide an organizing scheme for the arrangement of computer screens that eases clinicians' access for documentation. Likewise, the linkages offer greater efficiency by supplying groupings of diagnoses, interventions, and outcomes with a high probability of effective relationships for patient care. In a study evaluating the implementation, both teaching and

application, of nursing diagnoses, interventions, and outcomes, Muller-Staub (2009) concluded that "the use of NNN in the electronic nursing documentation is recommended" and the use of NNN in practice "led to higher quality of nursing documentation" (pp. 14–15).

An exemplar that fuses information technology and NNN linkages is the work of the team led by Keenan to develop the Hands-on Automated Nursing Data System (HANDS), which is an extensively tested user-friendly clinical nursing information system with embedded NANDA-I/NIC/NOC linkages. Research testing the HANDS tool in homecare and ambulatory settings provided evidence to its reliability, sensitivity, and usefulness in planning and documenting care and achieving desired patient outcomes (Westra, Delaney, Konicek, & Keenan, 2008).

NNN linkages also offer some decision support. A review of the outcomes and interventions that experienced nurses selected for a diagnosis will help clinicians consider possible treatments and responses that might be overlooked in the context of hectic and demanding clinical decision making. This decision support is likely to be even more helpful to novice nurses, who also need clinical reasoning options available for review but often have difficulty identifying the critical and priority outcomes and interventions for a diagnosis. A detailed description of design, implementation, and application of nursing computerized information systems using NNN is discussed in Chapter 3.

CLINICAL REASONING AND DECISION MAKING

Quality improvement rests on the foundation of patient-centered, competent, and effective clinical reasoning and decision making. Clinical decision making is based on clinical reasoning, which includes the use of knowledge, experience, and critical thinking. Nursing decision-making models are the engines of nursing practice (Butcher, 2004b). Since the 1950s, the nursing process has provided the structure facilitating clinical reasoning. Initially the nursing process consisted of four steps—assessment, planning, intervention, and evaluation. In 1973 the American Nurses Association modified the four-step nursing process by adding diagnosis as the second step in the decision-making model, thereby establishing the five-step model—assessment, diagnosis, planning, intervention, and evaluation (or **ADPIE**)—as a standard of nursing practice. The nursing process has been an organizing framework for professional nursing practice since the early 1960s. In the traditional nursing process, increasingly it has become standard practice to end the **A**ssessment process by identifying NANDA-I diagnoses in the **D**iagnostic phase; choosing relevant nursing-sensitive NOC outcomes and indicators when **P**lanning care for each diagnosis; selecting NIC interventions and activities for the **I**ntervention phase; and determining the changes in selected NOC indicators during **E**valuation. Thus NNN nursing languages provide the content or *knowledge* used in the nursing process.

Although the nursing process has demonstrated its usefulness as a clinical decision-making method, the traditional nursing process presents a number of limitations for contemporary nursing practice. Current nursing practice emphasizes knowing the patient's "story," thereby placing the patient's situation in a meaningful context and enabling creative and reflective thinking, theory-based practice, evidence-based practice, and consideration of desired patient outcomes. Pesut and Herman (1999) stated that the traditional nursing process does not explicitly focus on outcomes; instead, it deemphasizes reflective and concurrent creative thinking; is more procedure-oriented, rather than focused on the structures and processes of thinking; uses stepwise and linear thinking, which limits the relational thinking needed to understand the complex interconnections among the patient's presenting problems; and limits the development of the practice of relevant theory. In response to the need for a more contemporary model for clinical reasoning, Pesut and Herman developed the Outcome–Present State Test (OPT) model of reflective clinical reasoning. A significant strength of the OPT model is that it embraces a number of the types of thinking required in the emerging "conceptual age" or "big picture thinking" advocated by Pink (2005), including the emphasis on *story* or narrative, the use of *empathy* as a means to forge relationships through caring, and *symphony,* which is synthesizing elements into a whole.

The OPT model provides a major advancement in the teaching and practice of clinical decision making by using a clinical reasoning structure linking NANDA-I, NIC, and NOC. In fact, Pesut (2002) asserts "clinical thinking and reasoning presupposes the use of a standardized nursing language . . .

nursing knowledge classification systems provide the vocabulary for clinical thinking" (p. 3). The OPT model advances quality improvement by providing a structure for clinical reasoning that focuses on outcomes by using a *synthesizing* or systems' thinking approach about the relationships among nursing care problems associated with a particular client *story.* Contrary to the traditional nursing process, the OPT model of reflective clinical reasoning provides a structure for clinical thinking with a focus on outcomes and is not a stepwise linear process. Clinical reasoning that focuses on outcomes enhances quality improvement by optimizing the evaluation of effectiveness rather than focusing primarily on problems. In the OPT model of clinical reasoning, the nurse simultaneously focuses on problems and outcomes by juxtapositions of both problems and outcomes at the same time. The model requires nurses to simultaneously consider relationships among diagnoses, interventions, and outcomes with attention to the evidence used to make judgments. Rather than considering one problem at a time, the OPT requires nurses to consider several identified problems simultaneously and to discern which problem or issue is central and most important in relationship with all the other problems.

The OPT model provides a structure linking NANDA-I, NIC, and NOC and is a major advancement in the development of nursing practice decision-making models. The model's emphasis on eliciting the patient's story, framing the story in a discipline-specific theoretical context, incorporating reflective thinking, emphasizing nursing outcomes, identifying relationships among nursing diagnoses, and specifying the keystone issue provides a distinct advantage over the traditional nursing process. As an emerging clinical decision-making model, the OPT model is a new way for teaching, learning, and practicing nursing content–based care.

Pink (2005) explains that stories are important because they capture and encapsulate the context for understanding the assessment information and scientific knowledge. The OPT model (Figure 2-1) begins by listening to the **client-in-context story.** The OPT model uses listening to the "client-in-context story" to gather important information regarding the context, major issues, and insights about the patient's situation. It is through the telling and listening to stories that patients reveal their

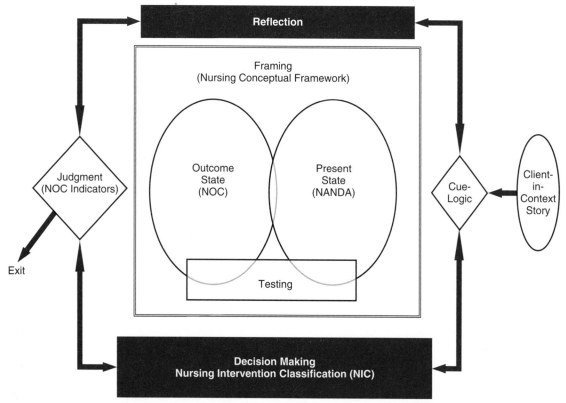

Figure 2-1 Integrating Outcome–Present State Test (OPT) model with NANDA, NIC, and NOC.

experiences and explore and make sense of the meaning of their health-illness experiences and that nurses learn about their patients' concerns, fears, hopes, and dreams. The story is not just expressed in words, but also in the silences, in what is not said, in the gaps between words, in the gestures or movements, and by the look in the eyes. Within the OPT model, assessing for the purpose of information gathering is replaced by attentively, empathetically, and compassionately listening to the patient's story, thereby extending diagnostic listening and privileging the person receiving care by attaining a fuller understanding of the patient's concerns. Attentive listening to the patient's story in context also can facilitate forming healing nurse-patient partnerships, meeting the patient's real concerns, and assisting the patient's ability to find meaning in the situation.

Client stories are complex and require "big picture thinking" using analysis and synthesis. To facilitate analysis and synthesis of the client story,

Pesut and Herman (1999) suggest the use of a "clinical reasoning web" worksheet, which is a pictorial representation of the functional relationships among the NANDA-I diagnoses describing the present state. Examining the relationships among the NANDA-I diagnoses using systems' thinking and synthesis enables nurses to identify the "keystone" issue. The keystone issue is the one or more diagnoses that are central to the patient's story and that support a majority of the other nursing diagnoses (Figure 2-2). In the clinical reasoning web worksheet, the diagnosis that has more relationships to other diagnoses (acute pain) will often be the keystone or priority nursing diagnosis. Keystone issues guide clinical reasoning by identifying the central NANDA-I diagnosis that needs to be addressed first and also contribute to **framing** the reasoning process. As the nurse elicits the client's story and constructs the clinical reasoning web, the theoretical framing of the story and relationships among

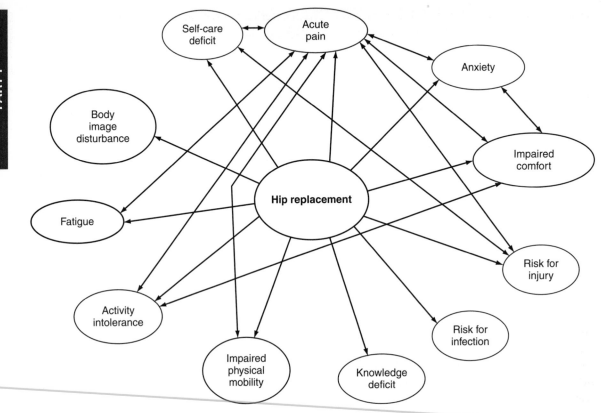

Figure 2-2 Sample clinical reasoning web.

diagnoses is elicited through the use of a mental model that gives meaning, language, clarity, and a way of organizing the information that is relevant to understanding the client's situation.

Framing an event, problem, or situation is analogous to using a lens through which one views and interprets the patient's story. The story may be framed by a specific nursing theory, a particular model, a developmental perspective, or a set of policies and procedures. Framing the patient's story by a particular nursing theory enables the nurse to "think nursing" rather than to think through a nonnursing perspective (e.g., medicine, psychology, or sociology) (Butcher, 2011). Framing the client's story helps the nurse focus on relevant information of the client's situation, guide the selection of relevant questions, organize the information gathered in a meaningful way, and provide a scientific understanding and rationale regarding why and how the client's concerns will be addressed.

Cue-logic is the deliberate structuring of the client-in-context data to discern the meaning for nursing care. Clinical evidence about the client-in-context is processed according to the nurse's cue-logic. Cue-logic via nursing theory contributes information that helps structure, or "frame," the particular situation. Cue-logic is also informed by memories or schema searches, that is, by patterns of past experiences that might be applied to the current situation. At the same time the nurse uses **reflection,** which is the process of observing oneself while simultaneously thinking about client situations. The goal of reflection is to achieve the best possible thought processes. Incorporating the ideas on guided reflective nursing practice according to Johns (2000, 2001) may be used to expand upon the original description of reflection by Pesut and Herman (1999). Reflective practice is a method of gaining access to a better understanding of the care experience, thereby enabling practitioners to develop increasing effectiveness of personal actions within the context of their work. Reflection during clinical decision making involves thinking about what you are doing while you are doing it by asking consciously or subconsciously questions such as the following (Johns, 1996): (1) What am I noticing here and what does it mean? (2) What judgment am I making and by what criteria? (3) What am I doing and why? (4) Is there an alternative course of action other than the one I am taking? The greater the reflection, the higher the quality of care delivered. As the nurse alternates between the client's story and the cue-logic guided by the particular frame that attributes meaning to the connections among the cues, the patient's present state or situation takes shape.

The **present state** is the description of the patient in context, or the initial condition. The present state will change with time as a result of both the nursing care and the changes in the nature of the patient's situation. The issues describing the present state may be organized by identifying the nursing diagnoses using the NANDA-I taxonomy (NANDA-I, 2009). NANDA-I diagnoses provide a structure and give meaning to the cues. Pesut and Herman (1999) describe in detail how the nurse creates a "clinical reasoning web" to describe the present state by identifying the relationship among and between the NANDA-I diagnoses associated with the patient's health condition. Informed by nursing knowledge and/or by the patient's direction, the outcomes are identified that indicate the client's desired condition. NOC outcomes (Moorhead et al., 2008) provide the means to determine the **outcome state** and are identified by juxtaposing, or making a side-by-side comparison, a specified outcome state with present state data. NOC outcomes are a state, behavior, or perception that is measured along a continuum in response to a nursing intervention. Each outcome has a group of indicators that are used to determine patient status in relation to the outcome. Therefore the indicators are more concrete and are measured along a 5-point Likert scale. There are currently 385 NOC outcomes, each with approximately 5 to 15 indicators. **Testing** is the process of thinking about how the gaps between the present state (NANDA-I diagnoses) and the desired state (NOC nursing-sensitive outcomes) will be filled. While testing, the nurse juxtaposes the present state and outcome state while

considering the NIC interventions that can be used to bridge the gap.

Decision making is the process of selecting and implementing the specific nursing interventions. The nurse identifies nursing interventions and the specific nursing actions that will help patients reach their desired outcomes. The taxonomy of NIC interventions (Bulechek et al., 2008) will facilitate the identification of standardized nursing interventions that are chosen based on their ability to help transition patients from problem states to more desirable outcome states. There are currently 542 NIC interventions. The following six factors discussed earlier in this chapter will facilitate the appropriate selection of an effective intervention: (1) desired patient outcomes (NOC); (2) characteristics of the nursing diagnoses (NANDA-I); (3) research base for the intervention; (4) feasibility for performing the intervention; (5) acceptability of the intervention to the patient; and (6) capability of the nurse. The nurse individualizes nursing care by selecting and implementing the specific nursing activities for each NIC intervention.

Judgment is the process of drawing conclusions based on actions taken. For example, the nurse may ask the following questions: How has the patient's present state changed based on the interventions? Does the present state now match the desired outcome state? The indicators for each of the NOC nursing-sensitive outcomes selected may be used to make judgments about the degree to which the desired state outcome achievement is met. A thinking strategy that supports judgment is reframing or attributing a different meaning to the acts and evidence. Judgments result in reflection and conclusions about the degree of match between the patient's present state and the outcome state. In addition, reflection about the entire process results in self-correction and contributes to the development of a schema for use with decision making in future similar patient situations. A reflection check involves the processes of self-monitoring, self-correcting, self-reinforcing, and self-evaluation of one's thinking about the task or situation.

Critical thinking is central to any clinical reasoning process, whether using the nursing process or the OPT model. Scheffer and Rubenfeld (2000) described critical thinking in nursing as consisting of a set of 7 cognitive skills and 10 interrelated "habits of mind." Cognitive skills include analyzing, applying standards, discriminating, information seeking, logical reasoning, predicting, and transforming knowledge; and habits of mind or intelligent nursing attributes include confidence, contextual perspective, creativity, flexibility, inquisitiveness, intellectual integrity, intuition, open-mindedness, perseverance, and reflection. Applying the NNN linkages presented in this text in teaching and practice enhances critical thinking because the linkages serve as a major enhancement of cognitive skills, particularly for applying standards, discriminating, and transforming knowledge.

Case studies and computer simulations have been developed based on the linkages in this book and appear in previous editions and increasingly in nursing textbooks. Faculty teaching clinical decision making can use the linkages to develop their own case studies and simulations. Discussion of cases can focus on the adequacy of the diagnosis selected to address the problem, the appropriateness of the outcomes and interventions selected, the rationale for their selection, and the identification of other outcomes or interventions that might be more appropriate in a given situation. A database with the linkages can be made available for students to use when planning care for a patient or a group of patients. Students can use the linkages to evaluate the relationship between the patient's signs and symptoms, the defining characteristics and related factors of the diagnosis, the outcome and its indicators, and the intervention and its activities. They can select the outcome indicators and intervention activities for a patient based on the patient's status and the elements of the nursing diagnosis.

The linkages will facilitate the teaching of clinical decision making through the application of teaching strategies such as the Outcome-Present State Test (OPT) model (Pesut & Herman, 1999). The linkages can be used in conjunction with the three languages (NANDA-I, NOC, and NIC) to assist students in developing the skills necessary for clinical decision making. Kautz and colleagues (2006) have conducted extensive research into the teaching of clinical reasoning using the NNN-standardized nursing languages within the OPT model. They note the many strengths in teaching clinical reasoning using NNN within the OPT model and request faculty to use NNN "linkage resources" with students. The researchers noted "that students who consistently used NNN language with the OPT model were the students who performed well in the clinical area and did better in completing their clinical reasoning webs" (Kautz et al., 2006, p. 137). Thus the linkages in this text can serve as a major resource in the teaching of clinical reasoning, whether using the OPT model or the traditional nursing process.

The linkages also can be used in planning content for the curriculum. They can assist the faculty in selecting a body of content and distributing the content among the various courses. The linkages between diagnoses, outcomes, and interventions can be a starting point to identify a body of content related to the nursing diagnoses and to determine when the content will be taught in the curriculum. For example, the faculty may choose to teach content related to the diagnosis *Anxiety* and the outcome *Anxiety Control*. Although these concepts may be covered in a number of courses, the interventions might be most appropriately distributed among courses. For example, *Active Listening, Calming Technique,* and *Exercise Promotion* might be presented early in the curriculum whereas *Hypnosis, Guided Imagery,* and *Therapeutic Touch* might be presented later in the curriculum or even in a graduate program. A publication describing a method to implement the three languages in an undergraduate curriculum (Finesilver & Metzler, 2002) is available through the Center for Nursing Classification and Clinical Effectiveness at the University of Iowa, College of Nursing.

There are a number of advantages to using NANDA-I/NOC/NIC vocabularies and linkages in a nursing curriculum. The vocabularies are comprehensive and can be used for patients across the continuum of care and in all settings in which care is provided. The terminology is useful for nurses in all nursing specialties and in various nursing roles. This makes the vocabularies and associated linkage work useful in both undergraduate and graduate curricula. As the electronic patient record becomes a reality, the use of standardized languages in the care setting will become commonplace and should be introduced to student nurses.

RESEARCH AND KNOWLEDGE DEVELOPMENT

Nursing classification systems—specifically nursing diagnoses (NANDA-I, 2009), nursing interventions classification (Bulechek et al., 2008), and nursing outcomes classification (Moorhead et al., 2008)—serve as *the* sources for knowledge development and provide the language of the nursing discipline (Butcher, 2011). NANDA-I/NIC/NOC (NNN) provides the concepts and language that enable nurses to work collaboratively with persons, families, communities, and members of other disciplines. Clark and Lang (1992) noted the importance of nursing taxonomies when stating, "If we cannot name it, we cannot control it, finance it, teach it, research it, or put it into public policy" (p. 27). Developments in the structure of nursing knowledge (NANDA-I/NIC/NOC) hold great promise for capturing the mid-range theories within a thorough and extensive framework of nursing knowledge. The taxonomies of nursing diagnoses, interventions, and outcomes and their linkages provide a full skeletal framework for nursing knowledge. In other words, the NNN linkages organize the substance of the discipline (Butcher, 2011). Professional practice languages and classification systems are the fundamental categories of thought that define a profession and its scope of practice. Although the nursing profession has made considerable progress in developing languages and classification systems, there is a need to use the languages to promote knowledge development. It is hoped that these linkages will suggest questions for study, including comparisons of the various languages currently used in nursing.

The development of nursing knowledge requires evaluation of the effectiveness of various nursing interventions and the appropriateness of the decision-making process in selecting interventions to resolve a diagnosis or to achieve a particular outcome. Kautz and Van Horn (2008) have cogently illustrated how NNN languages can be used in developing evidence-based practice guidelines for guiding practice and conducting research and conclude in asserting that "the use and continued development of uniform, standardized language capture the essence of nursing practice and help advance nursing knowledge in addition to providing the appropriate framework for evidence based practice" (p. 18).

Coherence among diagnoses, interventions, and outcomes displayed as evidence-based linkages is crucial to ensuring quality improvement and safety. The linkage work contained in this book provides numerous relationships that require testing and evaluation in a clinical setting. Questions about which of the suggested interventions achieve the best outcome

for a particular diagnosis, which of the outcomes are most achievable for a particular patient population, and which diagnoses and interventions are associated with specific medical diagnoses are just a sample of the questions that can be addressed. Studies, such as the one by Peters (2000), test the use of the outcomes and interventions with specific patient populations and add to the body of knowledge.

As well as studying the relationships between interventions and outcomes, the relationships among the environment, the structure of the health care organization, the processes of care, and patient outcomes need to be studied. Without these types of data, organizations have little information on which to adjust staff mix or determine the cost-effectiveness of structural or process changes in the nursing care delivery system. Issues related to the study of organizational factors that influence patient outcomes have gained increased emphasis in recent years.

Identification of patient factors that influence outcome attainment, referred to as risk factors, is another area that needs to be studied to carry out effectiveness research related to nursing interventions. Personal factors need to be identified to reduce or remove the effects of confounding factors in studies where the cases are not randomly assigned to different treatments, as is typical in most effectiveness research (Iezzoni, 1997). Identification of the personal factors that influence outcome achievement for a particular diagnosis or the effectiveness of an intervention for patients with varying personal characteristics and life circumstances will add to the body of nursing knowledge and allow nurses to provide the highest quality care possible. As effectiveness research and evidence-based practice gain momentum in nursing, both organizational and personal factors that need to be considered in the analysis of data are being identified in the literature (Johnson, 2002; Titler, Dochterman, & Reed, 2004).

CONCLUSION

The linkages provided in this text prepare nurses for the emerging conceptual age and are foundational to designing care, using computer-based electronic health care systems, teaching and practicing evidence-based clinical decision making, and developing and researching nursing's disciplinary knowledge. All four of these functions serve to enhance the safety and quality of nursing care. The public demands, requires, and deserves nothing less.

REFERENCES

Agency for Healthcare Research and Quality. (2008). *National healthcare quality report 2007* (AHRQ Pub. No. 08-0040). Rockville, MD: U.S. Department of Health and Human Services.

American Nurses Association. (1997). *Nursing informatics & data set evaluation center (NIDSEC) standards and scoring guidelines.* Washington, DC: Author.

Anderson, C. A., Keenan, G., & Jones, J. (2009). Using bibliometrics to support your selection of a nursing terminology set. *Computers, Informatics, Nursing, 27*(2), 82–90.

Bakken, S., & Currie, L. M. (2011). Standardized terminologies and integrated information systems: Building blocks for transforming data into nursing knowledge. In P. S. Cowen & S. Moorhead (Eds.), *Current issues in nursing* (8th ed., pp. 287–296). St. Louis: Mosby Elsevier.

Bulechek, G., Butcher, H. K., & Dochterman, J. M. (Eds.). (2008). *Nursing interventions classification (NIC)* (5th ed.). St. Louis: Mosby/Elsevier.

Butcher, H. K. (2004a). Nursing's distinctive knowledge base. In L. Haynes, H. K. Butcher, & T. Boese (Eds.), *Nursing in contemporary society: Issues, trends and transition into practice* (pp. 71–103). Upper Saddle River, NJ: Prentice Hall.

Butcher, H. K. (2004b, March). *Harmonizing nursing classification systems with nursing theories and narrative pedagogy using the Outcome–Present State Test (OPT) model of reflective clinical reasoning.* Presented at the NANDA, NIC, NOC 2004 Working together for quality nursing care: Striving toward harmonization, Chicago, IL.

Butcher, H. K. (2011). Creating the nursing theory-research-practice nexus. In P. S. Cowen & S. Moorhead (Eds.), *Current issues in nursing* (8th ed., pp. 123–135). St. Louis: Mosby Elsevier.

Chassin, M. R., Galvin, R. W., & the National Roundtable on Health Care Quality. (1988). The urgent need to improve health care quality. *Journal of the American Medical Association, 280*(11), 1000–1005.

Clancy, T., Delaney, C., Morrison, B., & Gunn, J. (2006). The benefits of standardized nursing languages in complex adaptive systems such as hospitals. *The Journal of Nursing Administration, 36*(9), 426–434.

Clark, J., & Lang, N. (1992). Nursing's next advance: An international classification for nursing practice. *International Nursing Review, 39*(4), 109–112.

Cronenwett, L., Sherwood, G., Barnsteiner, J., Disch, J., Johnson, J., Mitchell, P., Sullivan, D. T., & Warren, J. (2007). Quality and safety education for nurses. *Nursing Outlook, 55*(3), 122–131.

Dickerson, A. E. (2011). Why health information technology standards and harmonization are important. In P. S. Cowen & S. Moorhead (Eds.), *Current issues in nursing* (8th ed., pp. 311–330). St. Louis: Mosby Elsevier.

Drucker, P. (2001). The next society. *The Economist, 361*(8246), 3–5.

Finesilver, C., & Metzler, D. (Eds.). (2002). *Curriculum guide for implementation of NANDA, NIC, and NOC into an undergraduate nursing curriculum.* Iowa City, IA: College of Nursing, Center for Nursing Classification and Clinical Effectiveness.

Gardner, H. (2006). *Five minds for the future.* Boston: Harvard Business School Press.

Greiner, A. C., & Knebel, E. (Eds.). (2003). *Health professions education: A bridge to quality.* Washington, DC: The National Academies Press.

Iezzoni, L. I. (1997). Dimensions of risk. In L. I. Iezzoni (Ed.), *Risk adjustment for measuring healthcare outcomes* (2nd ed., pp. 43–115). Chicago: Health Administration Press.

Institute of Medicine (IOM). (2001). *Crossing the quality chasm: A new health system for the 21st century.* Washington, DC: The National Academies Press.

Iowa Intervention Project. (1997). Proposal to bring nursing into the information age. *Image: Journal of Nursing Scholarship, 29*(3), 275–281.

Johns, C. (1996). The benefits of a reflective model of nursing. *Nursing Times, 92*(27), 39–41.

Johns, C. (2000). *Becoming a reflective practitioner.* Oxford: Blackwell Science.

Johns, C. (2001). *Guided reflection: Advancing practice.* Oxford: Blackwell Science.

Johnson, M. (2002). Tools and systems for improved outcomes: Variables for outcomes analysis. *Outcomes Management, 6*(3), 95–98.

Jones, D. L. (1997). Building the information infrastructure required for managed care. *Image: Journal of Nursing Scholarship, 29*(4), 377–382.

Kautz, D. D., Kuiper, R., Pesut, D. J., & Williams, R. L. (2006). Using NANDA, NIC, and NOC (NNN) language for clinical reasoning with the Outcome-Present State (OPT) model. *International Journal of Nursing Terminologies and Classification, 17*, 129–138.

Kautz, D. D., & Van Horn, E. R. (2008). An exemplar of the use of NNN language in developing evidence-based practice guidelines. *International Journal of Nursing Terminologies and Classification, 19*(1), 14–19.

Keenan, G., & Aquilino, M. L. (1998). Standardized nomenclatures: Keys to continuity of care, nursing accountability and nursing effectiveness. *Outcomes Management for Nursing Practice, 2*(2), 81–85.

Kirchheimer, B. (2008). Overhaul this "broken system." *Modern Healthcare, 38*(16), 24–25.

Kohn, L. T., Corrigan, J. M., & Donaldson, M. S. (Eds.). (2000). *To err is human: Building a safer health system.* Washington, DC: The National Academies Press.

Lang, N. M. (2008). The promise of simultaneous transformation of practice and research with the use of clinical information systems. *Nursing Outlook, 56*(5), 232–236.

Lee, M. (2011). Personal health records as a tool for improving the delivery of health care. In P. S. Cowen & S. Moorhead (Eds.), *Current issues in nursing* (8th ed., pp. 331–339). St. Louis: Mosby Elsevier.

McBride, A. B. (2006). Informatics and the future of nursing practice. In C. A. Weaver, C. W. Delaney, P. Weber, & R. L. Carr (Eds.), *Nursing informatics for the 21st century: An international look at practice, trends and the future* (pp. 8–12). Chicago, IL: Healthcare Information and Management Systems Society.

Moorhead, S., & Johnson, M. (2004). Diagnostic-specific outcomes and nursing effectiveness research. *International Journal of Nursing Terminologies and Classifications, 15*(2), 49–57.

Moorhead, S., Johnson, M., Maas, M., & Swanson, E. (Eds.). (2008). *Nursing outcomes classification (NOC)* (4th ed.). St. Louis: Mosby/Elsevier.

Muller-Staub, M. (2009). Evaluation of the implementation of nursing diagnoses, interventions, and outcomes. *International Journal of Nursing Terminologies and Classifications, 20*(1), 9–15.

NANDA International. (2009). N*ursing diagnoses: Definitions and classification 2009-2011*. West Sussex, United Kingdom: Wiley-Blackwell.

National Center for Nursing Research. (1988, January 27–29). *Report on the national nursing research agenda for the participants in the conference on research priorities in nursing science.* Washington, DC: Author.

Page, A. (Ed.). (2003). *Keeping patients safe: Transforming the work environment of nurses.* Washington, DC: The National Academies Press.

Pesut, D. (2002). Nursing nomenclatures and eye-rolling anxiety control. *Journal of Professional Nursing, 18*(1), 2–4.

Pesut D. J., & Herman, J. (1999). *Clinical reasoning: The art and science of critical and creative thinking.* Albany, NY: Delmar.

Peters, R. M. (2000). Using NOC outcome of risk control in prevention, early detection, and control of hypertension. *Outcomes Management in Nursing Practice, 4*(1), 39–45.

Pink, D. H. (2005). *A whole new mind: Moving from the information age to the conceptual age.* New York: Riverhead Books.

Rubenfeld, M. G., & Scheffer, B. K. (1999). *Critical thinking in nursing: An interactive approach* (2nd ed.). Philadelphia: Lippincott, Williams & Wilkins.

Scheffer, B. K., & Rubenfeld, M. G. (2000). A consensus statement on critical thinking in nursing. *Journal of Nursing Education, 39*(8), 352–359.

Titler, M., Dochterman, J., & Reed, D. (2004). *Guideline for conducting effectiveness research in nursing & other health care services.* Iowa City, IA: Center for Nursing Classification & Clinical Effectiveness.

Westra, B. L., Delaney, C. W., Konicek, D., & Keenan, G. (2008). Nursing standards to support the electronic health record. *Nursing Outlook, 56*(5), 258–266.

Wilson, M. L. (2011). Nursing: A profession evolving with the use of informatics and technology. In P. S. Cowen & S. Moorhead (Eds.), *Current issues in nursing* (8th ed., pp. 281–286). St. Louis: Mosby Elsevier.

Yura, H., & Walsh, M. B. (1973). *The nursing process: Assessing, planning, implementing, evaluating* (2nd ed.). New York: Appleton-Century-Crofts.

CHAPTER 3

Use of NNN in Computerized Information Systems

Meridean Maas, Cindy Scherb, and Barbara Head

A number of hospitals and health care settings have developed nursing computerized information systems (CIS) and many more are developing CIS in response to available technology and the emergence of electronic health records (EHR). Many CIS, however, do not include standardized nursing nomenclatures. Furthermore, among those that do include standardized nursing terminologies, many systems are not designed to advantage the retrieval of nursing data for the development of nursing data repositories or warehouses. These data are necessary for the creation of useful reports for clinicians, nurse managers, and nurse executives. The result is that electronic clinical nursing practice data are minimally available in the United States for analyses that would benefit nursing, hospitals, and patients. This also impacts the type of information that can be shared as the patient moves among care settings and providers in the health care system.

When standardized nursing terminologies are not used, nurses cannot clearly and consistently communicate the meanings of the concepts they use with one another, with members of other disciplines, and with consumers. Furthermore, without standardized nursing terminologies electronic nursing data cannot be shared efficiently and directly with other settings. Most importantly, when standardized nursing terms for documenting nursing care are not used and therefore cannot be electronically retrieved, nursing data are not available to evaluate the quality of care. When the CIS is properly designed with standardized nursing terminologies, quality indicators can be downloaded directly from documented nursing practice data. Without the ability to electronically retrieve standardized nursing practice data, nursing data will not be included in large national EHR datasets that are analyzed to describe nursing contributions to health care and are used to inform policy makers.

Too often the main concern in CIS development is that nurses document the implementation of physician orders, actions for which there is a charge to the consumer, and other externally mandated data, such as national quality indicators, while limiting and compromising the documentation of meaningful nursing care data. Consequently, in many settings nursing electronic documentation does not truly represent the knowledge-based nursing care provided to patients and families that contributes to the quality of health care received by patients in our health care system. Furthermore, the development of many EHR systems continues to emphasize the documentation of nursing care plans and care delivered, but neglects standards to ensure that data are easily retrievable. Inattention to planning for data retrieval and data warehousing early in CIS development is a serious constraint on the use of electronic clinical nursing data. Because of this constraint, nursing data are not used to inform optimal decisions and quality evaluations by nursing administrators and clinicians; to support the ongoing development of nursing science and best practices; and to make local and national policy makers aware of the contributions and effectiveness of nursing care in providing health care to citizens (Barton, 1994). To enable these important uses of information generated by nursing CIS data, standardized nursing data must be retrieved and stored in common information tables within electronic data repositories and warehouses so that the data can be analyzed to answer specific queries.

This chapter outlines the characteristics of nursing CIS data that are required for clear representation, communication, and use of electronic nursing practice data. The development of data repositories and warehouses for the analysis of nursing data is described. Issues that constrain the retrieval of electronic nursing data and the development of data warehouses are discussed, and lessons learned from a pilot study are described. The chapter concludes with recommendations to address the issues that constrain the retrieval of nursing data that can be stored in data warehouses and analyzed for nursing effectiveness.

CHARACTERISTICS OF NURSING CIS DATA

Several characteristics of nursing data that are entered into CIS are essential for data to be used most advantageously. The data must meet the criteria for interoperability (Fetter, 2009). To be interoperable, the data must meet the following requirements:

- Functionally transferable, employing shared standards for character and file formats
- Transactional with a shared messaging format
- Semantically supported within a shared information model, such as HL7
- Built on a common procedural plan for execution support
- Implemented in an environment with an ergonomically shared work plan (Konstantas, Bourrières, Léonard, & Boudjlida, 2006)

To achieve interoperability, nurses and health information technology (HIT) specialists must work closely together. To be effective, nurses working with CIS development must understand the requirements to achieve each aspect of interoperability and help HIT specialists appreciate the importance of standardized nursing terminologies and their linkages in the electronic representation of nursing practice (Keenan, 1999). A foremost concern is the use of standardized terminologies in CIS to describe and document the nursing process elements of the Nursing Minimum Data Set (e.g., nursing diagnoses, nursing-sensitive outcomes, and nursing interventions) (Werley & Lang, 1988). Linkages among these elements and between terms documenting care planned and care actually delivered, however, are also critically important in order to evaluate the exact outcomes that result from specific interventions for each nursing diagnosis (Polk & Green, 2007).

Electronic nursing data must characterize identified individual patients and nurse providers, but also must be secure and protect the identity and privacy of individuals. Data security is regulated by the Health Insurance Portability and Accountability Act (HIPAA) of 1996. The HIPAA Privacy Rule establishes the conditions under which protected health information may be used for research purposes. Research is defined by HIPAA as "a systematic investigation, including research development, testing, and evaluation, designed to develop or contribute to generalizable knowledge" (U.S. Department of Health & Human Services, 2003). A covered entity may use, or disclose for research, health information that has been de-identified. Nursing data that are used for research purposes must meet these and other standards to protect the security and privacy of individuals.

More than 40 federal laws and regulations address privacy, security, and confidentiality of health information exchange, including HIPAA (U.S. Department of Health & Human Services, 2008). Recent updates within the Nationwide Privacy and Security Framework for Electronic Exchange of Individually Identifiable Health Information include interpretations of the law and guidelines from the multistate work of the Health Information Security and Privacy Collaborative (HISPC) (Dimitropoulos, 2009). These guidelines explicate the intrastate and interstate organizational standard agreements for data exchange and use. This work led to the Data Use and Reciprocal Support Agreement (DURSA) developed by the National Health Information Network (NHIN) Cooperative DURSA Team in November (2009).

Finally, the nursing data that are entered into a CIS must be retrievable. Unfortunately, in many CIS this is not the case, or the data are very labor-intensive and costly to retrieve. Many hospitals today consider downloading data of interest to nurses as low priority, compared to other types of data. This further reduces nurses' ability to enhance practice based on the evaluation of patient data. To ensure that nursing data are most efficiently retrievable, the structure of data in the operational CIS must be thoughtfully designed when the CIS is developed in anticipation of storage in multiple data repositories and warehouses. Data should be structured as a nursing data set (minimum to moderate) for inclusion in large and generic repositories to serve multiple purposes, such as storage of data from multiple operational CIS sources to be exported through the National Health Information Network to large, multisite, regional, national, and international data warehouses; as well as in specialized repositories for specific purposes internal and external to the organization. For example, nursing administrators and managers may want a smaller, specialized data warehouse so that real-time and retrospective data can be queried for program planning, resource distribution, and cost evaluation (Barton, 1994). Quality improvement officers and clinicians may need another type of warehouse to examine quality assessment and corrective actions. Clearly, with the advent of the EHR, data will become increasingly available in very large data warehouses to identify patterns of care provided and the outcomes that result for large groups of patients. Electronic nursing data must be retrievable for inclusion in these data warehouses if nurses are to participate in the research opportunities afforded to ensure that nursing's contributions to health care are known and used in health policy decisions (Bakken, 2003). Nursing effectiveness and cost-effectiveness studies with comparisons among many different health care settings will not be realized if electronic nursing data cannot be efficiently retrieved and stored in well-designed data warehouses.

DEVELOPING NURSING DATA REPOSITORIES AND WAREHOUSES

Nursing CIS that are properly designed store data generated by the operational EHR system for each variable, describing each patient separately in data repositories and warehouses with a relational or multidimensional database design. A relational database organizes a group of data items as a set of tables rather than one large table. The set of tables includes parent and child tables that are hierarchical. That is, any child table has only one parent table, but a parent table can have multiple child tables, and a child table can also be a parent table for other child tables (Gilfillan, 2002). The term "child" used in this manner refers to a subset of data from the "parent category." Data can be retrieved or reassembled in a variety of ways without needing to revise the database structure or reconstruct the tables. By using linking variables among the tables, the relationships among tables allow data to be drawn from several tables for querying and reporting. Advantages of relational databases are that they are relatively easy to construct, access, and extend. Once a relational database is developed, additional data categories can be inserted without requiring revision of previous applications. A complete explanation of a relational database is complex and beyond the scope of this chapter;

however, a brief description is provided for a beginning understanding of this process.

The tables in a relational database contain data in defined categories (Gilfillan, 2002). Each of one or more columns in a table contains data for a category, such as patient demography. Rows contain single instances of data, or single-entry descriptions, for the category defined by each column, such as date of birth, marital status, and education. When multiple entries for a category are required, such as the nursing diagnoses of the patient, a sub or child table is created. In this example, the patient table is the parent table and the nursing diagnoses table is the child table. In turn, the nursing diagnoses table will be a parent table for the child tables of defining characteristics and related factors.

Data stored in the data warehouse will come from several different data sets in the operational side of the CIS in the organization. For example, a nursing care database will include a table of patients with columns for name, identification (ID) code, age, gender, race/ethnicity, marital status, and occupation. Another table will be for admissions, containing columns for admission ID code, patient ID code, date of admission, time of admission, reason for admission, and unit of admission. Other tables would describe nursing care planned and care delivered. The source of patient and admission data will be from generic modules in the organization's CIS. Separate tables in a nursing data warehouse contain nursing diagnoses, nursing interventions, and nursing-sensitive outcomes. Separate tables are also constructed for each of the structural elements of nursing diagnoses, outcomes, and interventions, with NANDA-I defining characteristics and related factors, NOC indicators and measurement scales, and NIC activities. Columns for nursing diagnoses should be devoted to patient admission ID code, diagnosis code, date of diagnosis, and time of diagnosis. Columns for nursing-sensitive outcomes should include outcome code, date of outcome rating, and time of outcome rating with a linking variable to nursing diagnosis, nursing intervention, outcome, outcome indicator(s), measurement scale(s), and rating tables. Columns for interventions should include admission ID code, intervention code, date of intervention delivered, and time of intervention delivered with linking variable to nursing diagnosis, nursing intervention activities, and outcome tables. Other columns can be added to the tables to describe additional characteristics of each. As many separate tables as needed can be designed as long as the appropriate linking variables are included in each table. The linking variables must be designed so that the data describing outcomes to be monitored for specific interventions to treat precise nursing diagnoses for each identifiable patient on a certain date and/or specified time in a plan can be retrieved, as well as the dates and times documented when outcomes are measured or interventions are implemented for the patient.

The data in the database tables are linked by specific variables in each table and constrained by others. These linkages are necessary to capture all of the data that describe a specific patient or unit of data, such as a nursing diagnosis. Linkages of particular importance for analyzing the effectiveness of nursing interventions are among specific diagnoses, the outcomes that are monitored to assess the effect of specific interventions, and the nursing interventions that are selected to treat the diagnosis and achieve the desired outcomes. Figure 3-1 is a simple illustration of how the tables in relational databases are structured.

CONSTRAINTS ON NURSING DATA RETRIEVAL AND THE DEVELOPMENT OF DATA WAREHOUSES

There are a variety of constraints on nursing data retrieval and subsequent development of data warehouses. Vendor systems are repeatedly a significant constraint. Most vendors' first priority in developing an EHR is usually for purposes other than electronic nursing documentation. The EHR is more likely developed for billing, abstracting, provider order entry, admissions, laboratory, or x-ray as the main product priorities, but with the added need to market the product as a "total" package HIT. The development of the nursing portion of the "total" package is often a shell and not as robust as other applications within the EHR. In addition to low marketing priority, vendors and system developers tend to be inadequately informed about data that are optimally required for nursing. Likewise, many nurses, even those who are actively involved with system development, too often do not fully know what is required and/or do not adequately understand CIS structure, capabilities, and development. At minimum, nurses need to know CIS requirements for optimum efficiency to support

nurses' ability to document using standardized concepts for continuity of care exchange and to use nursing evidence-based resources within CIS to support the decisions of clinicians, administrators, and policy makers. Nurses need to pressure vendors to produce a product that meets these needs. To more fully understand CIS nursing needs, the view of desired output must be expanded to include the retrieval of data for populating data warehouses. Nurses need to understand that it is from these warehouses that data can be analyzed and reports generated to support decisions and fully describe the contribution of nursing to the effectiveness, or lack of effectiveness, of health care.

The use of nonstandardized terms in nursing CIS is a second issue that constrains data retrieval and the building of data warehouses, especially those that are interoperable among multiple organizations. Even when standardized nursing languages are used within a system, organizations frequently also use some nonstandardized terms. This is an issue for interoperability of nursing data, but also for the refinement of the nursing classifications. The primary reason given for the use of some nonstandardized nursing terms is that the standardized languages do not have some terms that fit the organization's needs. This is likely true because all of the nursing standardized terminologies are continually being refined. Terms are added or revised to describe patient conditions (diagnoses and outcomes) and nursing interventions as needed. When a new term is needed, nurses in the organization are helpful to nursing classification development and refinement if they submit suggestions for new or revised terms to the appropriate developers. All suggestions will be considered to refine or extend the respective classification. It is also important that organizations update and add new terms to their CIS as new editions are published.

When nonstandardized terms are used that describe the same nursing phenomenon as described by an existing standardized nursing term, the nonstandardized term will need to be mapped to a standardized term for coherent, nonredundant data retrieval and data warehousing. Although reference models are touted as enabling the use of uniform rather than standardized nursing terminologies, they will not solve the problem of accurate use of meaningful terms that have not been mapped before being

Table 1. Patients

PatientID	LastName	FirstName	BirthDate	Gender	MaritalStatus	NextofKin

Table 2. Admission

AdmissionID	PatientID	Date	TimeDay	AdmitUnitID

Table 3. Nursing Diagnoses

NrsDxID	AdmissionID	NurseID	DxDate	DxTime

Table 4. Defining Characteristics

DefCharID	NrsDxID

Table 5. Related Factors

RelatedFactorID	NrsDxID

Figure 3-1 Illustration of relational database tables.

applied to the reference model. Furthermore, no nursing reference information model (RIM) is yet operational. Mapping of terms is highly time-consuming and may not be possible with a large dataset. This issue underscores the folly of the use of nonstandardized terms—it either partially or completely compromises the analysis and reporting of nursing care and its effectiveness. Use of nonstandardized terms limits the interoperability of data across settings and the development of large, multiorganizational datasets.

A third issue is that nursing CIS designs are frequently not fully integrated in regard to (1) one to one linkages of nursing-sensitive outcomes to specific nursing interventions that are used to treat specific nursing diagnoses and (2) linkage of documented care planned and documented care delivered. When one to one linkages among nursing diagnoses, outcomes, and interventions are not explicitly identified by nurses and hardwired in the operational CIS, the specific outcomes that are measured to assess the response to specific interventions that are used to treat specific nursing diagnoses cannot be determined. Unless the linkages among only one outcome, one intervention, and one diagnosis are documented, the data retrieved are groups of diagnoses, outcomes, and interventions. This is a serious constraint on the ability to analyze nursing clinical data to evaluate effectiveness and to conduct clinical research.

Systems tend to separate nursing documentation of care provided from documentation of the plan of care. Although an increasing number of organizations are using standardized nursing terminologies in their care planning systems, most still do not fully integrate and maintain the use of the languages in the documentation of actual care provided. Because standardized nursing terminologies that are used in the care planning modules of operational CIS are often not used or carried through to documentation of care delivered in the operational CIS, retrieval of data to build a data warehouse that enables the evaluation of actual nursing care that is received by patients is also often not possible. This lack of integration further reflects the need for vendors and nurses to fully understand needed nursing output and CIS design.

When a system is designed with documentation of care planned and care delivered in separate unconnected parts of the CIS, it requires nurses to document the care planned in one place and the actual care delivered in another. Nurses often voice that they spend too much time documenting. To decrease this time, it is often the documentation of nursing care delivered that is deemed "necessary" versus updating the plan of care. Some settings use NANDA-I, NOC, and NIC standardized nursing labels to document the diagnosis, intervention, and outcome labels for care planning, but still fail to link them directly to documentation of actual care that is delivered using the same standardized terms. Systems need branching capabilities as a prerequisite for linking care planning with care delivered. Actual care delivered tends to be documented as flow sheets and with

discrete intervention activities and outcome indicators that are not hardwired to respective NIC interventions and NOC outcomes from which they are extracted. These more discrete terms are usually at the level of NOC indicators and NIC activities; however, these terms could be standardized and connected to the appropriate standardized NOC outcome(s) and NIC intervention(s) along with date and time assessed or delivered for a specific patient. Because some outcome indicators and intervention activities are associated with more than one outcome and intervention label, each must be unambiguously linked to the exact outcome(s) being monitored and intervention(s) and also linked to the specific nursing diagnosis being treated.

Integration of the documentation of care planned and actual care delivered, including flow sheet documentation, must maintain the nurse clinician's associations among standardized nursing terminologies that accurately represent practice decisions and actions throughout explicit episodes of each patient's care. If not completely linked in the system design, solutions are possible. For example, when a piece of patient data is on the flow sheet but not reflected on the plan of care, a decision support trigger can be added to alert the nurse to add the appropriate nursing diagnosis, nursing-sensitive patient outcome, and/or nursing intervention to the plan of care. Conversely, if a new nursing diagnosis, nursing-sensitive patient outcome, or nursing intervention is added to the plan of care, triggers can be used to alert the nurse to document the appropriate nursing care delivered. If the CIS is designed properly, however, such triggers will not be needed because the documentation of care planned and care delivered will be integrated so that new data added to one will automatically be added to the other. If the CIS does not explicitly integrate the connections among specific standardized nursing diagnoses, nursing-sensitive outcomes, and nursing interventions, the ability to retrieve and analyze the effect of specific nursing diagnoses on specific patient outcomes will continue to be compromised.

Illustration from a Pilot Study

Some of these issues are illustrated by a pilot study conducted to prepare for a larger nursing effectiveness study conducted by a team of researchers in association with the University of

Iowa College of Nursing Center for Nursing Classification and Clinical Effectiveness. The pilot study, *An Example of Electronic Nursing Clinical Data Retrieval for Data Warehouse Development and Research,* was conducted to evaluate the feasibility of a future large, multisite nursing effectiveness study with hospitalized older persons who were discharged with pneumonia or heart failure (Head et al., in press; Head et al., 2010; Scherb et al., in press).

The aims of the study were to use hospital CIS nursing clinical data to do the following:

1. Describe the 10 most frequent NANDA-I diagnoses, NIC interventions, and NOC outcomes documented by nurses for patients ≥60 years of age with a primary discharge diagnosis of pneumonia (diagnosis-related groups [DRGs] 89 and 90) or heart failure (DRG 127).
2. Describe the process of data retrieval for all variables needed to analyze the clinical and cost-effectiveness of nursing interventions.
3. Evaluate the development of a data warehouse needed for future study of the effectiveness of nursing interventions for hospitalized older adults.

Patient and hospital unit level variables that were requested to be collected from each hospital site are listed in Table 3-1.

The statistician converted the data into a uniform format allowing for a description of patient and unit demographics and the frequency and ranking of nursing diagnoses, nursing interventions, and nursing-sensitive patient outcomes documented in the sample of patient records. The data were reviewed by the research team members, including members from each hospital, for congruency and implications for practice.

After the preliminary data were reported and discussed, further data analyses were completed. Results of the data analyses describing patient and unit demographics and the frequency of nursing diagnoses, nursing interventions, and nursing-sensitive patient outcomes for patients discharged with heart failure and pneumonia and compared across sites are reported elsewhere (Head et al., 2010; Scherb et al., in press). Analysis showed greater variations in the nursing diagnoses, interventions, and patient outcomes among sites than expected. Some of the reasons for this variation may have been differences in patient populations

TABLE 3-1	Variables Collected from Hospital CIS
Patient Level	**Hospital Unit Level**
Patient identifier	Unit identifier
Age	Unit name
Gender	Unit size
Marital status	Unit type
Occupation	Unit occupancy rate
Nursing diagnoses	Nurse staff to patient ratio
Nursing interventions	Nurse staff skill mix
Nursing-sensitive patient outcomes	Nursing delivery model
Nursing acuity	Unit nurse hours per patient day
Nursing intensity	
Medical diagnoses	
Severity of illness	
Medical treatments	
Other treatments	
Medications	
Discharge disposition	
Number of readmissions	
Length of stay	
Primary language	

attributable to the prevalence of co-morbid conditions and patient demographics; geographic variations in practice; the use of locally developed care plan templates; the lack of research evidence available to develop care plans; differences in the length of time that each site had been using their CIS and NANDA-I, NIC, and NOC terminologies; and the tendency of some organizations to focus on national quality standards in their care plans, even if there was little relevance for the specific population, versus population-specific plans of care (Head et al., 2010; Scherb et al., in press)

The findings prompted two of the organizations to reevaluate and change their care plan templates to a population-specific focus and to further educate and discuss with the staff nurses care planning and documentation with standardized nursing terminologies. One year later, a 3-month period of data was recollected and analyzed, indicating improvement of appropriate care planning and documentation. The analysis of CIS nursing clinical data and the feedback of results to nurse administrators and nursing staff helped them understand the critical importance of documentation and standardized CIS nursing data for the analysis of nursing care effectiveness and ultimately quality improvement of patient care.

DATA RETRIEVAL ISSUES AND LESSONS LEARNED

As noted earlier, the pilot study was conducted to prepare for a larger nursing effectiveness study and was the first time that the study hospitals had attempted to retrieve the variables listed in Table 3-1 from their CIS. Several problems were encountered, including the following:

1. Data for some variables were not available from all hospitals' CIS because they were not documented electronically.
2. Data for some variables were available electronically, but were in other systems.
3. Data for some variables were not available because the data were not documented electronically or in paper forms.

Because of these problems complete data could not be retrieved for co morbid conditions, medications, race/ethnicity, nursing acuity, severity of illness, occupation, medical and other treatments, and primary language spoken by the patient (Head et al.,

in press). Three primary lessons were learned from this study:

Lesson 1: You cannot depend on electronic retrieval of data for all variables that are needed to evaluate nursing effectiveness.

Lesson 2: Nurses and vendors need to correct limitations in nursing clinical data in many hospital CIS before nursing effectiveness can be evaluated with data from these settings.

Lesson 3: Nurses must demand that vendors design systems to enable data retrieval with these linkages (Head et al., 2010).

The pilot study affirmed the necessity of knowing which variables are actually included in the CIS before designing a data warehouse for research or for queries and reports within the hospital. Although the research team knew this and asked the hospital representatives to confirm that the data for all variables were available and retrievable electronically, it was surprising that the nurse representatives who were working with the CIS usually were unaware of this information. Determining if variables were available in the CIS and if the data for each variable were retrievable took a significant amount of time and required consultation with a data retrieval specialist in each hospital. Further, because the data did not originate from a single system or CIS application, it was also necessary to have an experienced data retrieval specialist within the organization who understood the various CIS applications to assist with downloading the data. There is a crucial need to be specific with variable definitions, a major advantage of standardized nursing terminologies, and the format for data transfer. Very clear and complete variable definitions and formats are important for retrieval of all data, but were especially important because of the competing demands on the data retrieval specialist's time. Use of the data retrieval specialist underscores the importance of hospital organizational support for retrieving and analyzing clinical nursing data. The assistance of the data retrieval specialist was costly for the hospitals and would not have been possible without substantial organizational commitment. The data for some variables had to be extracted from documentation on paper forms. Retrieving these variables was also time and cost intensive for the hospital and for the research team. When the CIS is designed, nurses must carefully consider the data that will be needed to answer nursing effectiveness questions and the retrievability of these data.

The second lesson learned was that nursing data that can be retrieved have more limitations than anticipated. It was not a surprise that the clinical data documented by practicing nurses was less rigorous than the data collected specifically for a research study. The amount of time spent documenting; the nurses' knowledge of the standardized languages; and the accuracy of nursing diagnoses, interventions, and patient outcomes all affect the quality of clinical data (Head et al., 2010). These limitations can be partially reduced, as they were by the three clinical sites, by ensuring adequate ongoing education about the use of standardized nursing terminologies for clinical decision making and its application to the documentation system (Head et al., in press). A surprising lesson, however, was the difference between the documented care actually delivered versus the documented care planned in some systems. Many systems use flow sheet type charting for the actual care provided and have a separate module for the care plan. This was true in two of the three study hospitals. When NANDA-I, NIC, and NOC only existed in the care plan module and were not linked to the documentation of actual care provided, the data retrieved for evaluating care might not be a true reflection of the care delivered (Head et al., in press). The need for nurses and vendors to understand the importance of integrating the documentation of care planned and the documentation of care delivered using standardized nursing nomenclatures as well as the importance of designing decision support mechanisms that will enable simultaneous updating of both types of documentation is a lesson that cannot be ignored if nursing data are to be used to evaluate the effectiveness of nursing care.

Linkages between the nursing diagnoses, interventions, and outcomes data in the CIS were also not operationalized in all of the study hospitals. In the pilot study, the linkages were not necessary because the purpose was to describe the ten most frequently documented nursing diagnoses, interventions, and outcomes. It was clear to the researchers, however, that future nursing effectiveness research was severely limited without electronic linkages of a nursing diagnosis with a specific patient outcome(s) and a specific nursing intervention(s) used to treat the diagnosis and achieve a desired outcome(s).

The pilot study demonstrated the ability to obtain most of the variables necessary for larger nursing effectiveness studies. Some variables, however, were not available or were very difficult to obtain, and critical limitations of the CIS nursing data were revealed. The lessons learned about data retrieval and necessary linkages among CIS nursing data will help researchers develop a data warehouse and prepare for future studies. The lessons learned from the pilot study should also convince nurses in all settings to heed the following recommendations in order to make electronic nursing clinical data most advantageous both for nurses and for their patients.

RECOMMENDATIONS FOR ADDRESSING ISSUES THAT CONSTRAIN RETRIEVAL AND WAREHOUSING OF NURSING DATA

Nurses' lack of knowledge regarding the role of nursing classifications in the development of the knowledge base of the discipline and regarding CIS and data warehouse development is a fundamental, significant issue. Unlike disciplines that have a more mature science supporting their scholarship and practice, the curriculum in many nursing programs is not anchored in a standardized set of concepts that are the basis of their science. For example, every undergraduate student of chemistry immediately encounters the periodic table of the elements and first-year medical students learn standardized terms contained in the International Classification of Diseases (ICD) and the Diagnostic and Statistical Manual of Mental Disorders (DSM). While the inclusion of nursing standardized nomenclatures in nursing undergraduate programs is increasing, the rationale for the importance of nursing nomenclatures and their classification is not clearly provided. Many nursing graduate programs also do not include this content, including advanced practice nursing programs and doctoral programs. If the issues that hamper nursing data retrieval and warehousing are to be addressed, all nursing programs should strengthen curriculum content regarding the role of standardized nursing terminologies for building the knowledge base of the discipline and the importance of their inclusion in nursing CIS. Nursing continuing education programs should also offer this content for the many nurses who are currently practicing. As more nurses understand the importance of standardized nursing terms that describe nursing phenomena that are the building blocks of nursing knowledge and evidence-based practices, more will insist that nursing CIS are designed to benefit nurses and nursing. More nurses will realize the importance of retrieving data for storage in repositories and warehouses so that they can be analyzed to determine nursing's effectiveness and contribution to health care. Without nursing intervention effectiveness data to improve the delivery of patient care and to describe when patient outcomes do not reach desired levels, nurses and nursing will remain ignorant of the changes that need to be enacted to improve quality as well as the nursing interventions that are most successful for achieving optimal results. Armed with an understanding of the role of standardized nursing terminologies for building the knowledge base of the discipline and of the importance of data for determining the effectiveness of nursing care, nurses will be better equipped to communicate the importance of nursing to vendors, to organization system developers, and to organization policy makers.

Programs that prepare nursing informatics specialists are also increasing, but more are needed. These programs often neglect emphasizing the role and importance of nursing classifications. Many nurses who are assisting in developing electronic nursing documentation systems are nursing experts in clinical practice. These expert clinicians often do not have formal education in informatics and thus have a very steep learning curve to acquire sufficient understanding of CIS development. The expertise these clinicians bring to system development is invaluable to building a system that will meet the needs of the staff nurses using the system. Unfortunately, limited knowledge about standardized nursing terminologies, data structure, relational databases, data retrieval, and nursing effectiveness research often dilutes their influence and success in achieving a system that is most advantageous for evaluating nursing practice. Nursing clinical experts are also often hired by information technology departments and system vendors to provide input on nursing documentation and to learn how to build computer screens. These individuals, however, tend to lack knowledge about specific questions to ask the vendor about the system and its operation.

These experts often have limited understanding of the data, information, knowledge, and decision making needs of professional nurses and the skills for data retrieval and analyses that provide information to improve patient care and to develop nursing knowledge. Without such knowledge, nurse informatics specialists are insufficiently equipped to influence software development and purchases. A frequent result is that systems are purchased and documentation systems are built that do not meet the needs of nurse clinicians or nurse managers. If an organization cannot hire a nursing informatics specialist who fully understands the importance of standardized nursing languages and classification, a mentoring program with a qualified nursing informatics specialist and a classification developer is recommended. This mentoring can be supported by networking with other nursing informatics specialists, classification developers, and nurse researchers; by contacting nurses in organizations that have effective electronic nursing systems; and by joining informatics listserves and informatics-related organizations.

CONCLUSION

It is the responsibility and obligation of the profession and nurses to ensure that nursing CIS are designed to benefit nursing practice and enable the use of clinical nursing data to evaluate quality and effectiveness of the nursing care provided to patients. These systems should also inform clinical decision making, support evidence-based practice, and advance nursing science. To accomplish these ends, clinical nursing data must be documented in a properly integrated operational CIS and must be retrievable and stored in data repositories and warehouses for analysis. Advancing nurses' knowledge of the importance of standardized nursing terminologies and CIS development is the principal strategy recommended to address the issues that constrain nursing data retrieval and the development of data warehouses. Nurses who are armed with more knowledge will insist that EHR systems are properly designed to benefit their practice and use of nursing clinical data. If these knowledge issues are not addressed, nursing will not capture and use its clinical data to benefit the profession and nursing data will remain a neglected resource in the provision of quality health care to the patients nursing serves.

REFERENCES

Bakken, S. (2003). Building nursing knowledge through informatics: From concept representation to data mining. *Journal of Biomedical Informatics, 36*(4–5), 229–231.

Barton, A. J. (1994). Data needs for decision support of chief nurse executives. *Journal of Nursing Administration, 24*(4 Suppl.), 19–25.

Dimitropoulos, L. L. (2009). Health information security and privacy collaboration: Action and implementation manual. Retrieved September 24, 2010, from http://healthit.hhs.gov/html/hispc/AIMReport.pdf

Fetter, M. S. (2009). Using case studies to define nursing informatics interoperability. *Issues in Mental Health Nursing, 30*(8), 524–525.

Gilfillan, I. (2002, June). Introduction to relational databases. *Database Journal, 1.*

Head, B. J., Scherb, C. A., Maas, M. L., Swanson, E. A., Moorhead, S., Reed, D., et al. (in press). Clinical documentation data retrieval for hospitalized older adults with heart failure: Part 2. *International Journal of Nursing Terminologies and Classifications.*

Head, B. J., Scherb, C. A., Reed, D., Conley, D. M., Weinberg, B., Kozel, M., et al. (2010). Nursing diagnoses, nursing interventions, and patient outcomes of hospitalized older adults with pneumonia. *Research in Gerontological Nursing.* Advance online publication. doi:10.3928/19404921-20100601-99.

Keenan, G. (1999). Use of standardized nursing language will make nursing visible. *Michigan Nurse, 72*(2), 12–13.

Konstantas, D., Bourrières, J., Léonard, M., & Boudjlida, N. (Eds.). (2006). *Interoperability of enterprise software and applications.* London: Springer-Verlag.

Nationwide Health Information Network Cooperative DURSA Workgroup. (2009). Data use and reciprocal support agreement (DURSA). Retrieved September 24, 2010, from healthit.hhs.gov/. . ./DURSA_2009_VersionforProductionPilots_20091123.pdf

Polk, L. V., & Green, P. M. (2007). Contamination: Nursing diagnoses with outcome and intervention linkages. *International Journal of Nursing Terminologies and Classifications, 18*(2), 37–44.

Scherb, C. A., Head, B. J., Maas, M. L., Swanson, E. A., Moorhead, S., Reed, D., et al. (in press). Most frequent nursing diagnoses, nursing interventions, and nursing-sensitive patient outcomes of hospitalized older adults with heart failure: Part 1. *International Journal of Nursing Terminologies and Classifications.*

U.S. Department of Health & Human Services. (2003). *Health information privacy: Research.* Retrieved March 22, 2010, from www.hhs.gov/ocr/privacy/hipaa/understanding/special/research/index.html

U.S. Department of Health & Human Services. (2008). *National privacy and security framework for electronic exchange of individually identifiable health information.* Retrieved September 23, 2010 from http://healthit.hhs.gov/portal/server.pt/gateway/PTARGS_0_10731_848088_0_0_18/NationwidePS_Framework-5.pdf

Werley, H. H., & Lang, N. M. (Eds.). (1988). *Identification of the nursing minimum data set.* New York: Springer.

Introduction to Linkages for Actual and Health Promotion Diagnoses

This section of the book contains the linkages among NANDA-I, NOC, and NIC. **A number of changes have been made in how the linkages are constructed and presented.** Entry to the linkages continues to be through a NANDA-I diagnosis. The user will locate the diagnosis of interest, and suggested NOC outcomes and NIC interventions will appear with that diagnosis. The diagnoses are in alphabetical order; however, the first word represents the major concept in the diagnosis. For example, when looking for the NANDA-I diagnosis *Impaired Gas Exchange,* the user should search for *Gas Exchange, Impaired.* When the NANDA-I diagnosis begins with terms such as *impaired, ineffective,* or *imbalanced,* those terms will appear at the end of the label name rather than at the beginning. If the diagnosis begins with *Readiness for Enhanced,* again the concept will appear first, such as *Sleep, Readiness for Enhanced.* The diagnoses that depict the risk for developing a problem are not included in the alphabetical list of diagnoses that represent a patient/client state with defining characteristics. *Risk for Diagnoses* include only related factors and not defining characteristics; these diagnoses are handled as a group following the other diagnoses.

CONSTRUCTION OF THE LINKAGES

The NANDA-I diagnoses with defining characteristics include actual and health promotion diagnoses in which the defining characteristics are manifestations, signs, or symptoms of the patient/client state. The defining characteristics of health-promoting diagnoses support readiness to improve one's health status. The actual diagnoses also have related factors that describe conditions antecedent to, contributing to, or associated with the diagnosis (NANDA-International,

2009). The defining characteristics of the diagnosis and the indicators of the outcome describe the patient state that is to be improved or maintained by the nursing interventions.

In prior editions, linkages included some outcomes, but particularly interventions, that addressed the related factors as well as the defining characteristics. The authors recognize that the related factors may be of utmost importance in selecting interventions for a patient/client, but they often present a new diagnosis to be addressed. For example, the defining characteristics of the diagnosis *Ineffective Peripheral Tissue Perfusion* and the indicators of the outcome, *Tissue Perfusion: Peripheral,* are measures to assess actual tissue perfusion. Although related factors, such as deficient knowledge, diabetes mellitus, hypertension, and sedentary lifestyle, may be antecedent to or associated with inadequate tissue perfusion, they often represent another nursing diagnosis that must be considered. NANDA-I diagnoses that could be considered are *Deficient Knowledge* and *Sedentary Lifestyle.*

We have made every attempt to select outcomes and interventions that address the defining characteristics of the diagnosis or the indicators of the outcome that are pertinent given the diagnosis. To facilitate consideration of interventions that are crucial for treating the related factors, we have included with each nursing diagnosis the major interventions that can be used to address the related factors. Making these changes has decreased the number of interventions and, in some cases, the number of outcomes provided for each diagnosis; in other instances additional outcomes or interventions have been added.

PRESENTATION OF THE LINKAGES

The changes made in the construction of the linkages have allowed for changes in formatting of the linkages. The NIC interventions that are listed for the related factors with actual diagnoses are presented in alphabetical order before the table presenting the outcomes and interventions associated with the defining characteristics. Although the interventions are not linked to specific related factors, it is readily apparent which related factors have been considered when selecting interventions. For example, nursing interventions to treat the related factors of *Ineffective Peripheral Tissue Perfusion,* as described previously, include teaching interventions, exercise promotion, and health education. Related factors, such as aging and surgical procedures, cannot be resolved by nursing interventions, but need to be considered when planning care. In these instances, the important considerations are the effects of aging or surgery on the patient/client and the diagnoses, outcomes, and interventions that would address these effects.

The table linking the diagnoses, outcomes, and interventions now contains three columns: "Outcome," "Major Interventions," and "Suggested Interventions." The outcomes continue to be listed alphabetically with the outcome definition provided. The interventions are also listed alphabetically, thereby allowing the user to determine those most appropriate for the patient

situation. Many of the interventions previously in the "Optional Interventions" column addressed related factors and therefore have been moved to "NICs Associated with Diagnosis Related Factors" or have been deleted. In other instances, the interventions in the suggested column address both the related factors and the defining characteristics and are included in both sections.

The changes not only continue to require the nurse to make clinical judgments about the outcomes and interventions for the individual patient but also may assist in identifying additional diagnoses for consideration. The changes have also helped the developers of NOC and NIC identify new outcomes and interventions that are needed as well as those that need further refinement. These changes, hopefully, will increase the usefulness of the linkages for clinicians, students, nurse informaticists and health information technology specialist.

The two case studies that follow illustrate the use of NOC and NANDA-I linkages with two NANDA-I diagnoses. One is a case study using two actual diagnoses, and the other case study is for the health promotion diagnosis *Readiness for Enhanced Childbearing Process.* Other case studies using NNN can be found in the second edition of *NANDA, NOC, and NIC Linkages: Nursing Diagnoses, Outcomes, & Interventions* (Johnson et al., 2006) and in the critical thinking book written by Lunney (2009).

CASE STUDY 1

NANDA-I Actual Diagnosis

Karl L. is an 80-year-old man, widowed for 10 years, who resides in his own home. Karl had a cholecystectomy when he was 65 and a transurethral resection of the prostate for benign prostatic hypertrophy when he was 70. He has been treated for congestive heart failure for the past 5 years, and during the past 3 months he has been taking 80 mg of Lasix each morning. Karl has reduced his activity level because of his cardiac decompensation and has experienced loss of strength and compromised mobility for self-care activities. He has particular difficulty with small motor tasks, particularly changing his clothing. He often does not remove his clothing at night and resists changing his clothing more than once or twice a week. Frequently, the home health nurse or aide finds his underwear and trousers wet with urine. His urinary output is usually over 1000 mL. He is a heavy coffee drinker and does not like decaffeinated coffee. Urinalysis revealed that the urine was clear of bacteria and fungi. Karl reports that he knows when he has to urinate, but that he cannot reach the toilet in time. He states that he has reduced his fluid intake, except for coffee, in an effort to decrease the need to urinate. Following a comprehensive assessment, the nurse documents the signs and symptoms (defining characteristics) for two priority nursing diagnoses: *Urge Urinary Incontinence* and *Toileting Self-Care Deficit.*

The nurse used several significant defining characteristics to rule out other urinary incontinence nursing diagnoses. Karl is aware of the need to void; therefore a diagnosis of *Reflex Urinary Incontinence* is eliminated. The observation that Karl voids in large amounts in fairly regular 2- to 3-hour intervals is not consistent with a diagnosis of *Stress Urinary Incontinence*.

The plan of care for Karl is based on the nursing diagnoses and the desired nursing-sensitive patient outcomes, and includes the nursing interventions selected to achieve the outcomes. Karl and the nurse agreed that he should be able to consistently demonstrate urinary continence, maintain an adequate fluid intake, be completely independent with his toileting self-care, and be knowledgeable about his medications. The priority NOC outcome for Karl is *Urinary Continence*. Nursing interventions for his plan of care are selected to resolve or ameliorate the identified etiologies of his urinary incontinence diagnoses. The establishment of a predictable pattern of urination is most important to avoid an incontinent accident attributable to the inability to suppress urge. It is also important to monitor the timeliness of Karl's response to urge and the adequacy of time needed to reach the toilet in the event a predictable pattern of voiding is not attained. Assessment of dryness of undergarments during the day and of bedding at night provides data needed to determine if there are any incontinent episodes. Karl's ability to manage clothing independently is evaluated periodically to assess whether it continues to interfere with the time it takes him to respond to the urge to urinate. His self-care with toileting is monitored both to evaluate his abilities to get to and from the toilet and remove clothing and to determine if any interventions are needed to prevent the loss of these abilities. Fluid intake is an essential outcome indicator to measure the dilution of urine and decreased bladder irritation. The amount of oral intake and avoidance of fluids that contain caffeine are important indicators for the outcome *Urinary Continence*. Being knowledgeable about his medication is another essential outcome for Karl because of the effect of Lasix on urine output and urgency. Because Lasix plays an important role in the management of Karl's congestive heart failure, he should possess a thorough understanding of the medication and its effects. The other outcomes listed below for his plan of care should be measured weekly for the first month; depending on his progress, the outcomes could then potentially be measured monthly or at longer intervals.

The nurse discussed the nursing diagnoses of *Urge Urinary Incontinence*, and *Functional Urinary Incontinence* with Karl, explaining the factors that contributed to each, including the action of his medication. Karl agreed that he desired to be continent, and therefore was willing to become more knowledgeable about his medication and to improve his self-care in toileting. He and the nurse established the following plan to achieve the priority goal of reducing his incidents of incontinence.

CASE STUDY 1—cont'd

NANDA-I Diagnosis

Urge Urinary Incontinence
Defining Characteristics
Reports inability to reach toilet in time to avoid
   urine loss
Reports urinary urgency

NOC Outcomes	NIC Interventions
Urinary Continence	Urinary Habit Training
Indicators	Urinary Incontinence Care
Maintains predictable pattern of voiding	Pelvic Muscle Exercise
Responds to urge in timely manner	
Gets to toilet between urge and passage of urine	
Manages clothing independently	
Ingests adequate amount of fluid	
Identifies medication that interferes with	
urinary control	
Knowledge: Prescribed Medication	Teaching: Prescribed Medication
Indicators	
Medication therapeutic effects	
Medication side effects	
Medication adverse effects	
Correct use of prescribed medication	

NANDA-I Diagnosis

Toileting Self-Care Deficit
Defining Characteristics
Inability to get to toilet
Inability to carry out proper toilet hygiene
Inability to manipulate clothing for toileting

NOC Outcomes	NIC Interventions
Self-Care: Toileting	Self-Care Assistance: Toileting
Indicators	Fluid Monitoring
Responds to full bladder in timely manner	Urinary Elimination Management
Gets to toilet between urge and passage of urine	Urinary Incontinence Care
Removes clothing	
Adjusts clothing after toileting	

After Karl understood the impact of caffeine and reduced fluid intake in causing bladder irritation, he agreed to limit his coffee intake to 2 to 3 cups each day and to increase his total fluid intake to at least 1500 mL daily. He volunteered to try decaffeinated coffee and to drink noncitric juices and a beer with his evening meal. With his approval, the nurse sent a pair of his trousers to the local laundry to have Velcro fasteners placed on the fly instead of a zipper. Karl also agreed to toilet himself at least every 2 hours in an attempt to avoid urgency and precipitance of urination. The nurse also trained Karl to regularly perform pelvic floor exercises each time he toileted. The nurse reviewed Karl's outcomes and indicators with him and together they rated his progress at each weekly visit. They agreed to monitor his progress monthly thereafter until the diagnosis is resolved.

CASE STUDY 2

NANDA-I Health Promotion Diagnosis

Kate B., a 27-year-old married woman, is 9 weeks pregnant with her first child. She lives with her husband Ben and their two dogs in a three-bedroom townhouse. Both Kate and her husband are attorneys and looking forward to starting a family. Kate works full-time in a small firm specializing in environmental law; Ben works in a large practice as a trial lawyer and spends approximately 60 hours a week at work. Kate intends to take a 6 month leave of absence after the birth of her child and then return to work on a part-time basis. Because her husband works long hours, Kate's mother will come to help Kate when she and the baby return home after the delivery. Kate is presenting for her second prenatal visit to her obstetrician and nurse practitioner in a private obstetrical practice. Kate's general health is excellent; she does not smoke and is avoiding alcohol during her pregnancy. Her vital signs are within normal limits as are her laboratory test results. However, she is experiencing some nausea in the mornings and occasionally at other times of the day that is being controlled with medication. She is concerned that she might be gaining weight too rapidly and unsure about continuing with her exercise program and running. She also has some questions about the herbs and vitamins she normally takes; she is not sure which ones are safe. She is an only child and states she is somewhat worried about caring for an infant because of her limited contact with babies and small children. Kate indicated that both she and her husband plan to attend prenatal and parenting classes before the birth of their child. After her examination, the nurse practitioner identified the following diagnosis, outcomes, and interventions. The defining characteristics used to make the diagnosis are presented along with the outcome, outcome indicators and interventions that will be the nurse practitioner's focus during this and future visits until Kate reaches the third trimester.

NANDA-I Diagnosis

Readiness for Enhanced Childbearing Process
Defining Characteristics
Reports an appropriate prenatal lifestyle (has questions about controlling her weight gain, exercise limitations, and the safety of vitamins and herbs)
Reports managing unpleasant symptoms in pregnancy (nausea)
Seeks necessary knowledge (delivery and parenting)
Reports availability of support systems
Has regular prenatal visits

NOC Outcomes

Knowledge: Pregnancy
Indicators
Importance of prenatal education
Warning signs of pregnancy complications
Major fetal developmental milestones
Fetal movement pattern
Anatomic and physiologic changes in pregnancy
Psychological changes associated with pregnancy
Emotional changes associated with pregnancy
Proper body mechanics
Benefits of activity and exercise
Healthy nutritional practices
Healthy weight gain pattern
Correct use of nonprescription medication
Correct use of motor vehicle safety devices

NIC Interventions

Anticipatory Guidance
Body Mechanics Promotion
Childbirth Preparation
Energy Management
Medication Management
Nutritional Counseling
Teaching: Individual
Teaching: Group
Weight Management

Continued

CASE STUDY 2—cont'd

Prenatal Health Behavior
Indicators
Uses proper body mechanics
Keeps appointments for prenatal care
Maintains healthy weight gain pattern
Attends childbirth education classes
Participates in regular exercise
Maintains adequate nutrient intake for pregnancy
Uses medication as prescribed
Consults health professional about nonprescription
    medication use
Avoids environmental hazards

Body Mechanics Promotion
Environmental Management:
    Safety
Exercise Promotion
Medication Management
Nutritional Counseling
Prenatal Care
Risk Identification
Vehicle Safety Promotion
Weight Management

REFERENCES

Johnson, M., Bulechek, G., Butcher, H., Dochterman, J. M., Maas, M., Moorhead, S., & Swanson, E. (2006). *NANDA, NOC, and NIC linkages: Nursing diagnoses, outcomes, & interventions* (2nd ed.). Philadelphia: Mosby Elsevier.

Lunney, M. (Ed). (2009). *Critical thinking to achieve positive health outcomes: Nursing case studies and analyses* (2nd ed.). Ames, Iowa: Wiley-Blackwell.

NANDA-International. (2009). *Nursing diagnoses: Definitions and classification 2009-2011*. West Sussex, United Kingdom: Wiley-Blackwell.

NOC and NIC Linked to Nursing Diagnoses

NURSING DIAGNOSIS: Activity Intolerance

Definition: Insufficient physiological or psychological energy to endure or complete required or desired daily activities

NICS ASSOCIATED WITH DIAGNOSIS RELATED FACTORS

Activity Therapy
Bed Rest Care
	Cardiac Care:
	  Rehabilitative
	Exercise
	  Promotion
		Exercise Promotion: Strength
		  Training
		Exercise Therapy:
		  Ambulation
			Oxygen Therapy
			Ventilation Assistance

NOC-NIC LINKAGES FOR ACTIVITY INTOLERANCE

Outcome	Major Interventions	Suggested Interventions	

Activity Tolerance
 	
Definition:
Physiological
  response to
  energy-consuming
  movements with
  daily activities
	Cardiac Care:
	  Rehabilitative
	Exercise
	  Promotion:
	  Strength
	  Training
		Activity Therapy
		Asthma Management
		Autogenic Training
		Biofeedback
		Body Mechanics
		  Promotion
		Dysrhythmia
		  Management
		Energy Management
		Environmental
		  Management
		Exercise Promotion
		Exercise Promotion:
		  Stretching
		Exercise Therapy:
		  Ambulation
		Exercise Therapy: Balance
			Exercise Therapy: Joint
			  Mobility
			Exercise Therapy: Muscle
			  Control
			Medication
			  Management
			Nutrition
			  Management
			Oxygen Therapy
			Pain Management
			Respiratory
			  Monitoring
			Sleep Enhancement
			Smoking Cessation
			  Assistance
			Teaching: Prescribed
			  Activity/Exercise
			Vital Signs
			  Monitoring
			Weight Management

Continued

NOC-NIC LINKAGES FOR ACTIVITY INTOLERANCE

Outcome	Major Interventions	Suggested Interventions	
Endurance Definition: Capacity to sustain activity	Energy Management Exercise Promotion: Strength Training	Activity Therapy Cardiac Care: Rehabilitative Eating Disorders Management Environmental Management Environmental Management: Comfort Exercise Promotion Exercise Therapy: Ambulation Exercise Therapy: Balance	Exercise Therapy: Joint Mobility Exercise Therapy: Muscle Control Nutrition Management Oxygen Therapy Pain Management Sleep Enhancement Teaching: Prescribed Activity/Exercise Weight Management
Energy Conservation Definition: Personal actions to manage energy for initiating and sustaining activity	Energy Management Environmental Management	Activity Therapy Body Mechanics Promotion Environmental Management: Comfort Exercise Promotion Exercise Therapy: Ambulation Exercise Therapy: Balance Exercise Therapy: Joint Mobility	Exercise Therapy: Muscle Control Nutrition Management Self-Modification Assistance Sleep Enhancement Teaching: Prescribed Activity/Exercise Weight Management
Fatigue Level Definition: Severity of observed or reported pro-longed generalized fatigue	Energy Management Sleep Enhancement	Anxiety Reduction Massage Mood Management Nutrition Management Pain Management	Referral Self-Care Assistance Self-Care Assistance: IADL Teaching: Prescribed Activity/Exercise
Psychomotor Energy Definition: Personal drive and energy to maintain activities of daily living, nutrition, and personal safety	Energy Management Mood Management	Animal-Assisted Therapy Art Therapy Counseling Emotional Support Exercise Promotion Grief Work Facilitation Guilt Work Facilitation	Hope Inspiration Medication Management Music Therapy Recreation Therapy Self-Esteem Enhancement Spiritual Support Therapy Group
Rest Definition: Quantity and pattern of diminished activity for mental and physical rejuvenation	Energy Management	Aromatherapy Environmental Management: Comfort Massage Meditation Facilitation	Relaxation Therapy Respite Care Sleep Enhancement

NOC-NIC LINKAGES FOR ACTIVITY INTOLERANCE

Outcome	Major Interventions	Suggested Interventions	
Self-Care: Activities of Daily Living (ADL)			
Definition: Ability to perform the most basic physical tasks and personal care activities independently with or without assistive device	Self-Care Assistance	Body Mechanics Promotion Energy Management Exercise Promotion Exercise Promotion: Stretching Exercise Therapy: Ambulation Exercise Therapy: Balance Exercise Therapy: Joint Mobility Exercise Therapy: Muscle Control	Self-Care Assistance: Bathing/Hygiene Self-Care Assistance: Dressing/Grooming Self-Care Assistance: Feeding Self-Care Assistance: Toileting Self-Care Assistance: Transfer Teaching: Prescribed Activity/Exercise
Self-Care: Instrumental Activities of Daily Living (IADL)			
Definition: Ability to perform activities needed to function in the home or community independently with or without assistive device	Home Maintenance Assistance Self-Care Assistance: IADL	Body Mechanics Promotion Energy Management Environmental Management Environmental Management: Home Preparation	Exercise Promotion: Strength Training Financial Resource Assistance Referral

Critical reasoning note: A number of possible outcomes are provided because endurance and management of energy and fatigue are aspects of activity tolerance necessary for carrying out daily activities. The self-care outcomes are included because the definition identifies Activity Tolerance as energy needed to carry out desired daily living. Some chronic conditions increase the risk for experiencing this diagnosis, such as asthma, cardiac conditions, respiratory diseases, cancer, and depression, and are reflected in the interventions listed.

NURSING DIAGNOSIS: Activity Planning, Ineffective

Definition: Inability to prepare for a set of actions fixed in time and under certain conditions

NICS ASSOCIATED WITH DIAGNOSIS RELATED FACTORS

Decision-Making Support Delusion Management	Dementia Management Family Involvement Promotion	Family Mobilization Self-Efficacy Enhancement	Self-Responsibility Facilitation Support System Enhancement

NOC-NIC LINKAGES FOR ACTIVITY PLANNING, INEFFECTIVE

Outcome	Major Interventions	Suggested Interventions	
Anxiety Level			
Definition: Severity of manifested apprehension, tension, or uneasiness arising from an unidentifiable source	Anxiety Reduction	Active Listening Calming Technique Coping Enhancement Meditation Facilitation	Relaxation Therapy Resiliency Promotion Sleep Enhancement Vital Signs Monitoring

Continued

NOC-NIC LINKAGES FOR ACTIVITY PLANNING, INEFFECTIVE

Outcome	Major Interventions	Suggested Interventions	
Decision-Making			
Definition: Ability to make judgments and choose between two or more alternatives	Decision-Making Support Mutual Goal Setting	Coping Enhancement Dementia Management	Memory Training
Fear Level			
Definition: Severity of manifested apprehension, tension, or uneasiness arising from an identifiable source	Calming Technique	Active Listening Anticipatory Guidance Anxiety Reduction Coping Enhancement Counseling	Emotional Support Relaxation Therapy Resiliency Promotion Sleep Enhancement Vital Signs Monitoring
Health Beliefs: Perceived Ability to Perform			
Definition: Personal conviction that one can carry out a given health behavior	Self-Efficacy Enhancement Teaching: Individual	Anticipatory Guidance Culture Brokerage Health Education Health Literacy Enhancement	Learning Readiness Enhancement Self-Modification Assistance Self-Responsibility Facilitation
Motivation			
Definition: Inner urge that moves or prompts an individual to positive action(s)	Self-Efficacy Enhancement Self-Responsibility Facilitation	Decision-Making Support Financial Resource Assistance Mutual Goal Setting	Resiliency Promotion Self-Modification Assistance

NURSING DIAGNOSIS: Airway Clearance, Ineffective

Definition: Inability to clear secretions or obstructions from the respiratory tract to maintain a clear airway

NICS ASSOCIATED WITH DIAGNOSIS RELATED FACTORS

Artificial Airway Management Asthma Management	Chest Physiotherapy Cough Enhancement	Infection Control Smoking Cessation Assistance

NOC-NIC LINKAGES FOR AIRWAY CLEARANCE, INEFFECTIVE

Outcome	Major Interventions	Suggested Interventions	
Aspiration Prevention			
Definition: Personal actions to prevent the passage of fluid and solid particles into the lung	Airway Suctioning Aspiration Precautions Positioning	Airway Management Chest Physiotherapy Cough Enhancement Emergency Care Endotracheal Extubation	Respiratory Monitoring Resuscitation: Neonate Surveillance Swallowing Therapy

NOC-NIC LINKAGES FOR AIRWAY CLEARANCE, INEFFECTIVE

Outcome	Major Interventions	Suggested Interventions	
Respiratory Status: Airway Patency Definition: Open, clear tracheobronchial passages for air exchange	Airway Management Airway Suctioning	Airway Insertion and Stabilization Allergy Management Anaphylaxis Management Anxiety Reduction Artificial Airway Management Aspiration Precautions Asthma Management Chest Physiotherapy	Cough Enhancement Emergency Care Positioning Respiratory Monitoring Resuscitation Surveillance Vital Signs Monitoring
Respiratory Status: Ventilation Definition: Movement of air in and out of the lungs	Airway Management Respiratory Monitoring Ventilation Assistance	Acid-Base Monitoring Airway Insertion and Stabilization Airway Suctioning Allergy Management Anxiety Reduction Artificial Airway Management Aspiration Precautions Asthma Management Chest Physiotherapy Cough Enhancement Energy Management	Fluid Monitoring Infection Control Mechanical Ventilation Management: Invasive Mechanical Ventilatory Weaning Medication Administration: Inhalation Oxygen Therapy Positioning Smoking Cessation Assistance Tube Care: Chest

Critical reasoning note: A number of the interventions for related factors are also interventions for specific outcomes. This occurs because an obstructed airway (related factor) is the cause of many of the symptoms identified in the defining characteristics.

PART II - A

NURSING DIAGNOSIS: Anxiety

Definition: Vague uneasy feeling of discomfort or dread accompanied by an autonomic response (the source often nonspecific or unknown to the individual); a feeling of apprehension caused by anticipation of danger. It is an alerting signal that warns of impending danger and enables the individual to take measures to deal with threat

NICS ASSOCIATED WITH DIAGNOSIS RELATED FACTORS

Conflict Mediation
Crisis Intervention
Environmental Management: Safety

Environmental Risk Protection
Financial Resource Assistance
Grief Work Facilitation

Role Enhancement
Self-Awareness Enhancement

Substance Use Treatment
Values Clarification

Continued

NOC-NIC LINKAGES FOR ANXIETY

Outcome	Major Interventions	Suggested Interventions	

Anxiety Level
Definition:
Severity of manifested apprehension, tension, or uneasiness arising from an unidentifiable source
	Anxiety Reduction
	Calming Technique
		Active Listening
		Anger Control Assistance
		Aromatherapy
		Autogenic Training
		Coping Enhancement
		Crisis Intervention
		Decision-Making Support
		Dementia Management
		Dementia Management:
		  Bathing
			Distraction
			Medication
			  Administration
			Music Therapy
			Relaxation Therapy
			Relocation Stress
			  Reduction
			Security Enhancement
			Sleep Enhancement
			Vital Signs Monitoring

Anxiety Self-Control
Definition:
Personal actions to eliminate or reduce feelings of apprehension, tension, or uneasiness from an unidentifiable source
	Coping Enhancement
	Relaxation Therapy
		Animal-Assisted Therapy
		Anxiety Reduction
		Autogenic Training
		Biofeedback
		Diarrhea Management
		Distraction
		Environmental
		  Management
		Exercise Promotion
		Guided Imagery
		Medication Administration
		Meditation Facilitation
			Music Therapy
			Nausea Management
			Premenstrual
			  Syndrome (PMS)
			  Management
			Preparatory Sensory
			  Information
			Progressive Muscle
			  Relaxation
			Sleep Enhancement
			Support Group
			Teaching: Preoperative
			Therapeutic Play
			Therapy Group

Concentration
Definition:
Ability to focus on a specific stimulus
	Anxiety Reduction
	Calming Technique
		Autogenic Training
		Behavior Management:
		  Overactivity/Inattention
		Distraction
			Guided Imagery
			Learning Readiness
			  Enhancement
			Relaxation Therapy
			Reminiscence Therapy

Coping
Definition:
Personal actions to manage stressors that tax an individual's resources
	Anxiety Reduction
	Coping Enhancement
		Anticipatory Guidance
		Behavior Modification
		Childbirth Preparation
		Genetic Counseling
		Grief Work Facilitation
		Grief Work Facilitation:
		  Perinatal Death
		Guilt Work Facilitation
		Meditation Facilitation
		Preparatory Sensory
		  Information
			Recreation Therapy
			Relaxation Therapy
			Relocation Stress
			  Reduction
			Reminiscence Therapy
			Self-Awareness
			  Enhancement
			Spiritual Support
			Support Group
			Therapeutic Play

NURSING DIAGNOSIS: Autonomic Dysreflexia

Definition: Life-threatening, uninhibited sympathetic response of the nervous system to a noxious stimulus after a spinal cord injury at T7 or above

NICS ASSOCIATED WITH DIAGNOSIS RELATED FACTORS

Bowel Management
Medication
  Administration: Skin
Skin Care: Topical
  Treatments

Teaching: Disease
  Process
Teaching: Prescribed
  Medication
Teaching: Procedure/
  Treatment

Temperature Regulation
Urinary Catheterization

Urinary Catheterization:
  Intermittent
Urinary Elimination
  Management

NOC-NIC LINKAGES FOR AUTONOMIC DYSREFLEXIA

Outcome	Major Interventions	Suggested Interventions	
Neurological Status Definition: Ability of the peripheral and central nervous systems to receive, process, and respond to internal and external stimuli	Dysreflexia Management Vital Signs Monitoring	Code Management Emergency Care Medication Administration Neurological Monitoring Respiratory Monitoring Seizure Precautions	Surveillance Teaching: Disease Process Teaching: Prescribed Medication Teaching: Procedure/ Treatment Temperature Regulation
Neurological Status: Autonomic Definition: Ability of the autonomic nervous system to coordinate visceral and homeostatic functions	Dysreflexia Management Vital Signs Monitoring	Anxiety Reduction Code Management Emergency Care Infection Protection Intravenous (IV) Insertion Intravenous (IV) Therapy Medication Administration	Pain Management Neurological Monitoring Respiratory Monitoring Surveillance Technology Management Temperature Regulation
Vital Signs Definition: Extent to which temperature, pulse, respiration, and blood pressure are within normal range	Dysreflexia Management Vital Signs Monitoring	Airway Management Anxiety Reduction Cough Enhancement Emergency Care	Medication Administration Pain Management Shock Prevention

PART II - A

NURSING DIAGNOSIS: Body Image, Disturbed

Definition: Confusion in mental picture of one's physical self

NICS ASSOCIATED WITH DIAGNOSIS RELATED FACTORS

Cognitive Restructuring
Culture Brokerage
Delusion Management

Developmental
  Enhancement:
  Adolescent

Socialization
  Enhancement
Spiritual Support

NOC-NIC LINKAGES FOR BODY IMAGE, DISTURBED

Outcome	Major Interventions	Suggested Interventions	
Adaptation to Physical Disability Definition: Adaptive response to a significant functional challenge due to a physical disability	Body Image Enhancement Self-Esteem Enhancement	Active Listening Anticipatory Guidance Anxiety Reduction Coping Enhancement Counseling Emotional Support Grief Work Facilitation	Home Maintenance Assistance Self-Care Assistance: IADL Socialization Enhancement Support Group Support System Enhancement Teaching: Disease Process Teaching: Procedure/ Treatment
Body Image Definition: Perception of own appearance and body functions	Body Image Enhancement	Active Listening Amputation Care Anticipatory Guidance Cognitive Restructuring Coping Enhancement Counseling Eating Disorders Management Emotional Support Grief Work Facilitation Ostomy Care	Self-Awareness Enhancement Self-Esteem Enhancement Support Group Support System Enhancement Therapy Group Truth Telling Unilateral Neglect Management Values Clarification Weight Management
Child Development: Middle Childhood Definition: Milestones of physical, cognitive, and psychosocial progression from 6 years through 11 years of age	Developmental Enhancement: Child Parent Education: Childrearing Family	Abuse Protection Support: Child Behavior Management: Overactivity/ Inattention Body Image Enhancement Eating Disorders Management Exercise Promotion	Self-Awareness Enhancement Self-Esteem Enhancement Teaching: Sexuality Therapeutic Play Urinary Incontinence Care: Enuresis Weight Management

NOC-NIC LINKAGES FOR BODY IMAGE, DISTURBED		
Outcome	**Major Interventions**	**Suggested Interventions**
Child Development: Adolescence Definition: Milestones of physical, cognitive, and psychosocial progression from 12 years through 17 years of age	Body Image Enhancement Developmental Enhancement: Adolescent Self-Esteem Enhancement	Abuse Protection Support Counseling Eating Disorders Management Exercise Promotion Parent Education: Adolescent	Self-Awareness Enhancement Teaching: Safe Sex Teaching: Sexuality Values Clarification Weight Management
Heedfulness of Affected Side Definition: Personal actions to acknowledge, protect, and cognitively integrate body part(s) into self	Unilateral Neglect Management	Amputation Care Behavior Modification	Cognitive Restructuring Self-Modification Assistance
Self-Esteem Definition: Personal judgment of self-worth	Body Image Enhancement Self-Esteem Enhancement	Active Listening Bibliotherapy Coping Enhancement Counseling Developmental Enhancement: Adolescent Developmental Enhancement: Child Emotional Support	Journaling Parent Education: Adolescent Parent Education: Childrearing Family Security Enhancement Self-Awareness Enhancement Spiritual Support Support Group Weight Management

PART II - B

NURSING DIAGNOSIS: Bowel Incontinence

Definition: Change in normal bowel habits characterized by involuntary passage of stool

NICS ASSOCIATED WITH DIAGNOSIS RELATED FACTORS			
Allergy Management Anxiety Reduction Dementia Care	Environmental Management Exercise Therapy: Ambulation Medication Management	Nutritional Counseling Reality Orientation	Self-Care Assistance: Toileting Teaching: Prescribed Diet

Continued

NOC-NIC LINKAGES FOR BOWEL INCONTINENCE

Outcome	Major Interventions	Suggested Interventions	
Bowel Continence Definition: Control of passage of stool from the bowel	Bowel Incontinence Care	Anxiety Reduction Bowel Incontinence Care: Encopresis Bowel Management Bowel Training Constipation/Impaction Management Diarrhea Management Diet Staging Exercise Therapy: Ambulation	Flatulence Reduction Fluid Management Medication Management Nutrition Management Rectal Prolapse Management Self-Care Assistance: Toileting Teaching: Prescribed Diet
Tissue Integrity: Skin & Mucous Membranes Definition: Structural intactness and normal physiological function of skin and mucous membranes	Bowel Incontinence Care Perineal Care Skin Surveillance	Bathing Diarrhea Management	Medication Administration: Skin Medication Management

Critical reasoning note: The outcome Tissue Integrity: Skin & Mucous Membranes is included because red perianal skin is one of the defining characteristics and a potential complication of bowel incontinence that can be prevented with nursing care.

NURSING DIAGNOSIS: Breastfeeding, Effective

Definition: Mother-infant dyad/family exhibits adequate proficiency and satisfaction with breastfeeding process

NICS ASSOCIATED WITH DIAGNOSIS RELATED FACTORS

Childbirth Preparation Developmental Care	Family Involvement Promotion	Lactation Counseling	Parent Education: Infant

NOC-NIC LINKAGES FOR BREASTFEEDING, EFFECTIVE

Outcome	Major Interventions	Suggested Interventions	
Breastfeeding Establishment: Infant Definition: Infant attachment to and sucking from the mother's breast for nourishment during the first 3 weeks of breastfeeding	Breastfeeding Assistance Lactation Counseling	Attachment Promotion Infant Care	Newborn Care Parent Education: Infant
Breastfeeding Establishment: Maternal Definition: Maternal establishment of proper attachment of an infant to and sucking from the breast for nourishment during the first 3 weeks of breastfeeding	Breastfeeding Assistance Lactation Counseling	Anticipatory Guidance Childbirth Preparation Fluid Management Fluid Monitoring Infection Protection	Skin Surveillance Support Group Teaching: Individual Teaching: Psychomotor Skill

NOC-NIC LINKAGES FOR BREASTFEEDING, EFFECTIVE		
Outcome	**Major Interventions**	**Suggested Interventions**
Breastfeeding Maintenance Definition: Continuation of breastfeeding from establishment to weaning for nourishment of an infant/toddler	Lactation Counseling	Family Involvement Promotion Fluid Management Infant Care Infection Protection Skin Care: Topical Treatments Skin Surveillance	Support Group Teaching: Infant Nutrition 0-3 Months Teaching: Infant Nutrition 4-6 Months Teaching: Infant Nutrition 7-9 Months Teaching: Infant Nutrition 10-12 Months
Breastfeeding Weaning Definition: Progressive discontinuation of breastfeeding of an infant/toddler	Lactation Suppression	Anticipatory Guidance Breast Examination Heat/Cold Application Infection Protection Pain Management Skin Surveillance	Teaching: Infant Nutrition 0-3 Months Teaching: Infant Nutrition 4-6 Months Teaching: Infant Nutrition 7-9 Months Teaching: Infant Nutrition 10-12 Months

Clinical reasoning note: Although maternal nutrition is not addressed in the diagnosis, Nutritional Counseling should be considered as an intervention if maternal nutrition is inadequate. This diagnosis is unique in that it addresses the dyad of mother and baby.

NURSING DIAGNOSIS: Breastfeeding, Ineffective

Definition: Dissatisfaction or difficulty a mother, infant, or child experiences with the breastfeeding process

NICS ASSOCIATED WITH DIAGNOSIS RELATED FACTORS			
Anxiety Reduction	Developmental Care	Family Integrity Promotion: Childrearing Family	Family Involvement Promotion

NOC-NIC LINKAGES FOR BREASTFEEDING, INEFFECTIVE		
Outcome	**Major Interventions**	**Suggested Interventions**
Breastfeeding Establishment: Infant Definition: Infant attachment to and sucking from the mother's breast for nourishment during the first 3 weeks of breastfeeding	Breastfeeding Assistance Lactation Counseling	Attachment Promotion Calming Technique Infant Care Kangaroo Care	Newborn Monitoring Nonnutritive Sucking Parent Education: Infant Teaching: Infant Safety 0-3 Months

Continued

PART II - B

NOC-NIC LINKAGES FOR BREASTFEEDING, INEFFECTIVE

Outcome	Major Interventions	Suggested Interventions	
Breastfeeding Establishment: Maternal Definition: Maternal establishment of proper attachment of an infant to and sucking from the breast for nourishment during the first 3 weeks of breastfeeding	Breastfeeding Assistance Lactation Counseling	Anticipatory Guidance Anxiety Reduction Childbirth Preparation Coping Enhancement Discharge Planning Environmental Management: Attachment Process Family Involvement Promotion Family Support Fluid Management	Fluid Monitoring Infection Protection Pain Management Relaxation Therapy Skin Care: Topical Treatments Skin Surveillance Support Group Teaching: Individual Telephone Consultation
Breastfeeding Maintenance Definition: Continuation of breastfeeding from establishment to weaning for nourishment of an infant/toddler	Lactation Counseling	Active Listening Attachment Promotion Breastfeeding Assistance Coping Enhancement Family Integrity Promotion Family Involvement Promotion Fluid Management Infant Care Infection Protection Nonnutritive Sucking Parent Education: Infant	Relaxation Therapy Skin Care: Topical Treatments Skin Surveillance Support Group Teaching: Individual Teaching: Infant Nutrition 0-3 Months Teaching: Infant Nutrition 4-6 Months Teaching: Infant Nutrition 7-9 Months Teaching: Infant Nutrition 10-12 Months
Breastfeeding Weaning Definition: Progressive discontinuation of breastfeeding of an infant/toddler	Lactation Suppression	Anticipatory Guidance Heat/Cold Application Infection Protection Pain Management Skin Surveillance	Teaching: Infant Nutrition 0-3 Months Teaching: Infant Nutrition 4-6 Months Teaching: Infant Nutrition 7-9 Months Teaching: Infant Nutrition 10-12 Months
Knowledge: Breastfeeding Definition: Extent of understanding conveyed about lactation and nourishment of an infant through breastfeeding	Lactation Counseling	Anticipatory Guidance Breastfeeding Assistance Environmental Management: Attachment Process Health System Guidance Learning Facilitation Learning Readiness Enhancement Nonnutritive Sucking Parent Education: Infant Teaching: Individual Teaching: Infant Nutrition 0-3 Months	Teaching: Infant Nutrition 4-6 Months Teaching: Infant Nutrition 7-9 Months Teaching: Infant Nutrition 10-12 Months Teaching: Infant Stimulation 0-4 Months Teaching: Infant Stimulation 5-8 Months Teaching: Infant Stimulation 9-12 Months

NURSING DIAGNOSIS: Breastfeeding, Interrupted

Definition: Break in the continuity of the breastfeeding process as a result of inability or inadvisability to put baby to breast for feeding

NICS ASSOCIATED WITH DIAGNOSIS RELATED FACTORS		
Developmental Care	Infant Care	

NOC-NIC LINKAGES FOR BREASTFEEDING, INTERRUPTED		
Outcome	**Major Interventions**	**Suggested Interventions**
Breastfeeding Maintenance Definition: Continuation of breastfeeding from establishment to weaning for nourishment of an infant/toddler	Bottle Feeding Lactation Counseling	Anticipatory Guidance Anxiety Reduction Coping Enhancement Infant Care Infection Protection Nonnutritive Sucking Pain Management	Skin Care: Topical Treatments Skin Surveillance Support Group Teaching: Individual Teaching: Infant Nutrition 0-3 Months Teaching: Infant Nutrition 4-6 Months Teaching: Infant Nutrition 7-9 Months Teaching: Infant Nutrition 10-12 Months
Knowledge: Breastfeeding Definition: Extent of understanding conveyed about lactation and nourishment of an infant through breastfeeding	Lactation Counseling	Anticipatory Guidance Bottle Feeding Environmental Management: Attachment Process Learning Facilitation Learning Readiness Enhancement Nonnutritive Sucking	Parent Education: Infant Teaching: Individual Teaching: Infant Nutrition 0-3 Months Teaching: Infant Nutrition 4-6 Months Teaching: Infant Nutrition 7-9 Months Teaching: Infant Nutrition 10-12 Months
Parent-Infant Attachment Definition: Parent and infant behaviors that demonstrate an enduring affectionate bond	Attachment Promotion Environmental Management: Attachment Process	Anticipatory Guidance Anxiety Reduction Bottle Feeding Childbirth Preparation Coping Enhancement	Family Integrity Promotion Infant Care Kangaroo Care Parent Education: Infant Role Enhancement

PART II - B

NURSING DIAGNOSIS: Breathing Pattern, Ineffective

Definition: Inspiration and/or expiration that does not provide adequate ventilation

NICS ASSOCIATED WITH DIAGNOSIS RELATED FACTORS

Anxiety Reduction	Delirium Management	Pain Management	Sleep Enhancement
Cognitive Stimulation	Developmental Care	Positioning	Weight Reduction
			Assistance

NOC-NIC LINKAGES FOR BREATHING PATTERN, INEFFECTIVE

Outcome	Major Interventions	Suggested Interventions	
Allergic Response: Systemic Definition: Severity of systemic hypersensitive immune response to a specific environmental (exogenous) antigen	Allergy Management Anaphylaxis Management	Airway Insertion and Stabilization Airway Management Airway Suctioning Anxiety Reduction Asthma Management Emergency Care Fluid Monitoring Mechanical Ventilation Management: Invasive	Medication Administration Medication Administration: Nasal Presence Respiratory Monitoring Resuscitation Surveillance Ventilation Assistance Vital Signs Monitoring
Mechanical Ventilation Response: Adult Definition: Alveolar exchange and tissue perfusion are supported by mechanical ventilation	Artificial Airway Management Mechanical Ventilation Management: Invasive	Acid-Base Monitoring Airway Suctioning Anxiety Reduction Aspiration Precautions Emergency Care Emotional Support Endotracheal Extubation Energy Management Mechanical Ventilatory Weaning Medication Management	Neurological Monitoring Oxygen Therapy Pain Management Phlebotomy: Arterial Blood Sample Phlebotomy: Venous Blood Sample Positioning Respiratory Monitoring Surveillance Vital Signs Monitoring
Mechanical Ventilation Weaning Response: Adult Definition: Respiratory and psychological adjustment to progressive removal of mechanical ventilation	Mechanical Ventilation Management: Invasive Mechanical Ventilatory Weaning	Acid-Base Monitoring Airway Suctioning Anxiety Reduction Aspiration Precautions Cough Enhancement Emotional Support Energy Management Medication Management	Oxygen Therapy Pain Management Positioning Respiratory Monitoring Surveillance Swallowing Therapy Vital Signs Monitoring

NOC-NIC LINKAGES FOR BREATHING PATTERN, INEFFECTIVE

Outcome	Major Interventions	Suggested Interventions	
Respiratory Status: Airway Patency			
Definition: Open, clear tracheobronchial passages for air exchange	Airway Management Airway Suctioning	Airway Insertion and Stabilization Allergy Management Anaphylaxis Management Anxiety Reduction Artificial Airway Management Aspiration Precautions Chest Physiotherapy Cough Enhancement	Emergency Care Emotional Support Positioning Respiratory Monitoring Resuscitation Smoking Cessation Assistance Surveillance Vital Signs Monitoring
Respiratory Status: Ventilation			
Definition: Movement of air in and out of the lungs	Airway Management Asthma Management Ventilation Assistance	Acid-Base Monitoring Airway Insertion and Stabilization Airway Suctioning Allergy Management Analgesic Administration Anxiety Reduction Artificial Airway Management Aspiration Precautions Chest Physiotherapy Cough Enhancement	Energy Management Exercise Promotion Mechanical Ventilatory Weaning Oxygen Therapy Pain Management Positioning Progressive Muscle Relaxation Respiratory Monitoring Tube Care: Chest Vital Signs Monitoring
Vital Signs			
Definition: Extent to which temperature, pulse, respiration, and blood pressure are within normal range	Respiratory Monitoring Vital Signs Monitoring	Acid-Base Management Airway Management Allergy Management Anxiety Reduction Emergency Care Fluid Management Intravenous (IV) Insertion Intravenous (IV) Therapy Medication Management	Oxygen Therapy Pain Management Postanesthesia Care Resuscitation Surveillance Teaching: Prescribed Activity/Exercise Teaching: Prescribed Medication Teaching: Procedure/ Treatment Ventilation Assistance

Critical reasoning note: The outcomes and interventions are those that both maintain an open airway and foster the movement of oxygen and carbon dioxide in and out of the lungs. Patients with this diagnosis require many physiological support interventions based on the etiology of the problem and emotional support for the anxiety frequently experienced with inadequate ventilation when the patient is conscious.

PART II - B

NURSING DIAGNOSIS: Cardiac Output, Decreased

Definition: Inadequate blood pumped by the heart to meet metabolic demands of the body

NICS ASSOCIATED WITH DIAGNOSIS RELATED FACTORS		
Vital Signs Monitoring	Hemodynamic Regulation	

NOC-NIC LINKAGES FOR CARDIAC OUTPUT, DECREASED

Outcome	Major Interventions	Suggested Interventions	
Blood Loss Severity Definition: Severity of internal or external bleeding/hemorrhage	Bleeding Reduction Hemorrhage Control Shock Management: Volume	Bleeding Reduction: Antepartum Uterus Bleeding Reduction: Gastrointestinal Bleeding Reduction: Nasal Bleeding Reduction: Postpartum Uterus Bleeding Reduction: Wound Dysrhythmia Management Fluid Management Fluid Monitoring Fluid Resuscitation	Hemodynamic Regulation Intravenous (IV) Therapy Invasive Hemodynamic Monitoring Pneumatic Tourniquet Precautions Resuscitation Shock Management Shock Management: Cardiac Shock Prevention Surveillance Vital Signs Monitoring
Cardiac Pump Effectiveness Definition: Adequacy of blood volume ejected from the left ventricle to support systemic perfusion pressure	Cardiac Care Cardiac Care: Acute Shock Management: Cardiac	Acid-Base Management Acid-Base Monitoring Airway Management Bleeding Reduction Blood Products Administration Cardiac Care: Rehabilitative Cardiac Precautions Code Management Dysrhythmia Management Electrolyte Management Electrolyte Monitoring Electronic Fetal Monitoring: Antepartum Electronic Fetal Monitoring: Intrapartum Energy Management Fluid/Electrolyte Management Fluid Management Fluid Monitoring Hemodynamic Regulation	Intravenous (IV) Insertion Intravenous (IV) Therapy Invasive Hemodynamic Monitoring Medication Administration Medication Management Pacemaker Management: Permanent Pacemaker Management: Temporary Phlebotomy: Arterial Blood Sample Phlebotomy: Cannulated Vessel Phlebotomy: Venous Blood Sample Resuscitation Resuscitation: Fetus Resuscitation: Neonate Vital Signs Monitoring

NOC-NIC LINKAGES FOR CARDIAC OUTPUT, DECREASED		
Outcome	**Major Interventions**	**Suggested Interventions**
Circulation Status		
Definition: Unobstructed, unidirectional blood flow at an appropriate pressure through large vessels of the systemic and pulmonary circuits	Circulatory Care: Arterial Insufficiency Circulatory Care: Mechanical Assist Device Circulatory Care: Venous Insufficiency	Autotransfusion Bedside Laboratory Testing Bleeding Precautions Blood Products Administration Circulatory Precautions Fluid Monitoring Fluid Resuscitation Hemodynamic Regulation Hypervolemia Management Hypovolemia Management Intravenous (IV) Insertion Intravenous (IV) Therapy Invasive Hemodynamic Monitoring Laboratory Data Interpretation Lower Extremity Monitoring Mechanical Ventilation Management: Noninvasive Medication Management Peripherally Inserted Central (PIC) Catheter Care Pneumatic Tourniquet Precautions Shock Management: Vasogenic Shock Prevention Surveillance Vital Signs Monitoring
Tissue Perfusion: Abdominal Organs		
Definition: Adequacy of blood flow through the small vessels of the abdominal viscera to maintain organ function	Circulatory Care: Arterial Insufficiency Circulatory Care: Venous Insufficiency	Acid-Base Management Acid-Base Management: Metabolic Acidosis Acid-Base Management: Metabolic Alkalosis Acid-Base Monitoring Bedside Laboratory Testing Bleeding Precautions Bleeding Reduction: Antepartum Uterus Bleeding Reduction: Gastrointestinal Bleeding Reduction: Postpartum Uterus Bleeding Reduction: Wound Blood Products Administration Electrolyte Management Electrolyte Monitoring Emergency Care Fluid Management Fluid Monitoring Fluid Resuscitation Hemodialysis Therapy Hypovolemia Management Intravenous (IV) Insertion Intravenous (IV) Therapy Laboratory Data Interpretation Nausea Management Pain Management Shock Prevention Surveillance Urinary Elimination Management Vital Signs Monitoring Vomiting Management
Tissue Perfusion: Cardiac		
Definition: Adequacy of blood flow through the coronary vasculature to maintain heart function	Circulatory Care: Arterial Insufficiency Shock Management: Cardiac	Anxiety Reduction Bleeding Precautions Cardiac Care: Acute Circulatory Care: Venous Insufficiency Code Management Dysrhythmia Management Electrolyte Management Fluid Management Fluid Monitoring Hypoglycemia Management Invasive Hemodynamic Monitoring Medication Management Nausea Management Oxygen Therapy Pacemaker Management: Temporary Pain Management Shock Management: Vasogenic Shock Management: Volume Sleep Enhancement Surveillance Vital Signs Monitoring Vomiting Management

PART II - C

Continued

NOC-NIC LINKAGES FOR CARDIAC OUTPUT, DECREASED

Outcome	Major Interventions	Suggested Interventions	
Tissue Perfusion: Cellular Definition: Adequacy of blood flow through the vasculature to maintain function at the cellular level	Lower Extremity Monitoring Vital Signs Monitoring	Acid-Base Management Anxiety Reduction Fluid/Electrolyte Management Fluid Management Fluid Monitoring Fluid Resuscitation	Nausea Management Neurological Monitoring Pain Management Skin Surveillance Vomiting Management
Tissue Perfusion: Cerebral Definition: Adequacy of blood flow through the cerebral vasculature to maintain brain function	Cerebral Perfusion Promotion Neurological Monitoring	Anxiety Reduction Cerebral Edema Management Code Management Fluid Management Fluid Monitoring Fluid Resuscitation Hypoglycemia Management Hypovolemia Management	Intracranial Pressure (ICP) Monitoring Positioning: Neurological Seizure Management Seizure Precautions Shock Prevention Surveillance Vital Signs Monitoring Vomiting Management
Tissue Perfusion: Peripheral Definition: Adequacy of blood flow through the small vessels of the extremities to maintain tissue function	Circulatory Care: Arterial Insufficiency Circulatory Care: Venous Insufficiency Lower Extremity Monitoring	Bleeding Precautions Bleeding Reduction Blood Products Administration Cardiac Care: Acute Circulatory Care: Mechanical Assist Device Circulatory Precautions Embolus Care: Peripheral Fluid Management Fluid Monitoring Fluid Resuscitation Hemodynamic Regulation	Hypovolemia Management Intravenous (IV) Insertion Intravenous (IV) Therapy Pain Management Pneumatic Tourniquet Precautions Resuscitation Resuscitation: Fetus Resuscitation: Neonate Shock Prevention Skin Care: Topical Treatments Skin Surveillance Vital Signs Monitoring
Tissue Perfusion: Pulmonary Definition: Adequacy of blood flow through pulmonary vasculature to perfuse alveoli/ capillary unit	Circulatory Care: Arterial Insufficiency Embolus Care: Pulmonary	Acid-Base Management: Respiratory Acidosis Acid-Base Management: Respiratory Alkalosis Airway Management Anxiety Reduction Code Management Fluid Management	Fluid Monitoring Oxygen Therapy Pain Management Respiratory Monitoring Resuscitation Shock Management Vital Signs Monitoring

NOC-NIC LINKAGES FOR CARDIAC OUTPUT, DECREASED

Outcome	Major Interventions	Suggested Interventions	
Vital Signs			
Definition: Extent to which temperature, pulse, respiration, and blood pressure are within normal range	Hemodynamic Regulation Vital Signs Monitoring	Acid-Base Management Anxiety Reduction Blood Products Administration Cardiac Care Dysrhythmia Management Electrolyte Management Emergency Care Fluid Management Fluid Monitoring Fluid Resuscitation Hemorrhage Control Hypovolemia Management	Intravenous (IV) Therapy Malignant Hyperthermia Precautions Medication Administration Medication Management Medication Prescribing Postanesthesia Care Postpartal Care Resuscitation Shock Management Shock Prevention Surveillance

Critical reasoning note: Perfusion outcomes with related interventions are provided as measures of the adequacy of the blood being pumped to meet metabolic demands. The diagnostic related factors (altered heart rate/rhythm, altered preload, altered afterload, altered contractility) and behavioral/emotional aspects comprise the framework for the defining characteristics; therefore the interventions are provided with the outcomes and not repeated for the related factors.

NURSING DIAGNOSIS: Caregiver Role Strain

Definition: Difficulty in performing family caregiver role

NICS ASSOCIATED WITH DIAGNOSIS RELATED FACTORS

Abuse Protection Support Anger Control Assistance Conflict Mediation	Coping Enhancement Dementia Management	Discharge Planning Mood Management	Risk Identification Substance Use Prevention

NOC-NIC LINKAGES FOR CAREGIVER ROLE STRAIN

Outcome	Major Interventions	Suggested Interventions	
Caregiver Emotional Health			
Definition: Emotional well-being of a family care provider while caring for a family member	Caregiver Support Coping Enhancement	Anger Control Assistance Anxiety Reduction Emotional Support Grief Work Facilitation Guilt Work Facilitation Humor	Meditation Facilitation Mood Management Resiliency Promotion Spiritual Support Substance Use Prevention Support System Enhancement
Caregiver Lifestyle Disruption			
Definition: Severity of disturbances in the lifestyle of a family member due to caregiving	Caregiver Support Respite Care	Case Management Family Integrity Promotion Family Involvement Promotion Family Process Maintenance Health System Guidance Home Maintenance Assistance Insurance Authorization	Referral Resiliency Promotion Role Enhancement Sleep Enhancement Support Group Support System Enhancement

Continued

NOC-NIC LINKAGES FOR CAREGIVER ROLE STRAIN

Outcome	Major Interventions	Suggested Interventions	
Caregiver-Patient Relationship			
Definition: Positive interactions and connections between the caregiver and care recipient	Coping Enhancement Role Enhancement	Abuse Protection Support: Child Abuse Protection Support: Domestic Partner Abuse Protection Support: Elder Active Listening Anger Control Assistance Caregiver Support Conflict Mediation	Forgiveness Facilitation Grief Work Facilitation Guilt Work Facilitation Humor Reminiscence Therapy Respite Care Socialization Enhancement
Caregiver Performance: Direct Care			
Definition: Provision by family care provider of appropriate personal and health care for a family member	Teaching: Disease Process Teaching: Prescribed Diet Teaching: Prescribed Medication	Anticipatory Guidance Caregiver Support Environmental Management: Comfort Environmental Management: Home Preparation Environmental Management: Safety Infant Care Learning Facilitation Medication Management	Nutrition Management Pain Management Parent Education: Infant Parenting Promotion Role Enhancement Teaching: Prescribed Activity/Exercise Teaching: Procedure/ Treatment Teaching: Psychomotor Skill
Caregiver Performance: Indirect Care			
Definition: Arrangement and oversight by family care provider of appropriate care for a family member	Decision-Making Support Health System Guidance	Assertiveness Training Culture Brokerage Discharge Planning Environmental Management Family Involvement Promotion Family Process Maintenance Financial Resource Assistance	Insurance Authorization Mutual Goal Setting Parenting Promotion Referral Teaching: Individual Telephone Consultation
Caregiver Physical Health			
Definition: Physical well-being of a family care provider while caring for a family member	Energy Management Nutrition Management	Anxiety Reduction Body Mechanics Promotion Cardiac Precautions Exercise Promotion Fluid Management Health Screening Infection Protection Medication Management Oral Health Maintenance	Pain Management Premenstrual Syndrome (PMS) Management Respite Care Sleep Enhancement Substance Use Prevention Teaching: Individual Weight Management

NOC-NIC LINKAGES FOR CAREGIVER ROLE STRAIN

Outcome	Major Interventions	Suggested Interventions	

Caregiver Role Endurance
 	
Definition:
Factors that promote family care provider's capacity to sustain caregiving over an extended period of time
	Caregiver Support
	Respite Care
		Decision-Making Support
		Emotional Support
		Financial Resource
		  Assistance
		Health Literacy
		  Enhancement
		Health System Guidance
			Home Maintenance
			  Assistance
			Support Group
			Support System
			  Enhancement
			Telephone Consultation

Caregiver Well-Being
 	
Definition:
Extent of positive perception of primary care provider's health status
	Caregiver Support
	Respite Care
		Coping Enhancement
		Emotional Support
		Family Involvement
		  Promotion
		Family Mobilization
		Financial Resource
		  Assistance
		Home Maintenance
		  Assistance
			Normalization Promotion
			Resiliency Promotion
			Role Enhancement
			Socialization
			  Enhancement
			Support Group
			Support System
			  Enhancement

Parenting Performance
 	
Definition:
Parental actions to provide a child with a nurturing and constructive physical, emotional, and social environment
	Attachment
	  Promotion
	Parenting
	  Promotion
		Abuse Protection
		  Support: Child
		Behavior Management:
		  Overactivity/Inattention
		Bowel Incontinence Care:
		  Encopresis
		Developmental Care
		Developmental
		  Enhancement:
		  Adolescent
		Developmental
		  Enhancement: Child
		Family Integrity Promotion:
		  Childbearing Family
		Infant Care
		Kangaroo Care
		Lactation Counseling
		Normalization Promotion
		Parent Education: Adolescent
		Parent Education:
		  Childrearing Family
		Parent Education: Infant
		Resiliency Promotion
		Sibling Support
		Teaching: Infant Nutrition
		  0-3 Months
		Teaching: Infant Nutrition
		  4-6 Months
		Teaching: Infant Nutrition
		  7-9 Months
			Teaching: Infant Nutrition
			  10-12 Months
			Teaching: Infant Safety
			  0-3 Months
			Teaching: Infant Safety
			  4-6 Months
			Teaching: Infant Safety
			  7-9 Months
			Teaching: Infant Safety
			  10-12 Months
			Teaching: Infant
			  Stimulation 0-4 Months
			Teaching: Infant
			  Stimulation 5-8 Months
			Teaching: Infant Stimulation
			  9-12 Months
			Teaching: Toddler
			  Nutrition 13-18 Months
			Teaching: Toddler
			  Nutrition 19-24 Months
			Teaching: Toddler
			  Nutrition 25-36 Months
			Teaching: Toddler Safety
			  13-18 Months
			Teaching: Toddler Safety
			  19-24 Months
			Teaching: Toddler Safety
			  25-36 Months
			Teaching: Toilet Training
			Urinary Incontinence Care:
			  Enuresis

Continued

PART II - C

NOC-NIC LINKAGES FOR CAREGIVER ROLE STRAIN

Outcome	Major Interventions	Suggested Interventions	
Role Performance Definition: Congruence of an individual's role behavior with role expectations	Caregiver Support Role Enhancement	Active Listening Anticipatory Guidance Coping Enhancement Counseling Decision-Making Support Emotional Support Family Involvement Promotion	Family Integrity Promotion Parenting Promotion Respite Care Support System Enhancement Teaching: Disease Process Teaching: Individual Values Clarification

NURSING DIAGNOSIS: Childbearing Process, Readiness for Enhanced

Definition: A pattern of preparing for, maintaining, and strengthening a healthy pregnancy and childbirth process and care of newborn

NOC-NIC LINKAGES FOR CHILDBEARING PROCESS, READINESS FOR ENHANCED

Outcome	Major Interventions	Suggested Interventions	
Knowledge: Infant Care Definition: Extent of understanding conveyed about caring for a baby from birth to first birthday	Attachment Promotion Parent Education: Infant	Anticipatory Guidance Environmental Management: Attachment Process Bottle Feeding Circumcision Care Infant Care Lactation Counseling	Nonnutritive Sucking Teaching: Infant Nutrition 0-3 Months Teaching: Infant Safety 0-3 Months Teaching: Infant Stimulation 0-4 Months
Knowledge: Labor & Delivery Definition: Extent of understanding conveyed about labor and vaginal delivery	Childbirth Preparation	Anticipatory Guidance	Teaching: Individual
Knowledge: Postpartum Maternal Health Definition: Extent of understanding conveyed about maternal health in the period following birth of an infant	Postpartal Care	Anticipatory Guidance Body Mechanics Promotion Energy Management Exercise Promotion Family Planning: Contraception Fluid Management	Health System Guidance Lactation Counseling Mood Management Nutritional Counseling Teaching: Prescribed Activity/Exercise

NOC-NIC LINKAGES FOR CHILDBEARING PROCESS, READINESS FOR ENHANCED

Outcome	Major Interventions	Suggested Interventions	
Knowledge: Preconception Maternal Health			
Definition: Extent of understanding conveyed about maternal health prior to conception to ensure a healthy pregnancy	Preconception Counseling	Energy Management Environmental Management: Safety Family Planning: Infertility Fertility Preservation Genetic Counseling	Nutritional Counseling Risk Identification Substance Use Prevention Vehicle Safety Promotion
Knowledge: Pregnancy			
Definition: Extent of understanding conveyed about promotion of a healthy pregnancy and prevention of complications	Childbirth Preparation	Anticipatory Guidance Body Mechanics Promotion Energy Management Medication Management Mood Management Nutritional Counseling	Prenatal Care Relaxation Therapy Sexual Counseling Substance Use Prevention Weight Management
Knowledge: Pregnancy & Postpartum Sexual Functioning			
Definition: Extent of understanding conveyed about sexual function during pregnancy and postpartum	Prenatal Care Postpartal Care	Culture Brokerage Family Planning: Contraception Mood Management	Sexual Counseling Teaching: Individual Teaching: Safe Sex
Maternal Status: Antepartum			
Definition: Extent to which maternal well-being is within normal limits from conception to the onset of labor	Prenatal Care	Abuse Protection Support: Domestic Partner Attachment Promotion Bleeding Reduction: Antepartum Uterus Childbirth Preparation Coping Enhancement Energy Management High-Risk Pregnancy Care Labor Suppression Mood Management	Nausea Management Nutritional Counseling Pain Management Sleep Enhancement Surveillance: Late Pregnancy Teaching: Prescribed Activity/Exercise Ultrasonography: Limited Obstetric Vital Signs Monitoring Vomiting Management Weight Management
Maternal Status: Intrapartum			
Definition: Extent to which maternal well-being is within normal limits from onset of labor to delivery	Birthing Intrapartal Care	Amnioinfusion Calming Technique Intrapartal Care: High-Risk Delivery Labor Induction Massage	Neurological Monitoring Pain Management Relaxation Therapy Surveillance Vital Signs Monitoring

Continued

PART II - C

NOC-NIC LINKAGES FOR CHILDBEARING PROCESS, READINESS FOR ENHANCED		
Outcome	**Major Interventions**	**Suggested Interventions**
Maternal Status: Postpartum Definition: Extent to which maternal well-being is within normal limits from delivery of placenta to completion of involution	Postpartal Care	Bleeding Reduction: Postpartum Uterus Breastfeeding Assistance Cesarean Section Care Lactation Counseling	Mood Management Pain Management Surveillance Vital Signs Monitoring
Parent-Infant Attachment Definition: Parent and infant behaviors that demonstrate an enduring affectionate bond	Attachment Promotion Environmental Management: Attachment Process	Family Integrity Promotion: Childbearing Family Parent Education: Infant	Teaching: Infant Stimulation 0-4 Months
Postpartum Maternal Health Behavior Definition: Personal actions to promote health of a mother in the period following birth of infant	Postpartal Care	Attachment Promotion Anxiety Reduction Body Mechanics Promotion Breastfeeding Assistance Energy Management Exercise Promotion Family Planning: Contraception Fluid Monitoring Health System Guidance Infection Protection	Mood Management Nutritional Counseling Pain Management Pelvic Muscle Exercise Sleep Enhancement Support Group Support System Enhancement Surveillance Teaching: Prescribed Activity/Exercise
Prenatal Health Behavior Definition: Personal actions to promote a healthy pregnancy and a healthy newborn	Prenatal Care	Abuse Protection Support: Domestic Partner Body Mechanics Promotion Environmental Management: Safety Exercise Promotion Medication Management Nutritional Counseling	Oral Health Maintenance Risk Identification Sexual Counseling Substance Use Prevention Teaching: Safe Sex Vehicle Safety Promotion Weight Management

NURSING DIAGNOSIS: Comfort, Impaired

Definition: Perceived lack of ease, relief and transcendence in physical, psychospiritual, environmental and social dimensions

NOC-NIC LINKAGES FOR COMFORT, IMPAIRED

Outcome	Major Interventions	Suggested Interventions	
Agitation Level Definition: Severity of disruptive physiological and behavioral manifestations of stress or biochemical triggers	Calming Technique Dementia Management Dementia Management: Bathing	Anger Control Assistance Anxiety Reduction Behavior Management: Overactivity/Inattention Elopement Precautions Environmental Management: Safety	Environmental Management: Violence Prevention Fluid Monitoring Sleep Enhancement Vital Signs Monitoring Weight Management
Client Satisfaction: Physical Environment Definition: Extent of positive perception of living environment, treatment environment, equipment, and supplies in acute or long term care settings	Environmental Management: Comfort	Admission Care Examination Assistance	Home Maintenance Assistance
Comfort Status Definition: Overall physical, psychospiritual, sociocultural, and environmental ease and safety of an individual	Anxiety Reduction Culture Brokerage Environmental Management: Comfort Environmental Management: Safety Positioning Relaxation Therapy Spiritual Support Support System Enhancement	See critical reasoning note on p. 67	
Comfort Status: Environment Definition: Environmental ease, comfort, and safety of surroundings	Environmental Management: Comfort Environmental Management: Safety	Bed Rest Care Environmental Management Environmental Management: Home Preparation	Home Maintenance Assistance Patient Rights Protection

Continued

PART II - C

NOC-NIC LINKAGES FOR COMFORT, IMPAIRED		
Outcome	**Major Interventions**	**Suggested Interventions**
Comfort Status: Physical Definition: Physical ease related to bodily sensations and homeostatic mechanisms	Environmental Management: Comfort Positioning Relaxation Therapy	Acupressure Airway Management Aromatherapy Bed Rest Care Biofeedback Bowel Incontinence Care Constipation/Impaction Management Cutaneous Stimulation Diarrhea Management Dying Care	Energy Management Exercise Promotion: Stretching Fever Treatment Flatulence Reduction Fluid Management Heat/Cold Application Hypnosis Massage Nausea Management Vomiting Management
Comfort Status: Psychospiritual Definition: Psychospiritual ease related to self-concept, emotional well-being, source of inspiration, and meaning and purpose in one's life	Anxiety Reduction Spiritual Support	Aromatherapy Autogenic Training Calming Technique Emotional Support Forgiveness Facilitation Grief Work Facilitation Grief Work Facilitation: Perinatal Death Guided Imagery Guilt Work Facilitation Hope Inspiration	Humor Meditation Facilitation Mood Management Relaxation Therapy Religious Ritual Enhancement Self-Awareness Enhancement Self-Esteem Enhancement Spiritual Growth Facilitation Suicide Prevention Values Clarification
Comfort Status: Sociocultural Definition: Social ease related to interpersonal, family, and societal relationships within a cultural context	Culture Brokerage Support System Enhancement	Active Listening Conflict Mediation Family Involvement Promotion Patient Rights Protection	Socialization Enhancement Support Group Truth Telling Visitation Facilitation
Symptom Control Definition: Personal actions to minimize perceived adverse changes in physical and emotional functioning	Self-Efficacy Enhancement Self-Modification Assistance	Active Listening Coping Enhancement Self-Responsibility Facilitation Teaching: Prescribed Activity/Exercise	Teaching: Prescribed Diet Teaching: Prescribed Medication Teaching: Procedure/Treatment

NOC-NIC LINKAGES FOR COMFORT, IMPAIRED

Outcome	Major Interventions	Suggested Interventions	
Symptom Severity Definition: Severity of perceived adverse changes in physical, emotional, and social functioning	Medication Administration Pain Management Positioning	Anxiety Reduction Calming Technique Coping Enhancement Energy Management Guided Imagery Massage Medication Management	Mood Management Pain Management Positioning Progressive Muscle Relaxation Relaxation Therapy Sleep Enhancement

Critical reasoning note: Suggested interventions for the broad outcome Comfort Status could include any of the interventions suggested for the more specific comfort labels. The diagnosis identifies no related factors, thereby allowing for the identification of antecedent or contributing factors for each patient. The defining characteristics include distress caused by symptoms and symptoms related to illness; if these are the patient's symptoms, Symptom Control should be considered as a possible outcome. Symptom Severity: Perimenopause and Symptom Severity: Premenstrual Syndrome (PMS) should be considered if the discomfort is related to these problems.

NURSING DIAGNOSIS: Comfort, Readiness for Enhanced

Definition: A pattern of ease, relief, and transcendence in physical, psychospiritual, environmental, and/or social dimensions that can be strengthened

NOC-NIC LINKAGES FOR COMFORT, READINESS FOR ENHANCED

Outcome	Major Interventions	Suggested Interventions	
Comfort Status Definition: Overall physical, psychospiritual, sociocultural, and environmental ease and safety of an individual	Health Education Self-Awareness Enhancement Self-Efficacy Enhancement Self-Modification Assistance	Aromatherapy Autogenic Training Bibliotherapy Body Image Enhancement Culture Brokerage Energy Management Environmental Management: Comfort Exercise Promotion Forgiveness Facilitation Grief Work Facilitation Guided Imagery Guilt Work Facilitation Journaling	Meditation Facilitation Nutritional Counseling Premenstrual Syndrome (PMS) Management Progressive Muscle Relaxation Religious Ritual Enhancement Role Enhancement Self-Esteem Enhancement Self-Hypnosis Facilitation Sleep Enhancement Spiritual Growth Facilitation Socialization Enhancement
Personal Autonomy Definition: Personal actions of a competent individual to exercise governance in life decisions	Assertiveness Training Decision-Making Support	Genetic Counseling Health System Guidance Resiliency Promotion	Self-Efficacy Enhancement Self-Modification Assistance Self-Responsibility Facilitation

Critical reasoning note: A number of the interventions as well as the outcome, Personal Autonomy, focus on enabling the individual to improve his/her comfort. Any of the interventions used with Impaired Comfort could be considered for specific problems that decrease comfort.

NURSING DIAGNOSIS: Communication, Impaired Verbal

Definition: Decreased, delayed, or absent ability to receive, process, transmit, and/or use a system of symbols

NICS ASSOCIATED WITH DIAGNOSIS RELATED FACTORS

Airway Insertion and Stabilization	Culture Brokerage	Health Literacy Enhancement	Socialization Enhancement
Cerebral Edema Management	Delusion Management	Mood Management	Support System Enhancement
Cerebral Perfusion Promotion	Environmental Management	Self-Esteem Enhancement	Teaching: Individual

NOC-NIC LINKAGES FOR COMMUNICATION, IMPAIRED VERBAL

Outcome	Major Interventions	Suggested Interventions	
Cognition Definition: Ability to execute complex mental processes	Decision-Making Support Memory Training	Cognitive Stimulation Communication Enhancement: Speech Deficit Delirium Management	Dementia Management Learning Facilitation Reality Orientation
Communication Definition: Reception, interpretation, and expression of spoken, written, and nonverbal messages	Active Listening Communication Enhancement: Hearing Deficit Communication Enhancement: Speech Deficit	Anxiety Reduction Art Therapy Bibliotherapy	Communication Enhancement: Visual Deficit Culture Brokerage
Communication: Expressive Definition: Expression of meaningful verbal and/or nonverbal messages	Communication Enhancement: Speech Deficit	Active Listening Anxiety Reduction Assertiveness Training	Bibliotherapy Communication Enhancement: Hearing Deficit
Communication: Receptive Definition: Reception and interpretation of verbal and/or nonverbal messages	Communication Enhancement: Hearing Deficit Communication Enhancement: Visual Deficit	Active Listening Cognitive Stimulation Communication Enhancement: Speech Deficit	Culture Brokerage
Information Processing Definition: Ability to acquire, organize, and use information	Decision-Making Support Memory Training	Anxiety Reduction Delirium Management Dementia Management	Health Literacy Enhancement Learning Facilitation Learning Readiness Enhancement

NURSING DIAGNOSIS: Communication, Readiness for Enhanced

Definition: A pattern of exchanging information and ideas with others that is sufficient for meeting one's needs and life's goals, and can be strengthened

NOC-NIC LINKAGES FOR COMMUNICATION, READINESS FOR ENHANCED		
Outcome	**Major Interventions**	**Suggested Interventions**

Communication
 	
Definition:
Reception, interpretation, and expression of spoken, written, and nonverbal messages
	Complex Relationship Building
	Socialization Enhancement
		Active Listening
		Anxiety Reduction
		Assertiveness Training
		Bibliotherapy
		Communication Enhancement:
		  Hearing Deficit
			Communication Enhancement:
			  Speech Deficit
			Culture Brokerage
			Development Enhancement:
			  Adolescent
			Development Enhancement: Child
			Humor

Communication: Expressive
 	
Definition:
Expression of meaningful verbal and/or nonverbal messages
	Assertiveness Training
	Communication Enhancement:
	  Speech Deficit
		Anxiety Reduction
		Complex Relationship Building
		Culture Brokerage
			Development Enhancement:
			  Adolescent
			Development Enhancement:
			  Child
			Socialization Enhancement

Communication: Receptive
 	
Definition:
Reception and interpretation of verbal and/or nonverbal messages
	Anxiety Reduction
	Communication Enhancement:
	  Hearing Deficit
		Communication Enhancement:
		  Visual Deficit
		Culture Brokerage
			Development Enhancement:
			  Adolescent
			Development Enhancement: Child

Critical reasoning note: The diagnosis has two foci of defining characteristics: the ability to communicate and the ability to use communication to share thoughts and ideas; thus interventions that promote sharing and relationship building are used.

PART II - C

NURSING DIAGNOSIS: Community Coping, Ineffective

Definition: Pattern of community activities for adaptation and problem-solving that is unsatisfactory for meeting the demands or needs of the community

NICS ASSOCIATED WITH DIAGNOSIS RELATED FACTORS			
Community Disaster Preparedness	Community Health Development	Fiscal Resource Management	Program Development

NOC-NIC LINKAGES FOR COMMUNITY COPING, INEFFECTIVE		
Outcome	**Major Interventions**	**Suggested Interventions**
Community Competence Definition: Capacity of a community to collectively problem solve to achieve community goals	Community Health Development Environmental Management: Community	Conflict Mediation Environmental Risk Protection Fiscal Resource Management Health Education Health Policy Monitoring Program Development Resiliency Promotion Risk Identification Surveillance: Community Vehicle Safety Promotion
Community Disaster Readiness Definition: Community preparedness to respond to a natural or man-made calamitous event	Bioterrorism Preparedness Community Disaster Preparedness	Environmental Risk Protection Health Policy Monitoring Immunization/ Vaccination Management Program Development Risk Identification Surveillance: Community Triage: Disaster
Community Health Status Definition: General state of well-being of a community or population	Communicable Disease Management Community Health Development	Documentation Environmental Risk Protection Health Education Health Policy Monitoring Health Screening Immunization/ Vaccination Management Infection Control Risk Identification Social Marketing Surveillance: Community Vehicle Safety Promotion
Community Health Status: Immunity Definition: Resistance of community members to the invasion and spread of an infectious agent that could threaten public health	Communicable Disease Management Immunization/ Vaccination Management	Community Health Development Documentation Environmental Risk Protection Health Education Health Policy Monitoring Program Development Risk Identification Surveillance: Community

NOC-NIC LINKAGES FOR COMMUNITY COPING, INEFFECTIVE		
Outcome	**Major Interventions**	**Suggested Interventions**

Community Risk Control: Chronic Disease
 	
Definition:
Community actions to reduce the risk of chronic diseases and related complications
	Case Management
	Health Education
	Program
	  Development
		Documentation
		Environmental
		  Management:
		  Community
		Environmental Risk
		  Protection
			Health Policy Monitoring
			Health Screening
			Risk Identification
			Surveillance:
			  Community

Community Risk Control: Communicable Disease
 	
Definition:
Community actions to eliminate or reduce the spread of infectious agents that threaten public health
	Communicable
	  Disease
	  Management
		Documentation
		Health Education
		Health Policy
		  Monitoring
		Health Screening
		Immunization/
		  Vaccination
		  Management
			Infection Control
			Infection Protection
			Program Development
			Risk Identification
			Surveillance:
			  Community

Community Risk Control: Lead Exposure
 	
Definition:
Community actions to reduce lead exposure and poisoning
	Environmental
	  Management:
	  Community
	Environmental Risk
	  Protection
		Case Management
		Community Health
		  Development
		Documentation
		Environmental
		  Management:
		  Worker Safety
			Health Education
			Health Screening
			Program Development
			Risk Identification
			Surveillance:
			  Community

Community Risk Control: Violence
 	
Definition:
Community actions to eliminate or reduce intentional violent acts resulting in serious physical or psychological harm
	Environmental
	  Management:
	  Community
	Environmental
	  Management:
	  Violence Prevention
		Abuse Protection
		  Support
		Program Development
		Risk Identification
			Surveillance:
			  Community
			Vehicle Safety
			  Promotion

Community Violence Level
 	
Definition:
Incidence of violent acts compared with local, state, or national values
	Environmental
	  Management:
	  Violence Prevention
	Surveillance:
	  Community
		Abuse Protection
		  Support
		Environmental
		  Management:
		  Community
		Environmental Risk
		  Protection
			Health Policy Monitoring
			Program Development
			Vehicle Safety
			  Promotion

NURSING DIAGNOSIS: Community Coping, Readiness for Enhanced

Definition: Pattern of community activities for adaptation and problem-solving that is satisfactory for meeting the demands or needs of the community but can be improved for management of current and future problems/stressors

NOC-NIC LINKAGES FOR COMMUNITY COPING, READINESS FOR ENHANCED		
Outcome	**Major Interventions**	**Suggested Interventions**
Community Competence Definition: Capacity of a community to collectively problem solve to achieve community goals	Health Policy Monitoring Program Development	Community Health Development Environmental Risk Protection Fiscal Resource Management Health Education Health Screening	Resiliency Promotion Risk Identification Sports-Injury Prevention: Youth Vehicle Safety Promotion
Community Disaster Readiness Definition: Community preparedness to respond to a natural or man-made calamitous event	Bioterrorism Preparedness Community Disaster Preparedness	Fiscal Resource Management Health Policy Monitoring Immunization/Vaccination Management	Program Development Risk Identification
Community Health Status: Immunity Definition: Resistance of community members to the invasion and spread of an infectious agent that could threaten public health	Communicable Disease Management Immunization/ Vaccination Management	Community Health Development Documentation Environmental Risk Protection Health Education Health Policy Monitoring	Health Screening Program Development Risk Identification Surveillance: Community
Community Risk Control: Communicable Disease Definition: Community actions to eliminate or reduce the spread of infectious agents that threaten public health	Communicable Disease Management Program Development	Documentation Health Education Health Policy Monitoring Health Screening	Immunization/ Vaccination Management Risk Identification Surveillance: Community
Community Risk Control: Lead Exposure Definition: Community actions to reduce lead exposure and poisoning	Environmental Management: Community Environmental Risk Protection	Community Health Development Documentation Environmental Management: Worker Safety Health Education	Health Screening Program Development Referral Risk Identification Surveillance: Community

NOC-NIC LINKAGES FOR COMMUNITY COPING, READINESS FOR ENHANCED

Outcome	Major Interventions	Suggested Interventions	
Community Violence Level			
Definition: Incidence of violent acts compared with local, state, or national values	Environmental Management: Violence Prevention Surveillance: Community	Documentation Environmental Management: Community Health Policy Monitoring	Program Development Risk Identification Vehicle Safety Promotion

NURSING DIAGNOSIS: Confusion, Acute

Definition: Abrupt onset of reversible disturbances of consciousness, attention, cognition, and perception that develop over a short period of time

NICS ASSOCIATED WITH DIAGNOSIS RELATED FACTORS

Delirium Management Dementia Management	Sleep Enhancement Substance Use Treatment	Substance Use Treatment: Alcohol Withdrawal

NOC-NIC LINKAGES FOR CONFUSION, ACUTE

Outcome	Major Interventions	Suggested Interventions	
Acute Confusion Level			
Definition: Severity of disturbance in consciousness and cognition that develops over a short period of time	Delirium Management Reality Orientation	Calming Technique Delusion Management Environmental Management: Safety Fall Prevention Hallucination Management Medication Management Mood Management	Seizure Precautions Sleep Enhancement Substance Use Treatment: Alcohol Withdrawal Substance Use Treatment: Drug Withdrawal Substance Use Treatment: Overdose
Cognitive Orientation			
Definition: Ability to identify person, place, and time accurately	Reality Orientation	Anxiety Reduction Calming Technique Delirium Management Delusion Management	Hallucination Management Medication Administration Medication Management
Distorted Thought Self-Control			
Definition: Self-restraint of disruptions in perception, thought processes, and thought content	Delusion Management Hallucination Management	Anxiety Reduction Calming Technique Cognitive Restructuring	Delirium Management Medication Management Reality Orientation
Information Processing			
Definition: Ability to acquire, organize, and use information	Cognitive Stimulation Memory Training	Anxiety Reduction Delirium Management Delusion Management	Environmental Management Fluid/Electrolyte Management

Continued

NOC-NIC LINKAGES FOR CONFUSION, ACUTE

Outcome	Major Interventions	Suggested Interventions	
Substance Withdrawal Severity Definition: Severity of physical and psychological signs or symptoms caused by withdrawal from addictive drugs, toxic chemicals, tobacco, or alcohol	Substance Use Treatment: Alcohol Withdrawal Substance Use Treatment: Drug Withdrawal	Anxiety Reduction Calming Technique Delirium Management Diarrhea Management Environmental Management: Comfort Eye Care Hallucination Management Medication Administration Mood Management	Nausea Management Pain Management Seizure Precautions Sleep Enhancement Substance Use Treatment Surveillance Temperature Regulation Vital Signs Monitoring

Critical reasoning note: Interventions that can address acute confusion attributable to both physiological and psychological factors have been identified.

NURSING DIAGNOSIS: Confusion, Chronic

Definition: Irreversible, long-standing, and/or progressive deterioration of intellect and personality characterized by decreased ability to interpret environmental stimuli; decreased capacity for intellectual thought processes; and manifested by disturbances of memory, orientation, and behavior

NICS ASSOCIATED WITH DIAGNOSIS RELATED FACTORS

Cerebral Edema Management Cerebral Perfusion Promotion	Dementia Management Substance Abuse Treatment	Thrombolytic Therapy Management

NOC-NIC LINKAGES FOR CONFUSION, CHRONIC

Outcome	Major Interventions	Suggested Interventions	
Cognition Definition: Ability to execute complex mental processes	Dementia Management Reminiscence Therapy	Activity Therapy Anxiety Reduction Behavior Management Calming Technique Cognitive Stimulation	Decision-Making Support Environmental Management Fall Prevention Family Involvement Promotion
Cognitive Orientation Definition: Ability to identify person, place, and time accurately	Dementia Management Reality Orientation	Calming Technique Chemical Restraint Cognitive Stimulation Humor Medication Management	Memory Training Patient Rights Protection Relocation Stress Reduction Surveillance: Safety Visitation Facilitation
Decision-Making Definition: Ability to make judgments and choose between two or more alternatives	Decision-Making Support Family Involvement Promotion	Dementia Management Family Support Health System Guidance	Memory Training Patient Rights Protection Relocation Stress Reduction

NOC-NIC LINKAGES FOR CONFUSION, CHRONIC

Outcome	Major Interventions	Suggested Interventions	
Distorted Thought Self-Control Definition: Self-restraint of disruptions in perception, thought processes, and thought content	Delusion Management Hallucination Management	Activity Therapy Anxiety Reduction Art Therapy Behavior Management Cognitive Restructuring Cognitive Stimulation	Dementia Management Environmental Management Medication Management Milieu Therapy Reality Orientation Validation Therapy
Identity Definition: Distinguishes between self and non-self and characterizes one's essence	Dementia Management Reality Orientation	Abuse Protection Support: Elder Cognitive Stimulation Dementia Management Environmental Management Environmental Management: Violence Prevention	Hallucination Management Medication Management Socialization Enhancement
Memory Definition: Ability to cognitively retrieve and report previously stored information	Memory Training	Active Listening Cognitive Stimulation Coping Enhancement	Learning Facilitation Reality Orientation Reminiscence Therapy

Critical reasoning note: A number of outcomes are provided to assess the various dimensions of chronic confusion; an outcome to measure chronic confusion is currently under development and will be available in the 5th edition of NOC.

NURSING DIAGNOSIS: Constipation

Definition: Decrease in normal frequency of defecation accompanied by difficult or incomplete passage of stool and/or passage of excessively hard, dry stool

NICS ASSOCIATED WITH DIAGNOSIS RELATED FACTORS

Anxiety Reduction Bowel Training Dementia Management Electrolyte Management	Exercise Promotion Exercise Therapy: Muscle Control Fluid/Electrolyte Management Fluid Resuscitation	Medication Management Mood Management Nutrition Therapy Oral Health Restoration	Postpartal Care Prenatal Care Rectal Prolapse Management Teaching: Prescribed Activity/Exercise Teaching: Prescribed Diet Weight Reduction Assistance

Continued

PART II - C

NOC-NIC LINKAGES FOR CONSTIPATION

Outcome	Major Interventions	Suggested Interventions	

Bowel Elimination
Definition:
Formation and
  evacuation of stool
	Bowel Management
	Bowel Training
	Constipation/
	  Impaction
	  Management
		Anxiety Reduction
		Bowel Irrigation
		Exercise Therapy:
		  Ambulation
		Flatulence Reduction
		Fluid Management
		Medication Administration
		Medication Administration:
		  Oral
		Medication Administration:
		  Rectal
			Medication Management
			Nausea Management
			Nutrition Management
			Nutritional Counseling
			Pain Management
			Rectal Prolapse
			  Management
			Self-Care Assistance:
			  Toileting
			Vomiting Management

Ostomy Self-Care
Definition:
Personal actions to
  maintain ostomy
  for elimination
	Bowel Management
	Ostomy Care
		Fluid Management
		Fluid Resuscitation
		Nutrition Management
		Skin Care: Topical
		  Treatments
			Skin Surveillance
			Teaching: Individual
			Teaching: Psychomotor
			  Skill
			Wound Care

NURSING DIAGNOSIS: Constipation, Perceived

Definition: Self-diagnosis of constipation and abuse of laxatives, enemas, and/or suppositories to ensure a daily bowel movement

NICS ASSOCIATED WITH DIAGNOSIS RELATED FACTORS

Culture Brokerage Dementia Management	Family Support	Patient Rights Protection	Reality Orientation

NOC-NIC LINKAGES FOR CONSTIPATION, PERCEIVED

Outcome	Major Interventions	Suggested Interventions	

Bowel Elimination
Definition:
Formation and evacuation
  of stool
	Bowel Management	Behavior Modification
		Counseling
		Medication
		  Management
			Nutritional Counseling
			Teaching: Individual
			Teaching: Prescribed
			  Medication

Health Beliefs
Definition:
Personal convictions that
  influence health
  behaviors
	Active Listening
	Health Education
		Behavior Modification
		Counseling
		Culture Brokerage
			Learning Facilitation
			Learning Readiness
			  Enhancement
			Self-Modification
			  Assistance

Knowledge: Health Behavior
Definition:
Extent of understanding
  conveyed about the
  promotion and
  protection of health
	Health Education
	Teaching: Individual
		Active Listening
		Anxiety Reduction
		Learning Facilitation
		Learning Readiness
		  Enhancement
			Teaching: Prescribed
			  Activity/Exercise
			Teaching: Prescribed Diet
			Teaching: Prescribed
			  Medication

NURSING DIAGNOSIS: Contamination

Definition: Exposure to environmental contaminants in doses sufficient to cause adverse health effects

NICS ASSOCIATED WITH DIAGNOSIS RELATED FACTORS			
Bioterrorism Preparedness	Environmental Risk Protection	Home Maintenance Assistance	Prenatal Care Smoking Cessation
Environmental Management: Safety	Health Education	Nutrition Management	Assistance

NOC-NIC LINKAGES FOR CONTAMINATION			
Outcome	**Major Interventions**	**Suggested Interventions**	
Community Disaster Readiness Definition: Community preparedness to respond to a natural or man-made calamitous event	Community Disaster Preparedness	Environmental Risk Protection Fiscal Resource Management Health Policy Monitoring Immunization/ Vaccination Management	Product Evaluation Program Development Risk Identification
Community Disaster Response Definition: Community response following a natural or man-made calamitous event	Environmental Risk Protection Triage: Disaster	Environmental Management: Safety Immunization/ Vaccination Management Infection Control	Infection Protection Risk Identification
Gastrointestinal Function Definition: Extent to which foods (ingested or tube-fed) are moved from ingestion to excretion	Nutrition Therapy Surveillance	Bowel Management Diarrhea Management Diet Staging Enteral Tube Feeding Flatulence Reduction Gastrointestinal Intubation Medication Administration: Enteral	Medication Administration: Oral Medication Administration: Rectal Nutrition Management Nutritional Monitoring Total Parenteral Nutrition (TPN) Administration Weight Management
Immune Hypersensitivity Response Definition: Severity of inappropriate immune responses	Skin Care: Topical Treatments Skin Surveillance	Allergy Management Circulatory Precautions Exercise Therapy: Joint Mobility Medication Administration: Skin Medication Administration: Vaginal	Neurological Monitoring Oral Health Maintenance Pruritus Management Respiratory Monitoring Wound Care

PART II - C

Continued

NOC-NIC LINKAGES FOR CONTAMINATION		
Outcome	**Major Interventions**	**Suggested Interventions**

Immune Status
Definition:
Natural and acquired appropriately targeted resistance to internal and external antigens
	Energy Management
	Infection Protection
		Fever Treatment
		Immunization/
		  Vaccination
		  Management
		Respiratory Monitoring
		Skin Surveillance
			Specimen Management
			Surveillance
			Temperature Regulation
			Weight Gain Assistance

Kidney Function
Definition:
Filtration of blood and elimination of metabolic waste products through the formation of urine
	Fluid Management
	Specimen
	  Management
		Electrolyte Monitoring
		Energy Management
		Fluid/Electrolyte
		  Management
		Fluid Monitoring
			Nausea Management
			Surveillance
			Vital Signs Monitoring

Neurological Status
Definition:
Ability of the peripheral and central nervous systems to receive, process, and respond to internal and external stimuli
	Neurological
	  Monitoring
		Exercise Therapy:
		  Muscle Control
		Pain Management
		Peripheral Sensation
		  Management
		Reality Orientation
			Seizure Management
			Seizure Precautions
			Temperature Regulation
			Vital Signs Monitoring

Personal Health Status
Definition:
Overall physical, psychological, social, and spiritual functioning of an adult 18 years or older
	Surveillance
	Vital Signs
	  Monitoring
		Circulatory Precautions
		Energy Management
		Exercise Promotion
		Infection Protection
		Medication
		  Management
		Neurological Monitoring
		Nutrition Management
			Nutritional Monitoring
			Pain Management
			Peripheral Sensation
			  Management
			Respiratory Monitoring
			Self-Care Assistance
			Self-Care Assistance:
			  IADL
			Weight Management

Respiratory Status
Definition:
Movement of air in and out of the lungs and exchange of carbon dioxide and oxygen at the alveolar level
	Respiratory
	  Monitoring
	Ventilation
	  Assistance
		Airway Insertion and
		  Stabilization
		Airway Management
		Airway Suctioning
		Artificial Airway
		  Management
			Aspiration Precautions
			Chest Physiotherapy
			Cough Enhancement
			Oxygen Therapy

Tissue Integrity: Skin & Mucous Membranes
Definition:
Structural intactness and normal physiological function of skin and mucous membranes
	Skin Surveillance	Medication
		  Administration: Skin
		Pruritus Management
			Skin Care: Topical
			  Treatments
			Wound Care

Critical reasoning note: The outcomes listed above address the various effects of environmental contaminants listed in the defining characteristics and some of the related factors. The user will need to select those outcomes appropriate for a specific contaminant.

NURSING DIAGNOSIS: Coping, Defensive

DEFINITION: Repeated projection of falsely positive self-evaluation based on a self-protective pattern that defends against underlying perceived threats to positive self-regard

NICS ASSOCIATED WITH DIAGNOSIS RELATED FACTORS

Resiliency Promotion
Self-Efficacy
   Enhancement
	Self-Esteem
	   Enhancement
		Support System
		   Enhancement
			Values Clarification

NOC-NIC LINKAGES FOR COPING, DEFENSIVE

Outcome	Major Interventions	Suggested Interventions	

**Acceptance:
Health Status**
Definition:
Reconciliation to
   significant change in
   health circumstances
	Coping Enhancement
	Self-Esteem
	   Enhancement
		Active Listening
		Anticipatory Guidance
		Counseling
		Emotional Support
		Grief Work Facilitation
		Hope Inspiration
		Presence
			Self-Awareness
			   Enhancement
			Spiritual Support
			Support Group
			Support System
			   Enhancement
			Truth Telling
			Values Clarification

**Adaptation to Physical
Disability**
Definition:
Adaptive response to a
   significant functional
   challenge due to a
   physical disability
	Behavior Modification
	Coping Enhancement
		Active Listening
		Activity Therapy
		Anticipatory Guidance
		Behavior Modification:
		   Social Skills
		Body Image
		   Enhancement
		Cognitive Restructuring
		Counseling
		Emotional Support
			Grief Work Facilitation
			Hope Inspiration
			Mutual Goal Setting
			Self-Esteem Enhancement
			Self-Responsibility
			   Facilitation
			Sexual Counseling
			Support Group
			Therapy Group

Coping
Definition:
Personal actions to
   manage stressors
   that tax an
   individual's
   resources
	Coping Enhancement
	Counseling
		Anxiety Reduction
		Behavior Modification
		Delusion Management
		Emotional Support
		Medication Management
		Mood Management
		Normalization Promotion
		Relocation Stress
		   Reduction
		Reminiscence Therapy
			Self-Awareness
			   Enhancement
			Self-Esteem Enhancement
			Self-Responsibility
			   Facilitation
			Socialization
			   Enhancement
			Spiritual Support
			Support Group
			Therapy Group
			Truth Telling

**Participation in Health
Care Decisions**
Definition:
Personal involvement
   in selecting and
   evaluating health
   care options to
   achieve desired
   outcome
	Coping Enhancement
	Self-Responsibility
	   Facilitation
		Assertiveness Training
		Behavior Modification
		Decision-Making Support
		Health Literacy
		   Enhancement
			Health System Guidance
			Mutual Goal Setting
			Self-Efficacy
			   Enhancement

PART II - C

Continued

NOC-NIC LINKAGES FOR COPING, DEFENSIVE

Outcome	Major Interventions	Suggested Interventions	
Self-Esteem			
Definition: Personal judgment of self-worth	Self-Esteem Enhancement	Behavior Modification Behavior Modification: Social Skills Cognitive Restructuring Complex Relationship Building Coping Enhancement Counseling Developmental Enhancement: Adolescent Developmental Enhancement: Child	Eating Disorders Management Emotional Support Milieu Therapy Self-Awareness Enhancement Socialization Enhancement Spiritual Support Support Group Therapy Group
Social Interaction Skills			
Definition: Personal behaviors that promote effective relationships	Behavior Modification: Social Skills	Anger Control Assistance Anxiety Reduction Assertiveness Training Behavior Modification Coping Enhancement Counseling Culture Brokerage Developmental Enhancement: Adolescent	Developmental Enhancement: Child Humor Recreation Therapy Self-Awareness Enhancement Self-Esteem Enhancement Self-Modification Assistance Self-Responsibility Facilitation Socialization Enhancement

NURSING DIAGNOSIS: Coping, Ineffective

DEFINITION: Inability to form a valid appraisal of the stressors, inadequate choices of practiced responses, and/or inability to use available resources

NICS ASSOCIATED WITH DIAGNOSIS RELATED FACTORS

Anxiety Reduction Crisis Intervention	Decision-Making Support Financial Resource Assistance	Security Enhancement Self-Efficacy Enhancement	Self-Esteem Enhancement Support System Enhancement

NOC-NIC LINKAGES FOR COPING, INEFFECTIVE

Outcome	Major Interventions	Suggested Interventions	
Adaptation to Physical Disability			
Definition: Adaptive response to a significant functional challenge due to a physical disability	Behavior Modification Coping Enhancement	Anger Control Assistance Anticipatory Guidance Anxiety Reduction Behavior Management: Self-Harm Body Image Enhancement Counseling Decision-Making Support	Emotional Support Security Enhancement Self-Care Assistance Sleep Enhancement Substance Use Prevention Support Group

NOC-NIC LINKAGES FOR COPING, INEFFECTIVE		
Outcome	**Major Interventions**	**Suggested Interventions**
Caregiver Adaptation to Patient Institutionalization Definition: Adaptive response of family caregiver when the care recipient is moved to an institution	Coping Enhancement Emotional Support	Anger Control Assistance Conflict Mediation Decision-Making Support Family Integrity Promotion Family Support Guilt Work Facilitation Reminiscence Therapy Spiritual Support Support Group Truth Telling Visitation Facilitation
Child Adaptation to Hospitalization Definition: Adaptive response of a child from 3 years through 17 years of age to hospitalization	Anxiety Reduction Coping Enhancement	Active Listening Anger Control Assistance Anticipatory Guidance Calming Technique Distraction Emotional Support Environmental Management Family Involvement Promotion Family Presence Facilitation Mutual Goal Setting Preparatory Sensory Information Security Enhancement Sleep Enhancement Teaching: Disease Process Teaching: Procedure/Treatment
Coping Definition: Personal actions to manage stressors that tax an individual's resources	Coping Enhancement Decision-Making Support	Anticipatory Guidance Anger Control Assistance Anxiety Reduction Behavior Management: Self-Harm Behavior Modification Calming Technique Cognitive Restructuring Counseling Crisis Intervention Decision-Making Support Environmental Management: Violence Prevention Impulse Control Training Mood Management Mutual Goal Setting Relaxation Therapy Resiliency Promotion Sleep Enhancement Spiritual Support Substance Use Prevention Support Group Support System Enhancement Therapy Group
Decision-Making Definition: Ability to make judgments and choose between two or more alternatives	Coping Enhancement Decision-Making Support	Culture Brokerage Genetic Counseling Health Literacy Enhancement Health System Guidance Learning Facilitation Parent Education: Adolescent Parent Education: Childrearing Family Parent Education: Infant Patient Rights Protection Self-Responsibility Facilitation Sexual Counseling Support System Enhancement Teaching: Individual Teaching: Prescribed Medication Teaching: Safe Sex Values Clarification

PART II - C

Continued

NOC-NIC LINKAGES FOR COPING, INEFFECTIVE		
Outcome	**Major Interventions**	**Suggested Interventions**
Impulse Self-Control Definition: Self-restraint of compulsive or impulsive behaviors	Coping Enhancement Impulse Control Training	Anger Control Assistance Anxiety Reduction Behavior Management: Self-Harm Environmental Management: Violence Prevention Medication Administration Mood Management Mutual Goal Setting Patient Contracting	Risk Identification Self-Modification Assistance Self-Responsibility Facilitation Substance Use Prevention Substance Use Treatment Support Group Support System Enhancement Therapy Group
Knowledge: Health Resources Definition: Extent of understanding conveyed about relevant health care resources	Anticipatory Guidance Health System Guidance	Case Management Coping Enhancement Decision-Making Support Discharge Planning	Financial Resource Assistance Learning Facilitation Patient Rights Protection Teaching: Individual
Psychosocial Adjustment: Life Change Definition: Adaptive psychosocial response of an individual to a significant life change	Anticipatory Guidance Coping Enhancement	Decision-Making Support Emotional Support Mutual Goal Setting Relocation Stress Reduction Reminiscence Therapy Role Enhancement Security Enhancement	Self-Esteem Enhancement Sleep Enhancement Socialization Enhancement Substance Use Prevention Support Group Support System Enhancement
Risk Control: Alcohol Use Definition: Personal actions to prevent, eliminate, or reduce alcohol use that poses a threat to health	Coping Enhancement Substance Use Prevention	Behavior Management: Self-Harm Behavior Modification Health System Guidance Impulse Control Training Risk Identification Self-Esteem Enhancement	Self-Modification Assistance Self-Responsibility Facilitation Spiritual Support Substance Use Treatment Support Group Support System Enhancement
Risk Control: Drug Use Definition: Personal actions to prevent, eliminate, or reduce drug use that poses a threat to health	Coping Enhancement Substance Use Prevention	Behavior Management: Self-Harm Behavior Modification Health Screening Health System Guidance Impulse Control Training Risk Identification Self-Esteem Enhancement	Self-Modification Assistance Self-Responsibility Facilitation Spiritual Support Substance Use Treatment Support Group Support System Enhancement

NOC-NIC LINKAGES FOR COPING, INEFFECTIVE		
Outcome	**Major Interventions**	**Suggested Interventions**
Role Performance Definition: Congruence of an individual's role behavior with role expectations	Coping Enhancement Role Enhancement	Behavior Modification Childbirth Preparation Decision-Making Support Emotional Support Health Education Parent Education: Adolescent Parent Education: Childrearing Family Parent Education: Infant Parenting Promotion Resiliency Promotion Self-Awareness Enhancement Self-Esteem Enhancement Substance Use Prevention Substance Use Treatment Support Group Support System Enhancement

NURSING DIAGNOSIS: Coping, Readiness for Enhanced

DEFINITION: A pattern of cognitive and behavioral efforts to manage demands that is sufficient for well-being and can be strengthened

NOC-NIC LINKAGES FOR COPING, READINESS FOR ENHANCED		
Outcome	**Major Interventions**	**Suggested Interventions**
Acceptance: Health Status Definition: Reconciliation to significant change in health circumstances	Coping Enhancement	Decision-Making Support Financial Resource Assistance Genetic Counseling Role Enhancement Self-Awareness Enhancement Self-Efficacy Enhancement Self-Modification Assistance Self-Responsibility Facilitation Socialization Enhancement Spiritual Growth Facilitation Support System Enhancement
Adaptation to Physical Disability Definition: Adaptive response to a significant functional challenge due to a physical disability	Anticipatory Guidance Coping Enhancement	Body Image Enhancement Decision-Making Support Role Enhancement Self-Care Assistance Self-Modification Assistance Self-Responsibility Facilitation Teaching: Individual
Coping Definition: Personal actions to manage stressors that tax an individual's resources	Coping Enhancement Resiliency Promotion	Decision-Making Support Health Education Meditation Facilitation Relaxation Therapy Religious Ritual Enhancement Relocation Stress Reduction Role Enhancement Self-Awareness Enhancement Self-Modification Assistance Self-Responsibility Facilitation Spiritual Growth Facilitation System Support Enhancement Values Clarification

Continued

PART II - C

NOC-NIC LINKAGES FOR COPING, READINESS FOR ENHANCED

Outcome	Major Interventions	Suggested Interventions	
Personal Well-Being			

Definition:
Extent of positive
  perception of one's
  health status
	Coping
	  Enhancement
	Self-Awareness En-
	  hancement
		Aromatherapy
		Decision-Making
		  Support
		Family Integrity
		  Promotion
		Health Education
		Health System
		  Guidance
		Meditation Facilitation
			Relaxation Therapy
			Risk Identification
			Role Enhancement
			Self-Esteem Enhancement
			Self-Modification
			  Assistance
			Socialization Enhancement

Role Performance			

Definition:
Congruence of an
  individual's role
  behavior with role
  expectations
	Coping
	  Enhancement
	Role Enhancement
		Anticipatory Guidance
		Childbirth Preparation
		Decision-Making
		  Support
		Family Integrity
		  Promotion
		Health Education
		Parent Education:
		  Adolescent
			Parent Education:
			  Childrearing Family
			Parent Education: Infant
			Self-Awareness
			  Enhancement
			Self-Modification
			  Assistance
			Support System
			  Enhancement
			Values Clarification

Stress Level			

Definition:
Severity of manifested
  physical or mental
  tension resulting from
  factors that alter an
  existing equilibrium
	Anxiety Reduction
	Coping
	  Enhancement
		Aromatherapy
		Decision-Making
		  Support
		Distraction
		Humor
		Meditation Facilitation
		Relaxation Therapy
			Relocation Stress Reduction
			Security Enhancement
			Self-Hypnosis Facilitation
			Self-Modification
			  Assistance
			Spiritual Support
			Support Group

NURSING DIAGNOSIS: Death Anxiety

DEFINITION: Vague uneasy feeling of discomfort or dread generated by perceptions of real or imagined threat to one's existence

NICS ASSOCIATED WITH DIAGNOSIS RELATED FACTORS

Complex Relationship
  Building
	Environmental
	  Management:
	  Comfort
		Truth Telling

NOC-NIC LINKAGES FOR DEATH ANXIETY

Outcome	Major Interventions	Suggested Interventions	
Acceptance: Health Status			

Definition:
Reconciliation to
  significant change in
  health circumstances
	Anxiety Reduction
	Coping
	  Enhancement
		Active Listening
		Anticipatory Guidance
		Decision-Making Support
		Emotional Support
		Grief Work Facilitation
		Hope Inspiration
			Presence
			Referral
			Spiritual Support
			Support System
			  Enhancement
			Truth Telling
			Values Clarification

NOC-NIC LINKAGES FOR DEATH ANXIETY		
Outcome	**Major Interventions**	**Suggested Interventions**

Anxiety Level

Definition:
Severity of manifested apprehension, tension, or uneasiness arising from an unidentifiable source

Major Interventions: Anxiety Reduction

Suggested Interventions:
Active Listening
Animal-Assisted Therapy
Aromatherapy
Calming Technique
Coping Enhancement
Massage
Music Therapy
Presence
Relaxation Therapy
Sleep Enhancement
Spiritual Support
Touch

Comfortable Death

Definition:
Physical, psychospiritual, sociocultural, and environmental ease with the impending end of life

Major Interventions:
Anxiety Reduction
Dying Care

Suggested Interventions:
Analgesic Administration
Environmental Management: Comfort
Massage
Medication Management
Nausea Management
Nutrition Management
Nutritional Monitoring
Oral Health Maintenance
Pain Management
Patient-Controlled Analgesia (PCA) Assistance
Presence
Relaxation Therapy
Self-Care Assistance
Sleep Enhancement
Therapeutic Touch
Vomiting Management

Depression Level

Definition:
Severity of melancholic mood and loss of interest in life events

Major Interventions:
Hope Inspiration
Mood Management

Suggested Interventions:
Animal-Assisted Therapy
Anxiety Reduction
Dying Care
Emotional Support
Grief Work Facilitation
Medication Management
Music Therapy
Reminiscence Therapy
Sleep Enhancement
Spiritual Support
Support System Enhancement

Dignified Life Closure

Definition:
Personal actions to maintain control during approaching end of life

Major Interventions:
Decision-Making Support

Suggested Interventions:
Anxiety Reduction
Bibliotherapy
Coping Enhancement
Culture Brokerage
Dying Care
Emotional Support
Family Integrity Promotion
Family Involvement Promotion
Forgiveness Facilitation
Grief Work Facilitation
Organ Procurement
Patient Rights Protection
Reminiscence Therapy
Spiritual Growth Facilitation
Spiritual Support
Values Clarification
Visitation Facilitation

Fear Level

Definition:
Severity of manifested apprehension, tension, or uneasiness arising from an identifiable source

Major Interventions:
Anxiety Reduction
Coping Enhancement

Suggested Interventions:
Active Listening
Calming Technique
Decision-Making Support
Dying Care
Emotional Support
Family Mobilization
Guided Imagery
Music Therapy
Pain Management
Presence
Relaxation Therapy
Sleep Enhancement
Spiritual Support

Fear Level: Child

Definition:
Severity of manifested apprehension, tension, or uneasiness arising from an identifiable source in a child from 1 year through 17 years of age

Major Interventions:
Anxiety Reduction
Calming Technique

Suggested Interventions:
Active Listening
Anger Control Assistance
Animal-Assisted Therapy
Coping Enhancement
Diarrhea Management
Distraction
Family Involvement Promotion
Music Therapy
Nausea Management
Pain Management
Presence
Sleep Enhancement
Vital Signs Monitoring

PART II - D

Continued

NOC-NIC LINKAGES FOR DEATH ANXIETY		
Outcome	**Major Interventions**	**Suggested Interventions**

Hope
Definition:
Optimism that is
  personally satisfying
  and life-supporting
	Hope Inspiration
	Spiritual Support
		Anxiety Reduction
		Coping Enhancement
		Decision-Making Support
		Dying Care
			Emotional Support
			Grief Work Facilitation
			Presence
			Touch

Spiritual Health
Definition:
Connectedness with self,
  others, higher power,
  all life, nature, and the
  universe that tran-
  scends and
  empowers the self
	Religious Ritual
	  Enhancement
	Spiritual Growth
	  Facilitation
		Anxiety Reduction
		Dying Care
		Forgiveness Facilitation
		Grief Work Facilitation
		Guilt Work Facilitation
			Hope Inspiration
			Meditation Facilitation
			Self-Awareness
			  Enhancement
			Spiritual Support
			Values Clarification

Critical reasoning note: The interventions selected for the outcome Fear Level: Child will depend on both the severity of the symptoms and the age of the child.

NURSING DIAGNOSIS: Decision-Making, Readiness for Enhanced

Definition: A pattern of choosing courses of action that is sufficient for meeting short and long term health-related goals and can be strengthened

NOC-NIC LINKAGES FOR DECISION-MAKING, READINESS FOR ENHANCED		
Outcome	**Major Interventions**	**Suggested Interventions**

Adherence Behavior
Definition:
Self-initiated actions to
  promote optimal
  wellness, recovery,
  and rehabilitation
	Health Education	Decision-Making Support
		Health Screening
		Health System Guidance
			Risk Identification
			Teaching: Individual

Decision-Making
Definition:
Ability to make
  judgments and
  choose between two
  or more alternatives
	Decision-Making
	  Support
		Culture Brokerage
		Health Education
		Health Literacy
		  Enhancement
			Self-Awareness
			  Enhancement
			Teaching: Individual
			Values Clarification

Health Beliefs
Definition:
Personal convictions
  that influence health
  behaviors
	Decision-Making
	  Support
	Values
	  Clarification
		Active Listening
		Health Education
		Health Literacy Enhancement
		Self-Efficacy Enhancement
			Self-Responsibility
			  Facilitation
			Support Group
			Teaching: Individual

Personal Autonomy
Definition:
Personal actions of
  a competent
  individual to
  exercise governance
  in life decisions
	Decision-Making
	  Support
		Active Listening
		Assertiveness Training
		Patient Rights Protection
		Self-Efficacy Enhancement
			Self-Responsibility
			  Facilitation
			Teaching: Individual
			Values Clarification

NURSING DIAGNOSIS: Decisional Conflict

DEFINITION: Uncertainty about course of action to be taken when choice among competing actions involves risk, loss, or challenge to values and beliefs

NICS ASSOCIATED WITH DIAGNOSIS RELATED FACTORS

Decision-Making Support
Health Education

Patient Rights Protection
Support Group

Support System Enhancement
Values Clarification

NOC-NIC LINKAGES FOR DECISIONAL CONFLICT

Outcome	Major Interventions	Suggested Interventions	
Decision-Making Definition: Ability to make judgments and choose between two or more alternatives	Decision-Making Support Values Clarification	Anxiety Reduction Crisis Intervention Culture Brokerage Genetic Counseling Health Education	Health System Guidance Preconception Counseling Self-Awareness Enhancement Spiritual Support
Information Processing Definition: Ability to acquire, organize, and use information	Decision-Making Support Health Literacy Enhancement	Active Listening Anxiety Reduction Culture Brokerage Developmental Enhancement: Adolescent	Health Education Learning Facilitation Sleep Enhancement Teaching: Individual Values Clarification
Participation in Health Care Decisions Definition: Personal involvement in selecting and evaluating health care options to achieve desired outcome	Decision-Making Support Values Clarification	Active Listening Anticipatory Guidance Assertiveness Training Anxiety Reduction Coping Enhancement Counseling	Culture Brokerage Discharge Planning Family Involvement Promotion Health System Guidance Self-Responsibility Facilitation
Personal Autonomy Definition: Personal actions of a competent individual to exercise governance in life decisions	Decision-Making Support Health System Guidance	Anticipatory Guidance Assertiveness Training Emotional Support Health Education Learning Facilitation	Patients Rights Protection Resiliency Promotion Self-Awareness Enhancement Teaching: Individual

PART II - D

NURSING DIAGNOSIS: Denial, Ineffective

Definition: Conscious or unconscious attempt to disavow the knowledge or meaning of an event to reduce anxiety/fear, but leading to the detriment of health

NICS ASSOCIATED WITH DIAGNOSIS RELATED FACTORS

Anxiety Reduction	Coping Enhancement	Support System Enhancement

NOC-NIC LINKAGES FOR DENIAL, INEFFECTIVE

Outcome	Major Interventions	Suggested Interventions	
Acceptance: Health Status Definition: Reconciliation to significant change in health circumstances	Cognitive Restructuring Coping Enhancement	Counseling Decision-Making Support Emotional Support Hope Inspiration Mutual Goal Setting Reminiscence Therapy Self-Awareness Enhancement	Spiritual Support Support Group Support System Enhancement Therapy Group Truth Telling Values Clarification
Anxiety Level Definition: Severity of manifested apprehension, tension, or uneasiness arising from an unidentifiable source	Anxiety Reduction Self-Awareness Enhancement	Active Listening Coping Enhancement Counseling Decision-Making Support Medication Administration Milieu Therapy Presence Recreation Therapy	Relaxation Therapy Security Enhancement Spiritual Support Support Group Support System Enhancement Therapeutic Play Therapy Group Truth Telling
Compliance Behavior Definition: Personal actions to promote wellness, recovery, and rehabilitation recommended by a health professional	Coping Enhancement Self-Modification Assistance	Anticipatory Guidance Emotional Support Health System Guidance Self-Awareness Enhancement	Self-Responsibility Facilitation Teaching: Disease Process Teaching: Individual Teaching: Procedure/Treatment
Health Beliefs: Perceived Threat Definition: Personal conviction that a threatening health problem is serious and has potential negative consequences for lifestyle	Coping Enhancement Self-Efficacy Enhancement	Active Listening Anxiety Reduction Counseling Emotional Support Self-Awareness Enhancement Self-Modification Assistance	Self-Responsibility Facilitation Teaching: Disease Process Teaching: Individual Truth Telling Values Clarification

NOC-NIC LINKAGES FOR DENIAL, INEFFECTIVE

Outcome	Major Interventions	Suggested Interventions	
Symptom Control Definition: Personal actions to minimize perceived adverse changes in physical and emotional functioning	Self-Modification Assistance Self-Responsibility Facilitation	Anticipatory Guidance Behavior Modification Coping Enhancement Counseling Emotional Support Family Involvement Promotion Health Education Health System Guidance	Learning Facilitation Learning Readiness Enhancement Mutual Goal Setting Patient Contracting Self-Awareness Enhancement Teaching: Disease Process Teaching: Individual Teaching: Procedure/Treatment

NURSING DIAGNOSIS: Dentition, Impaired

Definition: Disruption in tooth development/eruption patterns or structural integrity of individual teeth

NICS ASSOCIATED WITH DIAGNOSIS RELATED FACTORS

Financial Resource Assistance Health Education Health System Guidance Insurance Authorization	Medication Management Nutrition Management Nutritional Counseling	Oral Health Maintenance Referral Self-Care Assistance: Bathing/Hygiene	Smoking Cessation Assistance Substance Use Treatment Teaching: Individual

NOC-NIC LINKAGES FOR DENTITION, IMPAIRED

Outcome	Major Interventions	Suggested Interventions	
Oral Hygiene Definition: Condition of the mouth, teeth, gums, and tongue	Oral Health Maintenance Oral Health Restoration	Medication Administration: Oral Oral Health Promotion Pain Management	Referral Teaching: Individual
Self-Care: Oral Hygiene Definition: Ability to care for own mouth and teeth independently with or without assistive device	Oral Health Maintenance Oral Health Restoration	Oral Health Promotion Self-Care Assistance: Bathing/Hygiene Self-Care Assistance: Feeding	Teaching: Individual Teaching: Psychomotor Skill

NURSING DIAGNOSIS: Diarrhea

Definition: Passage of loose, unformed stools

NICS ASSOCIATED WITH DIAGNOSIS RELATED FACTORS

Anxiety Reduction Communicable Disease Management Enteral Tube Feeding	Infection Control Medication Management	Radiation Therapy Management Substance Use Treatment	Substance Use Treatment: Alcohol Withdrawal

Continued

PART II - D

	**NOC-NIC LINKAGES FOR DIARRHEA**
Outcome	**Major Interventions**		**Suggested Interventions**

Bowel Continence

Definition: Control of passage of stool from the bowel

	Major Interventions	Suggested Interventions	
	Bowel Management Diarrhea Management	Bowel Incontinence Care Bowel Incontinence Care: Encopresis Fluid Management	Medication Management Medication Prescribing Nutrition Management Self-Care Assistance: Toileting

Bowel Elimination

Definition: Formation and evacuation of stool

	Bowel Management	Diarrhea Management Medication Management	Pain Management Specimen Management

Symptom Severity

Definition: Severity of perceived adverse changes in physical, emotional, and social functioning

	Diarrhea Management	Bowel Management Medication Administration	Medication Management Pain Management

Critical reasoning note: The diagnosis Diarrhea focuses on the passage of unformed stool, but severe and/or prolonged diarrhea can result in fluid and electrolyte imbalance. For these problems consider the following outcomes: Electrolyte & Acid/Base Balance, Fluid Balance, and Hydration. The following major interventions would address these outcomes: Acid-Base Management, Acid-Base Monitoring, Electrolyte Management, Electrolyte Management: Hypokalemia, Electrolyte Management: Hyponatremia, Electrolyte Monitoring, Fluid/Electrolyte Management, Fluid Resuscitation, and Intravenous (IV) Insertion.

NURSING DIAGNOSIS: Diversional Activity, Deficit

Definition: Decreased stimulation from (or interest or engagement in) recreational or leisure activities

NICS ASSOCIATED WITH DIAGNOSIS RELATED FACTORS

Environmental Management

	**NOC-NIC LINKAGES FOR DIVERSIONAL ACTIVITY, DEFICIT**
Outcome	**Major Interventions**		**Suggested Interventions**

Leisure Participation

Definition: Use of relaxing, interesting, and enjoyable activities to promote well-being

	Major Interventions	Suggested Interventions	
	Activity Therapy Recreation Therapy	Animal-Assisted Therapy Art Therapy Behavior Modification: Social Skills Bibliotherapy Exercise Promotion Family Mobilization Humor	Music Therapy Reminiscence Therapy Self-Responsibility Facilitation Socialization Enhancement Support System Enhancement Therapeutic Play

Motivation

Definition: Inner urge that moves or prompts an individual to positive action(s)

	Self-Modification Assistance Self-Responsibility Facilitation	Assertiveness Training Behavior Management Behavior Modification: Social Skills Mood Management Mutual Goal Setting	Patient Contracting Self-Awareness Enhancement Self-Esteem Enhancement Socialization Enhancement

NOC-NIC LINKAGES FOR DIVERSIONAL ACTIVITY, DEFICIT

Outcome	Major Interventions	Suggested Interventions	
Play Participation			
Definition: Use of activities by a child from 1 year through 11 years of age to promote enjoyment, entertainment, and development	Therapeutic Play	Activity Therapy Animal-Assisted Therapy Art Therapy Developmental Enhancement: Child Exercise Promotion	Music Therapy Recreation Therapy Socialization Enhancement Surveillance: Safety Visitation Facilitation
Social Involvement			
Definition: Social interactions with persons, groups, or organizations	Socialization Enhancement	Active Listening Activity Therapy Animal-Assisted Therapy Art Therapy Assertiveness Training Behavior Modification: Social Skills Communication Enhancement: Hearing Deficit Communication Enhancement: Speech Deficit Communication Enhancement: Visual Deficit Complex Relationship Building Counseling Culture Brokerage Developmental Enhancement: Adolescent	Developmental Enhancement: Child Family Integrity Promotion Family Mobilization Family Therapy Humor Milieu Therapy Mutual Goal Setting Presence Recreation Therapy Self-Awareness Enhancement Self-Esteem Enhancement Self-Responsibility Facilitation Support Group Support System Enhancement Therapeutic Play Visitation Facilitation

Critical reasoning note: Specific interventions that can increase diversional opportunities in the environment are included with the outcomes rather than with the diagnosis related factors.

NURSING DIAGNOSIS: Energy Field, Disturbed

Definition: Disruption of the flow of energy surrounding a person's being that results in disharmony of the body, mind, and/or spirit

NICS ASSOCIATED WITH DIAGNOSIS RELATED FACTORS

Anxiety Reduction Bed Rest Care Chemotherapy Management Developmental Enhancement: Adolescent	Developmental Enhancement: Child Grief Work Facilitation Grief Work Facilitation: Perinatal Death	High-Risk Pregnancy Care Intrapartal Care Pain Management	Prenatal Care Surgical Precautions

Continued

PART II - E

NOC-NIC LINKAGES FOR ENERGY FIELD, DISTURBED

Outcome	Major Interventions	Suggested Interventions	
Personal Well-Being Definition: Extent of positive perception of one's health status	Self-Awareness Enhancement Therapeutic Touch	Acupressure Aromatherapy	Environmental Management Temperature Regulation
Symptom Control Definition: Personal actions to minimize perceived adverse changes in physical and emotional functioning	Therapeutic Touch	Acupressure Aromatherapy Environmental Management: Comfort	Massage Surveillance

Critical reasoning note: There are a number of interventions to address the related factors. Therapeutic Touch is the major intervention to address a disturbance in the energy field.

NURSING DIAGNOSIS: Environmental Interpretation Syndrome, Impaired

Definition: Consistent lack of orientation to person, place, time, or circumstances over more than 3-6 months, necessitating a protective environment

NICS ASSOCIATED WITH DIAGNOSIS RELATED FACTORS

Dementia Management   Mood Management

NOC-NIC LINKAGES FOR ENVIRONMENTAL INTERPRETATION SYNDROME, IMPAIRED

Outcome	Major Interventions	Suggested Interventions	
Cognitive Orientation Definition: Ability to identify person, place, and time accurately	Dementia Management Reality Orientation	Anxiety Reduction Area Restriction Cognitive Stimulation Coping Enhancement	Emotional Support Environmental Management: Safety Patient Rights Protection
Concentration Definition: Ability to focus on a specific stimulus	Anxiety Reduction Cognitive Stimulation	Active Listening Calming Technique Cerebral Perfusion Promotion Communication Enhancement: Hearing Deficit	Communication Enhancement: Speech Deficit Communication Enhancement: Visual Deficit Dementia Management
Elopement Propensity Risk Definition: The propensity of an individual with cognitive impairment to escape a secure area	Elopement Precautions Risk Identification	Anxiety Reduction Area Restriction Environmental Management: Safety Grief Work Facilitation	Patient Rights Protection Relocation Stress Reduction Surveillance: Safety Visitation Facilitation

NOC-NIC LINKAGES FOR ENVIRONMENTAL INTERPRETATION SYNDROME, IMPAIRED		
Outcome	**Major Interventions**	**Suggested Interventions**
Memory Definition: Ability to cognitively retrieve and report previously stored information	Dementia Management Memory Training	Cognitive Stimulation Coping Enhancement Energy Management Learning Facilitation Medication Management	Milieu Therapy Patient Rights Protection Reality Orientation Reminiscence Therapy Sleep Enhancement
Safe Wandering Definition: Safe, socially acceptable moving about without apparent purpose in an individual with cognitive impairment	Elopement Precautions	Area Restriction Distraction Environmental Management: Safety	Fall Prevention Surveillance: Safety

Critical reasoning note: Safe Wandering and Elopement Propensity Risk are included as possible outcomes to provide a protective environment that allows patient movement when preventing elopement is a concern.

NURSING DIAGNOSIS: Failure to Thrive, Adult

Definition: Progressive functional deterioration of a physical and cognitive nature. The individual's ability to live with multisystem diseases, cope with ensuing problems, and manage his or her care is remarkably diminished

NICS ASSOCIATED WITH DIAGNOSIS RELATED FACTORS	
Mood Management	Suicide Prevention

NOC-NIC LINKAGES FOR FAILURE TO THRIVE, ADULT		
Outcome	**Major Interventions**	**Suggested Interventions**
Appetite Definition: Desire to eat when ill or receiving treatment	Nutrition Management Nutritional Monitoring	Diet Staging Fluid Monitoring Medication Management	Nausea Management Oral Health Maintenance Vomiting Management
Cognition Definition: Ability to execute complex mental processes	Decision-Making Support Dementia Management	Active Listening Cognitive Stimulation Patient Rights Protection	Presence Reality Orientation Reminiscence Therapy
Development: Late Adulthood Definition: Cognitive, psychosocial, and moral progression from 65 years of age and older	Nutrition Therapy Resiliency Promotion	Active Listening Activity Therapy Anger Control Assistance Decision-Making Support Dementia Management Diet Staging	Energy Management Home Maintenance Assistance Hope Inspiration Memory Training Self-Care Assistance

Continued

PART II - F

NOC-NIC LINKAGES FOR FAILURE TO THRIVE, ADULT

Outcome	Major Interventions	Suggested Interventions	
Nutritional Status Definition: Extent to which nutrients are available to meet metabolic needs	Fluid Monitoring Nutritional Monitoring	Eating Disorders Management Energy Management Enteral Tube Feeding Feeding Fluid/Electrolyte Management Nutrition Management	Nutrition Therapy Self-Care Assistance: Feeding Total Parenteral Nutrition (TPN) Administration Weight Gain Assistance Weight Maintenance
Nutritional Status: Food & Fluid Intake Definition: Amount of food and fluid taken into the body over a 24-hour period	Fluid Monitoring Nutritional Monitoring	Enteral Tube Feeding Feeding Intravenous (IV) Therapy Nutrition Management	Nutrition Therapy Self-Care Assistance: Feeding Total Parenteral Nutrition (TPN) Administration
Self-Care: Activities of Daily Living (ADL) Definition: Ability to perform the most basic physical tasks and personal care activities independently with or without assistive device	Self-Care Assistance	Energy Management Exercise Promotion Fall Prevention Self-Care Assistance: Bathing/Hygiene Self-Care Assistance: Dressing/Grooming	Self-Care Assistance: Feeding Self-Care Assistance: Toileting Self-Care Assistance: Transfer
Weight Gain Behavior Definition: Personal actions to gain weight following voluntary or involuntary significant weight loss	Weight Gain Assistance	Eating Disorders Management Enteral Tube Feeding Gastrointestinal Intubation Medication Administration Nutrition Therapy Nutritional Monitoring Oral Health Restoration	Self-Care Assistance: Feeding Support Group Swallowing Therapy Total Parenteral Nutrition (TPN) Administration Tube Care: Gastrointestinal
Will to Live Definition: Desire, determination, and effort to survive	Hope Inspiration Spiritual Support	Animal-Assisted Therapy Emotional Support Family Mobilization Patient Rights Protection	Religious Ritual Enhancement Relocation Stress Reduction Suicide Prevention Support System Enhancement

Critical reasoning note: The diagnosis is specific for adult failure to thrive attributable to multisystem disease. Other types of adult failure to thrive can occur (for example, with abuse). Although only Development: Late Adulthood has been selected as an outcome, failure to thrive can occur at a younger age, in which case Development: Young or Middle Adulthood would be used.

NURSING DIAGNOSIS: Family Coping, Compromised

Definition: Usually supportive primary person (family member or close friend) provides insufficient, ineffective, or compromised support, comfort, assistance, or encouragement that may be needed by the client to manage or master adaptive tasks related to his or her health challenge

NICS ASSOCIATED WITH DIAGNOSIS RELATED FACTORS

Crisis Intervention Respite Care	Support Group	Support System Enhancement	Teaching: Individual

NOC-NIC LINKAGES FOR FAMILY COPING, COMPROMISED

Outcome	Major Interventions	Suggested Interventions	
Caregiver Emotional Health Definition: Emotional well-being of a family care provider while caring for a family member	Caregiver Support Respite Care	Anger Control Assistance Coping Enhancement Emotional Support Forgiveness Facilitation Grief Work Facilitation Guilt Work Facilitation Health System Guidance	Referral Relaxation Therapy Resiliency Promotion Role Enhancement Spiritual Support Support Group Support System Enhancement

Caregiver-Patient Relationship
 	
Definition:
Positive interactions and connections between the caregiver and care recipient
	Caregiver Support	Conflict Mediation
		Emotional Support
		Environmental
		    Management:
		    Violence Prevention
		Home Maintenance
		    Assistance
			Mutual Goal Setting
			Respite Care
			Support Group
			Support System
			    Enhancement

Caregiver Performance: Direct Care
 	
Definition:
Provision by family care provider of appropriate personal and health care for a family member
	Caregiver Support
	Learning
	    Facilitation
		Environmental
		    Management: Comfort
		Health System Guidance
		Learning Readiness
		    Enhancement
		Normalization Promotion
		Respite Care
		Teaching: Disease
		    Process
			Teaching: Individual
			Teaching: Prescribed
			    Activity/Exercise
			Teaching: Prescribed
			    Diet
			Teaching: Prescribed
			    Medication
			Teaching: Procedure/
			    Treatment
			Teaching: Psychomotor
			    Skill

Caregiver Performance: Indirect Care
 	
Definition:
Arrangement and oversight by family care provider of appropriate care for a family member
	Health System
	    Guidance
		Decision-Making Support
		Discharge Planning
		Family Integrity
		    Promotion
		Family Involvement
		    Promotion
		Family Mobilization
			Financial Resource
			    Assistance
			Insurance Authorization
			Patient Rights Protection
			Referral
			Support Group

Continued

PART II - F

NOC-NIC LINKAGES FOR FAMILY COPING, COMPROMISED

Outcome	Major Interventions	Suggested Interventions	
Caregiver Role Endurance Definition: Factors that promote family care provider's capacity to sustain caregiving over an extended period of time	Caregiver Support Respite Care	Coping Enhancement Decision-Making Support Emotional Support Energy Management Environmental Management: Home Preparation Exercise Promotion Family Involvement Promotion	Family Mobilization Financial Resource Assistance Health System Guidance Recreation Therapy Spiritual Support Support Group Support System Enhancement
Family Coping Definition: Family actions to manage stressors that tax family resources	Coping Enhancement Family Involvement Promotion	Caregiver Support Case Management Conflict Mediation Decision-Making Support Family Integrity Promotion Family Mobilization Financial Resource Assistance Grief Work Facilitation	Guilt Work Facilitation Mutual Goal Setting Normalization Promotion Resiliency Promotion Respite Care Sibling Support Spiritual Support Trauma Therapy: Child
Family Normalization Definition: Capacity of the family system to develop strategies for optimal functioning when a member has a chronic illness or disability	Family Process Maintenance Normalization Promotion	Coping Enhancement Counseling Decision-Making Support Family Integrity Promotion Family Involvement Promotion Family Mobilization Family Support	Mutual Goal Setting Reminiscence Therapy Respite Care Role Enhancement Sibling Support Spiritual Support Sustenance Support

NURSING DIAGNOSIS: Family Coping, Disabled

Definition: Behavior of significant person (family member or other primary person) that disables his or her capacities and the client's capacities to effectively address tasks essential to either person's adaptation to the health challenge

NICS ASSOCIATED WITH DIAGNOSIS RELATED FACTORS

Anger Control Assistance Anxiety Reduction	Family Integrity Promotion	Guilt Work Facilitation	Mood Management

	NOC-NIC LINKAGES FOR FAMILY COPING, DISABLED		
Outcome	**Major Interventions**	**Suggested Interventions**	
Caregiver-Patient Relationship			
Definition: Positive interactions and connections between the caregiver and care recipient	Caregiver Support	Anger Control Assistance Counseling Environmental Management: Violence Prevention Family Involvement Promotion Family Mobilization	Home Maintenance Assistance Mutual Goal Setting Respite Care Self-Modification Assistance Support Group Support System Enhancement
Caregiver Performance: Direct Care			
Definition: Provision by family care provider of appropriate personal and health care for a family member	Caregiver Support	Case Management Family Involvement Promotion Health System Guidance Learning Facilitation Learning Readiness Enhancement Normalization Promotion Respite Care	Teaching: Disease Process Teaching: Individual Teaching: Prescribed Activity/Exercise Teaching: Prescribed Diet Teaching: Prescribed Medication Teaching: Procedure/ Treatment Teaching: Psychomotor Skill
Caregiver Performance: Indirect Care			
Definition: Arrangement and oversight by family care provider of appropriate care for a family member	Environmental Management: Home Preparation Health System Guidance	Decision-Making Support Discharge Planning Family Integrity Promotion Family Involvement Promotion Family Mobilization	Financial Resource Assistance Insurance Authorization Patient Rights Protection Referral Support Group
Caregiver Role Endurance			
Definition: Factors that promote family care provider's capacity to sustain caregiving over an extended period of time	Caregiver Support Coping Enhancement	Decision-Making Support Emotional Support Family Involvement Promotion Family Mobilization Financial Resource Assistance Health System Guidance	Recreation Therapy Relaxation Therapy Respite Care Support Group Support System Enhancement

Continued

PART II - F

PART II - F

NOC-NIC LINKAGES FOR FAMILY COPING, DISABLED

Outcome	Major Interventions	Suggested Interventions	
Caregiver Well-Being Definition: Extent of positive perception of primary care provider's health status	Caregiver Support Respite Care	Anger Control Assistance Coping Enhancement Emotional Support Family Involvement Promotion Family Mobilization Family Process Maintenance Guilt Work Facilitation	Mood Management Referral Role Enhancement Socialization Enhancement Spiritual Support Support Group Support System Enhancement
Family Coping Definition: Family actions to manage stressors that tax family resources	Coping Enhancement Family Involvement Promotion	Abuse Protection Support Abuse Protection Support: Child Abuse Protection Support: Domestic Partner Abuse Protection Support: Elder Anger Control Assistance Case Management Conflict Mediation Counseling Environmental Management: Violence Prevention	Family Integrity Promotion Family Mobilization Family Process Maintenance Family Support Family Therapy Financial Resource Assistance Normalization Promotion Resiliency Promotion Sustenance Support
Family Normalization Definition: Capacity of the family system to develop strategies for optimal functioning when a member has a chronic illness or disability	Family Support Normalization Promotion	Abuse Protection Support Coping Enhancement Counseling Environmental Management: Home Preparation	Family Integrity Promotion Family Involvement Promotion Family Mobilization Family Process Maintenance Role Enhancement
Neglect Cessation Definition: Evidence that the victim is no longer receiving substandard care	Abuse Protection Support Family Involvement Promotion	Anger Control Assistance Behavior Modification Caregiver Support Coping Enhancement Counseling Crisis Intervention Family Mobilization	Family Therapy Financial Resource Assistance Home Maintenance Assistance Spiritual Support Support System Enhancement Sustenance Support

NURSING DIAGNOSIS: Family Coping, Readiness for Enhanced

Definition: Effective management of adaptive tasks by family member involved with the client's health challenge, who now exhibits desire and readiness for enhanced health and growth in regard to self and in relation to the client

NOC-NIC LINKAGES FOR FAMILY COPING, READINESS FOR ENHANCED		
Outcome	**Major Interventions**	**Suggested Interventions**
Caregiver Well-Being		
Definition: Extent of positive perception of primary care provider's health status	Caregiver Support Respite Care	Coping Enhancement Family Integrity Promotion Family Involvement Promotion Family Mobilization Family Support / Home Maintenance Assistance Normalization Promotion Role Enhancement Support Group Support System Enhancement
Family Coping		
Definition: Family actions to manage stressors that tax family resources	Family Involvement Promotion Family Support	Coping Enhancement Family Integrity Promotion Family Mobilization Financial Resource Assistance Grief Work Facilitation / Normalization Promotion Preconception Counseling Resiliency Promotion Role Enhancement
Family Functioning		
Definition: Capacity of the family system to meet the needs of its members during developmental transitions	Family Support Normalization Promotion	Anticipatory Guidance Developmental Enhancement: Adolescent Developmental Enhancement: Child Family Integrity Promotion Family Involvement Promotion Family Planning: Contraception / Family Planning: Infertility Family Planning: Unplanned Pregnancy Parent Education: Adolescent Parent Education: Childrearing Family Parent Education: Infant Preconception Counseling Role Enhancement Sibling Support
Family Normalization		
Definition: Capacity of the family system to develop strategies for optimal functioning when a member has a chronic illness or disability	Family Involvement Promotion Normalization Promotion	Anticipatory Guidance Developmental Enhancement: Adolescent Developmental Enhancement: Child Family Integrity Promotion / Family Mobilization Family Support Respite Care Role Enhancement Sibling Support

Continued

PART II - F

NOC-NIC LINKAGES FOR FAMILY COPING, READINESS FOR ENHANCED

Outcome	Major Interventions	Suggested Interventions	
Family Resiliency Definition: Positive adaptation and function of the family following significant adversity or crisis	Coping Enhancement Resiliency Promotion	Caregiver Support Conflict Mediation Emotional Support Family Integrity Promotion Family Integrity Promotion: Childbearing Family Family Involvement Promotion Family Mobilization	Family Process Maintenance Family Support Health System Guidance Humor Respite Care Self-Efficacy Enhancement Support Group Support System Enhancement
Health-Promoting Behavior Definition: Personal actions to sustain or increase wellness	Health Education Self-Modification Assistance	Coping Enhancement Exercise Promotion Health Screening Nutritional Counseling Prenatal Care Risk Identification Self-Awareness Enhancement	Self-Efficacy Enhancement Smoking Cessation Assistance Substance Use Prevention Support Group Support System Enhancement Teaching: Safe Sex Weight Management
Health-Seeking Behavior Definition: Personal actions to promote optimal wellness, recovery, and rehabilitation	Health Education Teaching: Individual	Anticipatory Guidance Exercise Promotion Health Screening Health System Guidance Nutritional Counseling Parenting Promotion Self-Efficacy Enhancement Self-Modification Assistance Smoking Cessation Assistance	Substance Use Prevention Support Group Teaching: Prescribed Activity/Exercise Teaching: Prescribed Diet Teaching: Prescribed Medication Teaching: Procedure/ Treatment Vehicle Safety Promotion Weight Management

NURSING DIAGNOSIS: Family Processes, Dysfunctional

Definition: Psychosocial, spiritual, and physiological functions of the family unit are chronically disorganized, which leads to conflict, denial of problems, resistance to change, ineffective problem-solving, and a series of self-perpetuating crises

NICS ASSOCIATED WITH DIAGNOSIS RELATED FACTORS

Behavior Modification Coping Enhancement	Decision-Making Support Risk Identification	Self-Awareness Enhancement Substance Use Prevention	Substance Use Treatment

NOC-NIC LINKAGES FOR FAMILY PROCESSES, DYSFUNCTIONAL		
Outcome	**Major Interventions**	**Suggested Interventions**
Family Coping		
Definition: Family actions to manage stressors that tax family resources	Coping Enhancement Family Therapy	Abuse Protection Support Abuse Protection Support: Child Abuse Protection Support: Domestic Partner Abuse Protection Support: Elder Anger Control Assistance Anxiety Reduction Conflict Mediation Counseling Crisis Intervention	Decision-Making Support Family Integrity Promotion Family Process Maintenance Family Support Financial Resource Assistance Respite Care Spiritual Support Support Group Support System Enhancement
Family Functioning		
Definition: Capacity of the family system to meet the needs of its members during developmental transitions	Family Integrity Promotion: Childbearing Family Family Therapy	Caregiver Support Conflict Mediation Coping Enhancement Decision-Making Support Developmental Enhancement: Adolescent Developmental Enhancement: Child Family Integrity Promotion Family Mobilization Family Process Maintenance	Family Support Financial Resource Assistance Role Enhancement Self-Responsibility Facilitation Spiritual Support Substance Use Prevention Substance Use Treatment Support Group Support System Enhancement
Family Integrity		
Definition: Family members' behaviors that collectively demonstrate cohesion, strength, and emotional bonding	Family Integrity Promotion Family Integrity Promotion: Childbearing Family	Conflict Mediation Decision-Making Support Developmental Enhancement: Adolescent Developmental Enhancement: Child Family Support Family Therapy	Forgiveness Facilitation Role Enhancement Self-Awareness Enhancement Self-Esteem Enhancement Self-Responsibility Facilitation Substance Use Prevention Substance Use Treatment
Family Resiliency		
Definition: Positive adaptation and function of the family system following significant adversity or crises	Family Process Maintenance Resiliency Promotion	Conflict Mediation Coping Enhancement Crisis Intervention Decision-Making Support Emotional Support Family Integrity Promotion Family Integrity Promotion: Childbearing Family Family Support	Family Therapy Grief Work Facilitation Grief Work Facilitation: Perinatal Death Respite Care Sibling Support Spiritual Support Support System Enhancement Values Clarification

Continued

NOC-NIC LINKAGES FOR FAMILY PROCESSES, DYSFUNCTIONAL

Outcome	Major Interventions	Suggested Interventions	
Family Social Climate Definition: Supportive milieu as characterized by family member relationships and goals	Family Integrity Promotion Family Integrity Promotion: Childbearing Family	Abuse Protection Support Abuse Protection Support: Child Abuse Protection Support: Domestic Partner Abuse Protection Support: Elder Conflict Mediation Decision-Making Support	Family Support Family Therapy Substance Use Prevention Substance Use Treatment Support Group Support System Enhancement
Substance Addiction Consequences Definition: Severity of change in health status and social functioning due to substance addiction	Substance Use Treatment	Behavior Modification Complex Relationship Building Coping Enhancement Counseling Crisis Intervention Decision-Making Support Energy Management Exercise Promotion Family Involvement Promotion Family Therapy Impulse Control Training Infection Protection Patient Contracting	Role Enhancement Self-Awareness Enhancement Self-Esteem Enhancement Self-Modification Assistance Self-Responsibility Facilitation Socialization Enhancement Spiritual Support Substance Use Prevention Support Group Support System Enhancement Teaching: Disease Process Therapy Group

NURSING DIAGNOSIS: Family Processes, Interrupted

Definition: Change in family relationships and/or functioning

NICS ASSOCIATED WITH DIAGNOSIS RELATED FACTORS

Crisis Intervention Developmental Enhancement: Adolescent	Developmental Enhancement: Child Financial Resource Assistance Resiliency Promotion	Role Enhancement Social Marketing

NOC-NIC LINKAGES FOR FAMILY PROCESSES, INTERRUPTED		
Outcome	**Major Interventions**	**Suggested Interventions**

Family Coping

Definition:
Family actions to
   manage stressors
   that tax family
   resources
	Coping Enhancement
	Family Process
	   Maintenance
		Caregiver Support
		Conflict Mediation
		Counseling
		Decision-Making Support
		Family Integrity
		   Promotion
		Family Integrity
		   Promotion:
		     Childbearing Family
		Family Mobilization
			Family Support
			Family Therapy
			Grief Work Facilitation
			Grief Work Facilitation:
			   Perinatal Death
			Respite Care
			Support Group
			Support System
			   Enhancement
			Trauma Therapy: Child

Family Functioning

Definition:
Capacity of the family
   system to meet the
   needs of its
   members during
   developmental
   transitions
	Family Integrity
	   Promotion
	Family Integrity
	   Promotion:
	   Childbearing
	   Family
		Conflict Mediation
		Coping Enhancement
		Decision-Making Support
		Developmental
		   Enhancement:
		   Adolescent
		Developmental
		   Enhancement: Child
		Family Planning:
		   Contraception
		Family Planning:
		   Infertility
		Family Planning:
		   Unplanned Pregnancy
			Family Process
			   Maintenance
			Family Support
			Normalization
			   Promotion
			Parent Education:
			   Adolescent
			Parent Education:
			   Childrearing Family
			Parent Education: Infant
			Role Enhancement
			Support Group
			Support System
			   Enhancement

Family Normalization

Definition:
Capacity of the family
   system to develop
   strategies for
   optimal functioning
   when a member has
   a chronic illness or
   disability
	Family Process
	   Maintenance
	Normalization
	   Promotion
		Caregiver Support
		Coping Enhancement
		Counseling
		Dementia Management
		Emotional Support
		Family Involvement
		   Promotion
		Family Mobilization
		Family Therapy
			Grief Work Facilitation
			Guilt Work Facilitation
			Home Maintenance
			   Assistance
			Respite Care
			Role Enhancement
			Support System
			   Enhancement
			Trauma Therapy: Child

Family Resiliency

Definition:
Positive adaptation
   and function of the
   family system
   following significant
   adversity or crises
	Family Process
	   Maintenance
	Resiliency Promotion
		Conflict Mediation
		Coping Enhancement
		Counseling
		Decision-Making Support
		Emotional Support
		Family Planning:
		   Unplanned Pregnancy
			Family Support
			Family Therapy
			Normalization
			   Promotion
			Support Group
			Support System
			   Enhancement

Family Social Climate

Definition:
Supportive milieu as
   characterized by
   family member
   relationships and
   goals
	Family Integrity
	   Promotion
	Family Integrity
	   Promotion:
	   Childbearing
	   Family
	Family Support
		Behavior Modification
		Conflict Mediation
		Counseling
		Decision-Making Support
		Developmental
		   Enhancement:
		   Adolescent
			Developmental
			   Enhancement: Child
			Family Process
			   Maintenance
			Family Therapy
			Role Enhancement
			Spiritual Support

Continued

PART II - F

NOC-NIC LINKAGES FOR FAMILY PROCESSES, INTERRUPTED

Outcome	Major Interventions	Suggested Interventions	
Family Support During Treatment Definition: Family presence and emotional support for an individual undergoing treatment	Family Involvement Promotion Family Presence Facilitation	Case Management Culture Brokerage Discharge Planning Family Mobilization Health Care Information Exchange Health System Guidance	Pass Facilitation Spiritual Support Support Group Teaching: Disease Process Teaching: Procedure/ Treatment Visitation Facilitation

Clinical reasoning note: Some of the interventions to treat related factors are also used to achieve the desired outcomes. This is due to the fact that the related factors produce symptoms/changes that appear in the defining characteristics used to make the diagnosis.

NURSING DIAGNOSIS: Family Processes, Readiness for Enhanced

Definition: A pattern of family functioning that is sufficient to support the well-being of family members and can be strengthened

NOC-NIC LINKAGES FOR FAMILY PROCESSES, READINESS FOR ENHANCED

Outcome	Major Interventions	Suggested Interventions	
Family Functioning Definition: Capacity of the family system to meet the needs of its members during developmental transitions	Family Integrity Promotion Family Integrity Promotion: Childbearing Family	Developmental Enhancement: Adolescent Developmental Enhancement: Child Family Support Parent Education: Adolescent Parent Education: Childrearing Family	Parent Education: Infant Parenting Promotion Resiliency Promotion Role Enhancement Sibling Support
Family Health Status Definition: Overall health and social competence of family unit	Health Education Health Screening	Developmental Enhancement: Adolescent Developmental Enhancement: Child Exercise Promotion Family Integrity Promotion Family Integrity Promotion: Childbearing Family Family Support Genetic Counseling Health System Guidance	Home Maintenance Assistance Immunization/ Vaccination Management Parent Education: Adolescent Parent Education: Childrearing Family Parent Education: Infant Risk Identification: Childbearing Family Role Enhancement Support System Enhancement

PART II - F

NOC-NIC LINKAGES FOR FAMILY PROCESSES, READINESS FOR ENHANCED

Outcome	Major Interventions	Suggested Interventions	
Family Integrity Definition: Family members' behaviors that collectively demonstrate cohesion, strength, and emotional bonding	Family Integrity Promotion Family Integrity Promotion: Childbearing Family	Attachment Promotion Childbirth Preparation Developmental Enhancement: Adolescent Developmental Enhancement: Child Environmental Management: Attachment Process Family Process Maintenance Family Support	Forgiveness Facilitation Parent Education: Adolescent Parent Education: Childrearing Family Parent Education: Infant Parenting Promotion Resiliency Promotion Role Enhancement Sibling Support
Family Resiliency Definition: Positive adaptation and function of the family system following significant adversity or crises	Family Process Maintenance Resiliency Promotion	Coping Enhancement Decision-Making Support Family Support	Grief Work Facilitation Normalization Promotion Support System Enhancement
Family Social Climate Definition: Supportive milieu as characterized by family member relationships and goals	Family Integrity Promotion Family Integrity Promotion: Childbearing Family	Developmental Enhancement: Adolescent Developmental Enhancement: Child Family Support Resiliency Promotion	Role Enhancement Sibling Support Socialization Enhancement Values Clarification

NURSING DIAGNOSIS: Family Therapeutic Regimen Management, Ineffective

Definition: Pattern of regulating and integrating into family processes a program for treatment of illness and its sequelae that is unsatisfactory for meeting specific health goals

NICS ASSOCIATED WITH DIAGNOSIS RELATED FACTORS

Caregiver Support Case Management Conflict Mediation	Decision-Making Support Financial Resource Assistance	Health System Guidance Patient Rights Protection	Referral Telephone Consultation

NOC–NIC LINKAGES FOR FAMILY THERAPEUTIC REGIMEN MANAGEMENT, INEFFECTIVE

Outcome	Major Interventions	Suggested Interventions	
Caregiver Home Care Readiness Definition: Preparedness of a caregiver to assume responsibility for the health care of a family member in the home	Caregiver Support Self-Efficacy Enhancement	Family Involvement Promotion Respite Care Role Enhancement Teaching: Prescribed Activity/Exercise	Teaching: Prescribed Diet Teaching: Prescribed Medication Teaching: Procedure/ Treatment Teaching: Psychomotor Skill

Continued

NOC–NIC LINKAGES FOR FAMILY THERAPEUTIC REGIMEN MANAGEMENT, INEFFECTIVE			
Outcome	**Major Interventions**	**Suggested Interventions**	

Family Normalization
Definition:
Capacity of the family system to develop strategies for optimal functioning when a member has a chronic illness or disability
	Family Mobilization
	Normalization
	Promotion
		Family Involvement
		  Promotion
		Family Process
		  Maintenance
		Role Enhancement
			Sibling Support
			Support Group
			Support System
			  Enhancement

Family Participation in Professional Care
Definition:
Family involvement in decision-making, delivery, and evaluation of care provided by health care personnel
	Family Involvement
	  Promotion
		Assertiveness Training
		Coping Enhancement
		Culture Brokerage
			Decision-Making
			  Support
			Discharge Planning
			Family Presence
			  Facilitation

Family Resiliency
Definition:
Positive adaptation and function of the family system following significant adversity or crises
	Coping
	  Enhancement
	Resiliency
	  Promotion
		Conflict Mediation
		Counseling
		Crisis Intervention
		Decision-Making
		  Support
		Environmental
		  Management: Home
		  Preparation
		Family Integrity
		  Promotion
		Family Involvement
		  Promotion
		Family Process
		  Maintenance
			Family Support
			Financial Resource
			  Assistance
			Hope Inspiration
			Humor
			Respite Care
			Sibling Support
			Support Group
			Support System
			  Enhancement

Critical reasoning note: Interventions for the outcome Caregiver Home Care Readiness will be directed at the primary caregiver(s) rather than the patient.

NURSING DIAGNOSIS: Fatigue

Definition: An overwhelming sustained sense of exhaustion and decreased capacity for physical and mental work at usual level

NICS ASSOCIATED WITH DIAGNOSIS RELATED FACTORS			

Anxiety Reduction
Chemotherapy
  Management
Coping Enhancement
	Environmental
	  Management
	Exercise Promotion
	High-Risk Pregnancy
	  Care
		Medication
		  Management
		Mood Management
			Nutrition Management
			Prenatal Care

NOC-NIC LINKAGES FOR FATIGUE

Outcome	Major Interventions	Suggested Interventions	

Endurance
Definition:
Capacity to sustain activity
	Energy Management	Electrolyte Monitoring
		Exercise Promotion
		Exercise Promotion:
		  Strength Training
		Guilt Work Facilitation
		Medication
		  Management
			Nutrition Management
			Sleep Enhancement
			Teaching: Prescribed
			  Activity/Exercise
			Teaching: Prescribed
			  Diet

Energy Conservation
Definition:
Personal actions to manage energy for initiating and sustaining activity
	Energy Management
	Environmental
	  Management
		Body Mechanics
		  Promotion
		Exercise Promotion
		Nutrition Management
			Sleep Enhancement
			Teaching: Prescribed
			  Activity/Exercise

Fatigue Level
Definition:
Severity of observed or reported prolonged generalized fatigue
	Energy Management	Anxiety Reduction
		Environmental
		  Management
		Guilt Work Facilitation
		Laboratory Data
		  Interpretation
		Medication
		  Management
		Mood Management
			Nutritional Monitoring
			Pain Management
			Self-Care Assistance
			Self-Care Assistance:
			  IADL
			Sleep Enhancement
			Surveillance

Nutritional Status: Energy
Definition:
Extent to which nutrients and oxygen provide cellular energy
	Energy Management
	Nutrition
	  Management
		Eating Disorders
		  Management
		Enteral Tube Feeding
		  Feeding
		Nutrition Therapy
		Nutritional Counseling
		Nutritional Monitoring
			Self-Care Assistance:
			  Feeding
			Sustenance Support
			Teaching: Prescribed
			  Diet
			Total Parenteral
			  Nutrition (TPN)
			  Administration

Psychomotor Energy
Definition:
Personal drive and energy to maintain activities of daily living, nutrition, and personal safety
	Energy Management
	Mood Management
		Exercise Promotion
		Grief Work Facilitation
		Guilt Work Facilitation
		Medication
		  Management
			Music Therapy
			Self-Awareness
			  Enhancement
			Sleep Enhancement

PART II - F

NURSING DIAGNOSIS: Fear

Definition: Response to a perceived threat that is consciously recognized as a danger

NICS ASSOCIATED WITH DIAGNOSIS RELATED FACTORS

Communication
  Enhancement:
  Hearing Deficit
Communication
  Enhancement:
  Speech Deficit
	Communication
	  Enhancement:
	  Visual Deficit
	Environmental
	  Management:
	  Comfort
		Environmental
		  Management:
		  Safety
		Environmental
		  Management:
		  Violence Prevention
			Support System
			  Enhancement

Continued

NOC-NIC LINKAGES FOR FEAR

Outcome	Major Interventions	Suggested Interventions	

Fear Level
 	
Definition:
Severity of manifested apprehension, tension, or uneasiness arising from an identifiable source
	Anxiety Reduction
	Calming Technique
	Presence
		Abuse Protection
		  Support: Domestic
		  Partner
		Abuse Protection
		  Support: Elder
		Active Listening
		Anticipatory Guidance
		Childbirth Preparation
		Coping Enhancement
		Crisis Intervention
		Decision-Making
		  Support
		Diarrhea Management
		Environmental
		  Management: Safety
			Nausea Management
			Preparatory Sensory
			  Information
			Relocation Stress
			  Reduction
			Security Enhancement
			Support Group
			Teaching: Disease
			  Process
			Teaching: Preoperative
			Teaching: Procedure/
			  Treatment
			Therapy Group
			Vital Signs Monitoring

Fear Level: Child
 	
Definition:
Severity of manifested apprehension, tension, or uneasiness arising from an identifiable source in a child from 1 year through 17 years of age
	Calming Technique
	Presence
	Security
	  Enhancement
		Abuse Protection
		  Support: Child
		Active Listening
		Animal-Assisted
		  Therapy
		Art Therapy
		Distraction
		Emotional Support
		Environmental
		  Management: Safety
		Family Presence
		  Facilitation
			Pain Management
			Preparatory Sensory
			  Information
			Substance Use
			  Prevention
			Teaching: Individual
			Therapeutic Play
			Truth Telling
			Vital Signs Monitoring

Fear Self-Control
 	
Definition:
Personal actions to eliminate or reduce disabling feelings of apprehension, tension, or uneasiness from an identifiable source
	Anxiety Reduction
	Coping
	  Enhancement
		Anticipatory Guidance
		Autogenic Training
		Biofeedback
		Childbirth Preparation
		Counseling
		Decision-Making
		  Support
		Dying Care
		Guided Imagery
		Meditation Facilitation
			Pain Management
			Progressive Muscle
			  Relaxation
			Rape-Trauma Treatment
			Relaxation Therapy
			Role Enhancement
			Self-Esteem
			  Enhancement
			Self-Hypnosis
			  Facilitation
			Support Group
			Support System
			  Enhancement

NURSING DIAGNOSIS: Fluid Balance, Readiness for Enhanced

Definition: A pattern of equilibrium between fluid volume and chemical composition of body fluids that is sufficient for meeting physical needs and can be strengthened

NOC-NIC LINKAGES FOR FLUID BALANCE, READINESS FOR ENHANCED

Outcome	Major Interventions	Suggested Interventions	
Fluid Balance Definition: Water balance in the intracellular and extracellular compartments of the body	Fluid Management	Fluid/Electrolyte Management Fluid Monitoring	Vital Signs Monitoring Weight Management
Hydration Definition: Adequate water in the intracellular and extracellular compartments of the body	Fluid Management Fluid Monitoring	Electrolyte Management Fluid/Electrolyte Management Medication Management	Nutritional Counseling Urinary Elimination Management Weight Management
Kidney Function Definition: Filtration of blood and elimination of metabolic waste products through the formation of urine	Fluid Management Fluid Monitoring	Fluid/Electrolyte Management Health Education	Teaching: Individual

NURSING DIAGNOSIS: Fluid Volume, Deficient

Definition: Decreased intravascular, interstitial, and/or intracellular fluid. This refers to dehydration, water loss alone without change in sodium

NICS ASSOCIATED WITH DIAGNOSIS RELATED FACTORS

Bleeding Reduction Bleeding Reduction: Antepartum Uterus Bleeding Reduction: Gastrointestinal	Bleeding Reduction: Postpartum Uterus Bleeding Reduction: Wound Diarrhea Management	Fever Treatment Fluid Management Hemorrhage Control	Hyperglycemia Management Urinary Elimination Management Vomiting Management

NOC-NIC LINKAGES FOR FLUID VOLUME, DEFICIENT

Outcome	Major Interventions	Suggested Interventions	
Fluid Balance Definition: Water balance in the intracellular and extracellular compartments of the body	Fluid Management Fluid Monitoring	Enteral Tube Feeding Fluid Resuscitation Hypovolemia Management Intravenous (IV) Insertion Intravenous (IV) Therapy Laboratory Data Interpretation Medication Administration Medication Management Medication Prescribing	Peripherally Inserted Central (PIC) Catheter Care Shock Prevention Total Parenteral Nutrition (TPN) Administration Venous Access Device (VAD) Maintenance Vital Signs Monitoring

PART II - F

Continued

NOC-NIC LINKAGES FOR FLUID VOLUME, DEFICIENT

Outcome	Major Interventions	Suggested Interventions	
Hydration Definition: Adequate water in the intracellular and extracellular compartments of the body	Fluid Monitoring Hypovolemia Management	Bottle Feeding Diarrhea Management Fluid Management Fluid Resuscitation Intravenous (IV) Insertion Intravenous (IV) Therapy Peripherally Inserted Central (PIC) Catheter Care	Temperature Regulation Urinary Elimination Management Venous Access Device (VAD) Maintenance Vital Signs Monitoring Vomiting Management
Nutritional Status: Food & Fluid Intake Definition: Amount of food and fluid taken into the body over a 24-hour period	Fluid Management Fluid Monitoring	Bottle Feeding Breastfeeding Assistance Enteral Tube Feeding Feeding	Intravenous (IV) Therapy Swallowing Therapy Total Parenteral Nutrition (TPN) Administration

Critical reasoning note: As well as fluid loss, a substantial decrease in fluid intake might lead to fluid deficiency; therefore we have included fluid intake as a possible outcome. Attention should also be paid to the potential for electrolyte imbalances if fluid loss results in dehydration.

NURSING DIAGNOSIS: Fluid Volume, Excess

Definition: Increased isotonic fluid retention

NICS ASSOCIATED WITH DIAGNOSIS RELATED FACTORS

Electrolyte Management: Hypernatremia	Fluid Management	Hemodialysis Therapy	Peritoneal Dialysis Therapy

NOC-NIC LINKAGES FOR FLUID VOLUME, EXCESS

Outcome	Major Interventions	Suggested Interventions	
Fluid Balance Definition: Water balance in the intracellular and extracellular compartments of the body	Fluid Management Fluid Monitoring	Hypervolemia Management Laboratory Data Interpretation Medication Administration	Medication Management Vital Signs Monitoring Weight Management
Fluid Overload Severity Definition: Severity of excess fluids in the intracellular and extracellular compartments of the body	Fluid/Electrolyte Management Hypervolemia Management	Anxiety Reduction Capillary Blood Sample Cerebral Edema Management Dialysis Access Maintenance Electrolyte Management Electrolyte Monitoring Fluid Management Fluid Monitoring Hemodialysis Therapy	Medication Administration Medication Management Neurological Monitoring Peritoneal Dialysis Therapy Respiratory Monitoring Skin Surveillance Temperature Regulation Urinary Elimination Management Vital Signs Monitoring

NOC-NIC LINKAGES FOR FLUID VOLUME, EXCESS		
Outcome	**Major Interventions**	**Suggested Interventions**
Kidney Function		
Definition: Filtration of blood and elimination of metabolic waste products through the formation of urine	Fluid/Electrolyte Management Fluid Management	Acid-Base Management Bedside Laboratory Testing Dialysis Access Maintenance Electrolyte Monitoring Fluid Monitoring Hemodialysis Therapy	Laboratory Data Interpretation Peritoneal Dialysis Therapy Self-Care Assistance: Toileting Specimen Management Urinary Elimination Management Weight Management

NURSING DIAGNOSIS: Gas Exchange, Impaired

Definition: Excess or deficit in oxygenation and/or carbon dioxide elimination at the alveolar-capillary membrane

NICS ASSOCIATED WITH DIAGNOSIS RELATED FACTORS		
Mechanical Ventilation Management: Noninvasive	Medication Management	Oxygen Therapy

NOC-NIC LINKAGES FOR GAS EXCHANGE, IMPAIRED		
Outcome	**Major Interventions**	**Suggested Interventions**
Mechanical Ventilation Response: Adult		
Definition: Alveolar exchange and tissue perfusion are supported by mechanical ventilation	Mechanical Ventilation Management: Invasive Respiratory Monitoring	Airway Management Airway Suctioning Anxiety Reduction Artificial Airway Management Aspiration Precautions Bedside Laboratory Testing Family Presence Facilitation Infection Control	Laboratory Data Interpretation Medication Management Oxygen Therapy Phlebotomy: Arterial Blood Sample Positioning Surveillance Vital Signs Monitoring
Respiratory Status: Gas Exchange		
Definition: Alveolar exchange of carbon dioxide and oxygen to maintain arterial blood gas concentrations	Oxygen Therapy Respiratory Monitoring	Airway Insertion and Stabilization Airway Management Anxiety Reduction Artificial Airway Management Bedside Laboratory Testing Chest Physiotherapy Cough Enhancement	Laboratory Data Interpretation Mechanical Ventilation Management: Noninvasive Neurological Monitoring Phlebotomy: Arterial Blood Sample Positioning Surveillance

Continued

NOC-NIC LINKAGES FOR GAS EXCHANGE, IMPAIRED

Outcome	Major Interventions	Suggested Interventions	
Tissue Perfusion: Pulmonary Definition: Adequacy of blood flow through pulmonary vasculature to perfuse alveoli/capillary unit	Phlebotomy: Arterial Blood Sample Respiratory Monitoring	Bedside Laboratory Testing Embolus Care: Pulmonary Laboratory Data Interpretation Mechanical Ventilation Management: Invasive Medication Administration	Medication Management Oxygen Therapy Pain Management Surveillance Ventilation Assistance Vital Signs Monitoring
Vital Signs Definition: Extent to which temperature, pulse, respiration, and blood pressure are within normal range	Respiratory Monitoring Vital Signs Monitoring	Airway Management Medication Administration Medication Management	Medication Prescribing Oxygen Therapy Ventilation Assistance

Critical reasoning note: Although the diagnosis is focused on gas exchange at the alveolar-capillary membrane, interventions aimed at facilitating ventilation are provided as appropriate. Patients with respiratory problems frequently experience anxiety and are helped by basic interventions such as positioning and pain management.

NURSING DIAGNOSIS: Gastrointestinal Motility, Dysfunctional

Definition: Increased, decreased, ineffective, or lack of peristaltic activity within the gastrointestinal system

NICS ASSOCIATED WITH DIAGNOSIS RELATED FACTORS

Allergy Management Anxiety Reduction Bed Rest Care	Communicable Disease Management Diet Staging Enteral Tube Feeding	Exercise Promotion Medication Management Newborn Monitoring	Teaching: Prescribed Diet Tube Care: Gastrointestinal

NOC-NIC LINKAGES FOR GASTROINTESTINAL MOTILITY, DYSFUNCTIONAL

Outcome	Major Interventions	Suggested Interventions	
Bowel Elimination Definition: Formation and evacuation of stool	Bowel Management	Diarrhea Management Flatulence Reduction Fluid Management	Medication Management Pain Management
Gastrointestinal Function Definition: Extent to which foods (ingested or tube-fed) are moved from ingestion to excretion	Bowel Management Gastrointestinal Intubation	Anxiety Reduction Constipation/Impaction Management Diarrhea Management Flatulence Reduction Medication Management Nausea Management	Nutrition Management Pain Management Teaching: Prescribed Diet Tube Care: Gastrointestinal Vomiting Management

NURSING DIAGNOSIS: Grieving

Definition: A normal complex process that includes emotional, physical, spiritual, social, and intellectual responses and behaviors by which individuals, families, and communities incorporate an actual, anticipated, or perceived loss into their daily lives

NICS ASSOCIATED WITH DIAGNOSIS RELATED FACTORS

The related factors are personal actual or anticipated losses, such as loss of significant object, significant other, or anticipatory loss of a significant other, that are not preventable by nursing interventions

NOC-NIC LINKAGES FOR GRIEVING

Outcome	Major Interventions	Suggested Interventions	
Adaptation to Physical Disability Definition: Adaptive response to a significant functional challenge due to a physical disability	Coping Enhancement	Active Listening Amputation Care Anticipatory Guidance Decision-Making Support Grief Work Facilitation Hope Inspiration Mood Management	Relocation Stress Reduction Role Enhancement Spiritual Support Support Group Support System Enhancement Truth Telling
Coping Definition: Personal actions to manage stressors that tax an individual's resources	Coping Enhancement Grief Work Facilitation Grief Work Facilitation: Perinatal Death	Animal-Assisted Therapy Anxiety Reduction Counseling Emotional Support Family Integrity Promotion Forgiveness Facilitation Hope Inspiration Mood Management Normalization Promotion	Presence Reminiscence Therapy Resiliency Promotion Sibling Support Spiritual Support Support Group Support System Enhancement Truth Telling
Family Coping Definition: Family actions to manage stressors that tax family resources	Grief Work Facilitation Grief Work Facilitation: Perinatal Death	Coping Enhancement Counseling Culture Brokerage Family Integrity Promotion Family Process Maintenance Normalization Promotion	Resiliency Promotion Sibling Support Spiritual Support Support Group Support System Enhancement
Grief Resolution Definition: Adjustment to actual or impending loss	Grief Work Facilitation Grief Work Facilitation: Perinatal Death	Active Listening Anger Control Assistance Anticipatory Guidance Bibliotherapy Coping Enhancement Dying Care Emotional Support Exercise Promotion Guilt Work Facilitation	Hope Inspiration Mood Management Pregnancy Termination Care Reminiscence Therapy Sibling Support Sleep Enhancement Spiritual Support Support Group Support System Enhancement

Continued

PART II - G

NOC-NIC LINKAGES FOR GRIEVING

Outcome	Major Interventions	Suggested Interventions	
Psychosocial Adjustment: Life Change Definition: Adaptive psychosocial response of an individual to a significant life change	Anticipatory Guidance Coping Enhancement	Active Listening Counseling Decision-Making Support Dying Care Emotional Support Grief Work Facilitation Hope Inspiration	Reminiscence Therapy Self-Esteem Enhancement Self-Modification Assistance Socialization Enhancement Spiritual Support Support Group Truth Telling

NURSING DIAGNOSIS: Grieving, Complicated

Definition: A disorder that occurs after the death of a significant other, in which the experience of distress accompanying bereavement fails to follow normative expectations and manifests in functional impairment

NICS ASSOCIATED WITH DIAGNOSIS RELATED FACTORS

Mood Management	Support Group	Support System Enhancement

NOC-NIC LINKAGES FOR GRIEVING, COMPLICATED

Outcome	Major Interventions	Suggested Interventions	
Coping Definition: Personal actions to manage stressors that tax an individual's resources	Coping Enhancement Grief Work Facilitation Grief Work Facilitation: Perinatal Death	Anxiety Reduction Art Therapy Counseling Crisis Intervention Emotional Support Forgiveness Facilitation Guilt Work Facilitation Hope Inspiration	Relaxation Therapy Spiritual Support Support Group Support System Enhancement Therapeutic Play Therapy Group Truth Telling Values Clarification
Grief Resolution Definition: Adjustment to actual or impending loss	Grief Work Facilitation Grief Work Facilitation: Perinatal Death	Active Listening Anger Control Assistance Anxiety Reduction Coping Enhancement Counseling Culture Brokerage Emotional Support Family Integrity Promotion	Guilt Work Facilitation Hope Inspiration Mood Management Role Enhancement Spiritual Support Support Group Support System Enhancement
Role Performance Definition: Congruence of an individual's role behavior with role expectations	Grief Work Facilitation Role Enhancement Self-Awareness Enhancement	Behavior Modification Counseling Emotional Support Family Integrity Promotion Parenting Promotion	Resiliency Promotion Self-Esteem Enhancement Sibling Support Support Group

NURSING DIAGNOSIS: Growth and Development, Delayed

Definition: Deviations from age-group norms

NICS ASSOCIATED WITH DIAGNOSIS RELATED FACTORS

Abuse Protection
  Support
Abuse Protection
  Support: Child
Abuse Protection Support:
  Domestic Partner

Abuse Protection
  Support: Elder
Anticipatory Guidance
Family Integrity
  Promotion:
  Childbearing Family

Family Process
  Maintenance
Parent Education:
  Infant
Parenting Promotion

NOC-NIC LINKAGES FOR GROWTH AND DEVELOPMENT, DELAYED

Outcome	Major Interventions	Suggested Interventions	
Child Development: 1 Month Definition: Milestones of physical, cognitive, and psychosocial progression by 1 month of age	Attachment Promotion Parent Education: Infant Teaching: Infant Stimulation 0-4 Months	Anticipatory Guidance Environmental Management: Attachment Process Family Integrity Promotion: Childbearing Family Family Process Maintenance	Infant Care Newborn Care Nonnutritive Sucking Parenting Promotion Teaching: Infant Safety 0-3 Months Touch
Child Development: 2 Months Definition: Milestones of physical, cognitive, and psychosocial progression by 2 months of age			
Child Development: 4 Months Definition: Milestones of physical, cognitive, and psychosocial progression by 4 months of age	Parent Education: Infant Teaching: Infant Stimulation 0-4 Months Teaching: Infant Stimulation 5-8 Months	Anticipatory Guidance Attachment Promotion Family Integrity Promotion: Childbearing Family Family Process Maintenance	Infant Care Nonnutritive Sucking Parenting Promotion Teaching: Infant Safety 4-6 Months Touch
Child Development: 6 Months Definition: Milestones of physical, cognitive, and psychosocial progression by 6 months of age			
Child Development: 12 Months Definition: Milestones of physical, cognitive, and psychosocial progression by 12 months of age	Parent Education: Childrearing Family Teaching: Infant Simulation: 9-12 Months	Anticipatory Guidance Family Integrity Promotion: Childbearing Family Family Process Maintenance	Parenting Promotion Security Enhancement Teaching: Infant Safety 10-12 Months Teaching: Toddler Safety 13-18 Months Therapeutic Play

Continued

PART II - G

NOC-NIC LINKAGES FOR GROWTH AND DEVELOPMENT, DELAYED		
Outcome	**Major Interventions**	**Suggested Interventions**
Child Development: 2 Years		
Definition: Milestones of physical, cognitive, and psychosocial progression by 2 years of age	Developmental Enhancement: Child Parent Education: Childrearing Family	Anticipatory Guidance Bowel Training Family Integrity Promotion Family Process Maintenance Parenting Promotion Security Enhancement Teaching: Toddler Safety 19-24 Months	Teaching: Toddler Safety 25-36 Months Teaching: Toilet Training Therapeutic Play Urinary Habit Training
Child Development: 3 Years		
Definition: Milestones of physical, cognitive, and psychosocial progression by 3 years of age	Developmental Enhancement: Child Parent Education: Childrearing Family	Anticipatory Guidance Bowel Training Family Integrity Promotion Family Process Maintenance Parenting Promotion Security Enhancement	Teaching: Toddler Safety 25-36 Months Teaching: Toilet Training Therapeutic Play Urinary Habit Training
Child Development: 4 Years		
Definition: Milestones of physical, cognitive, and psychosocial progression by 4 years of age	Developmental Enhancement: Child Parent Education: Childrearing Family	Anticipatory Guidance Bowel Incontinence Care: Encopresis Family Integrity Promotion Family Process Maintenance	Parenting Promotion Security Enhancement Therapeutic Play Urinary Habit Training
Child Development: 5 Years		
Definition: Milestones of physical, cognitive, and psychosocial progression by 5 years of age	Developmental Enhancement: Child	Anticipatory Guidance Bowel Incontinence Care: Encopresis Family Integrity Promotion Parent Education: Childrearing Family	Parenting Promotion Security Enhancement Therapeutic Play Urinary Incontinence Care: Enuresis

NOC-NIC LINKAGES FOR GROWTH AND DEVELOPMENT, DELAYED		
Outcome	**Major Interventions**	**Suggested Interventions**
Child Development: Middle Childhood Definition: Milestones of physical, cognitive, and psychosocial progression from 6 years through 11 years of age	Developmental Enhancement: Child	Anticipatory Guidance Behavior Management: Overactivity/Inattention Behavior Modification: Social Skills Parent Education: Childrearing Family Parenting Promotion	Security Enhancement Self-Awareness Enhancement Self-Esteem Enhancement Self-Responsibility Facilitation Sports-Injury Prevention: Youth Urinary Incontinence Care: Enuresis
Child Development: Adolescence Definition: Milestones of physical, cognitive, and psychosocial progression from 12 years through 17 years of age	Developmental Enhancement: Adolescent Parent Education: Adolescent	Anger Control Assistance Anticipatory Guidance Behavior Modification: Social Skills Coping Enhancement Family Integrity Promotion Impulse Control Training	Parenting Promotion Substance Use Prevention Teaching: Safe Sex Teaching: Sexuality Values Clarification
Development: Late Adulthood Definition: Cognitive, psychosocial, and moral progression from 65 years of age and older	Anticipatory Guidance Coping Enhancement	Active Listening Activity Therapy Anger Control Assistance Animal-Assisted Therapy Behavior Management Communication Enhancement: Hearing Deficit Conflict Mediation Decision-Making Support Emotional Support Energy Management Family Integrity Promotion Family Process Maintenance Family Support Grief Work Facilitation	Hope Inspiration Learning Facilitation Learning Readiness Enhancement Memory Training Mood Management Recreation Therapy Religious Ritual Enhancement Reminiscence Therapy Role Enhancement Self-Care Assistance Sexual Counseling Socialization Enhancement Spiritual Growth Facilitation Substance Use Prevention Values Clarification

Continued

PART II - G

NOC-NIC LINKAGES FOR GROWTH AND DEVELOPMENT, DELAYED		
Outcome	**Major Interventions**	**Suggested Interventions**
Development: Middle Adulthood Definition: Cognitive, psychosocial, and moral progression from 40 through 64 years of age	Resiliency Promotion Role Enhancement	Anger Control Assistance Coping Enhancement Decision-Making Support Family Integrity Promotion Family Support Hope Inspiration Humor Impulse Control Training Learning Facilitation Learning Readiness Enhancement Mood Management Self-Awareness Enhancement Self-Efficacy Enhancement Self-Modification Assistance Socialization Enhancement Teaching: Safe Sex Values Clarification
Development: Young Adulthood Definition: Cognitive, psychosocial, and moral progression from 18 through 39 years of age	Resiliency Promotion Self-Responsibility Facilitation	Anger Control Assistance Coping Enhancement Decision-Making Support Family Integrity Promotion Family Integrity Promotion: Childbearing Family Family Support Impulse Control Training Learning Facilitation Learning Readiness Enhancement Mood Management Parent Education: Childrearing Family Role Enhancement Self-Esteem Enhancement Socialization Enhancement Substance Use Prevention Teaching: Safe Sex Values Clarification
Growth Definition: Normal increase in bone size and body weight during growth years	Health Screening Nutrition Management	Bottle Feeding Breastfeeding Assistance Eating Disorders Management Lactation Counseling Newborn Monitoring Nutritional Monitoring Sustenance Support Teaching: Infant Nutrition 0-3 Months Teaching: Infant Nutrition 4-6 Months Teaching: Infant Nutrition 7-9 Months Teaching: Infant Nutrition 10-12 Months Teaching: Infant Safety 0-3 Months Teaching: Infant Safety 4-6 Months Teaching: Infant Safety 7-9 Months Teaching: Infant Safety 10-12 Months Teaching: Toddler Nutrition 13-18 Months Teaching: Toddler Nutrition 19-24 Months Teaching: Toddler Nutrition 25-36 Months Weight Gain Assistance Weight Management Weight Reduction Assistance

NOC-NIC LINKAGES FOR GROWTH AND DEVELOPMENT, DELAYED		
Outcome	**Major Interventions**	**Suggested Interventions**

Physical Aging
 	
Definition:
Normal physical
  changes that occur
  with the natural
  aging process
	Body Mechanics
	  Promotion
	Exercise Promotion
		Anticipatory Guidance
		Biofeedback
		Cardiac Precautions
		Cognitive Stimulation
		Exercise Promotion:
		  Strength Training
		Exercise Promotion:
		  Stretching
		Exercise Therapy:
		  Balance
		Exercise Therapy:
		  Joint Mobility
			Hormone Replacement
			  Therapy
			Infection Protection
			Laboratory Data
			  Interpretation
			Memory Training
			Oral Health Maintenance
			Sexual Counseling
			Vital Signs Monitoring
			Weight Management

Physical Maturation: Female
 	
Definition:
Normal physical
  changes in the female
  that occur with the
  transition from child-
  hood to adulthood
	Developmental
	  Enhancement:
	  Adolescent
		Anticipatory Guidance
		Body Image
		  Enhancement
		Health Screening
			Parent Education:
			  Adolescent
			Teaching: Sexuality

Physical Maturation: Male
 	
Definition:
Normal physical
  changes in the male
  that occur with the
  transition from child-
  hood to adulthood
	Developmental
	  Enhancement:
	  Adolescent
		Anticipatory Guidance
		Body Image
		  Enhancement
		Health Screening
			Parent Education:
			  Adolescent
			Teaching: Sexuality

Preterm Infant Organization
 	
Definition:
Extrauterine integration
  of physiological and
  behavioral function
  by the infant born
  24 to 37 (term) weeks
  gestation
	Developmental Care	Environmental
		  Management
		Environmental
		  Management:
		  Attachment Process
		Kangaroo Care
		Newborn Monitoring
			Nonnutritive Sucking
			Phototherapy: Neonate
			Touch
			Vital Signs Monitoring

Critical reasoning note: Child Development outcomes for 1 and 2 months and for 4 and 6 months were grouped together because many interventions are appropriate for these combined age-groups. The NANDA-I diagnosis includes both growth and development while the NOC outcomes focus on development and growth separately. During the early years of life, interventions focus on assisting the parents/ caregiver to meet the needs of the infant/child; thus the majority of the interventions are directed at the parents rather than the child. You will notice that with age, interventions begin to focus on the older child/adult.

NURSING DIAGNOSIS: Health Behavior, Risk-Prone

Definition: Impaired ability to modify lifestyle/behaviors in a manner that improves health status

NICS ASSOCIATED WITH DIAGNOSIS RELATED FACTORS

Anxiety Reduction
Learning Facilitation
	Self-Efficacy
	  Enhancement
	Smoking Cessation
	  Assistance
		Substance Use
		  Treatment
			Support System
			  Enhancement

NOC-NIC LINKAGES FOR HEALTH BEHAVIOR, RISK-PRONE

Outcome	Major Interventions	Suggested Interventions	

Acceptance: Health Status
Definition:
Reconciliation to
  significant
  change in health
  circumstances
	Anticipatory
	  Guidance
	Coping
	  Enhancement
		Anxiety Reduction
		Counseling
		Decision-Making
		  Support
		Emotional Support
		Grief Work Facilitation
		Hope Inspiration
		Resiliency Promotion
			Self-Esteem Enhancement
			Self-Modification
			  Assistance
			Spiritual Support
			Support Group
			Support System
			  Enhancement
			Truth Telling
			Values Clarification

Adaptation to Physical Disability
Definition:
Adaptive response to a
  significant functional
  challenge due to a
  physical disability
	Anticipatory
	  Guidance
	Coping
	  Enhancement
		Counseling
		Emotional Support
		Grief Work Facilitation
		Home Maintenance
		  Assistance
		Hope Inspiration
		Learning Facilitation
		Self-Care Assistance
			Self-Care Assistance: IADL
			Self-Esteem Enhancement
			Self-Modification
			  Assistance
			Self-Responsibility
			  Facilitation
			Support Group
			Support System
			  Enhancement
			Values Clarification

Compliance Behavior
Definition:
Personal actions to
  promote wellness,
  recovery, and
  rehabilitation
  recommended by a
  health professional
	Mutual Goal Setting
	Patient Contracting
		Behavior Modification
		Case Management
		Coping Enhancement
		Counseling
		Culture Brokerage
		Decision-Making
		  Support
		Health System
		  Guidance
		Learning Readiness
		  Enhancement
		Self-Modification
		  Assistance
		Self-Responsibility
		  Facilitation
			Support Group
			Teaching: Disease Process
			Teaching: Individual
			Teaching: Prescribed
			  Activity/Exercise
			Teaching: Prescribed Diet
			Teaching: Prescribed
			  Medication
			Teaching: Procedure/
			  Treatment
			Teaching: Psychomotor
			  Skill
			Values Clarification

PART II - H

NOC-NIC LINKAGES FOR HEALTH BEHAVIOR, RISK-PRONE

Outcome	Major Interventions	Suggested Interventions	
Coping			
Definition: Personal actions to manage stressors that tax an individual's resources	Coping Enhancement Counseling	Anticipatory Guidance Anxiety Reduction Behavior Modification Decision-Making Support Emotional Support Grief Work Facilitation Health System Guidance Hope Inspiration	Mood Management Mutual Goal Setting Relaxation Therapy Support Group Support System Enhancement Truth Telling Values Clarification
Health-Seeking Behavior			
Definition: Personal actions to promote optimal wellness, recovery, and rehabilitation	Health Education Values Clarification	Bibliotherapy Culture Brokerage Health System Guidance Learning Facilitation Learning Readiness Enhancement Mutual Goal Setting Patient Contracting Self-Efficacy Enhancement Self-Modification Assistance Self-Responsibility Facilitation	Smoking Cessation Assistance Substance Use Prevention Support Group Teaching: Disease Process Teaching: Prescribed Activity/Exercise Teaching: Prescribed Diet Teaching: Prescribed Medication Teaching: Procedure/ Treatment Teaching: Safe Sex Weight Management
Motivation			
Definition: Inner urge that moves or prompts an individual to positive action(s)	Self-Efficacy Enhancement Self-Responsibility Facilitation	Decision-Making Support Family Involvement Promotion Financial Resource Assistance Meditation Facilitation Mutual Goal Setting Resiliency Promotion Self-Awareness Enhancement	Self-Esteem Enhancement Self-Modification Assistance Spiritual Support Support Group Support System Enhancement Values Clarification
Psychosocial Adjustment: Life Change			
Definition: Adaptive psychosocial response of an individual to a significant life change	Anticipatory Guidance Coping Enhancement	Activity Therapy Decision-Making Support Emotional Support Hope Inspiration Humor Mutual Goal Setting Relocation Stress Reduction	Role Enhancement Self-Awareness Enhancement Self-Esteem Enhancement Socialization Enhancement Spiritual Support Support System Enhancement

PART II - H

Continued

NOC-NIC LINKAGES FOR HEALTH BEHAVIOR, RISK-PRONE

Outcome	Major Interventions	Suggested Interventions	

Risk Control
 	
Definition:
Personal actions to
  prevent, eliminate, or
  reduce modifiable
  health threats
	Risk Identification	Behavior Modification
		Breast Examination
		Environmental
		  Management: Safety
		Health Education
			Health Screening
			Immunization/Vaccination
			  Management
			Infection Control
			Self-Efficacy Enhancement

Clinical reasoning note: Any of the risk related outcomes would be appropriate if the goal is to control a specific risk and prevent the occurrence of a health problem. Risk outcomes that might be considered include Risk Control for the following conditions: Alcohol Use, Cancer, Cardiovascular Health, Drug Use, Hearing Impairment, Sexually Transmitted Diseases (STDs), and Visual Impairment.

NURSING DIAGNOSIS: Health Maintenance, Ineffective

Definition: Inability to identify, manage, and/or seek out help to maintain health

NICS ASSOCIATED WITH DIAGNOSIS RELATED FACTORS

Cognitive Stimulation
Communication
  Enhancement:
  Hearing Deficit
Communication
  Enhancement:
  Speech Deficit
	Communication
	  Enhancement:
	  Visual Deficit
	Coping Enhancement
	Decision-Making
	  Support
	Delusion Management
		Exercise Therapy:
		  Muscle Control
		Family Involvement
		  Promotion
		Financial Resource
		  Assistance
		Grief Work Facilitation
			Grief Work Facilitation:
			  Perinatal Death
			Reality Orientation
			Spiritual Support
			Sustenance Support

NOC-NIC LINKAGES FOR HEALTH MAINTENANCE, INEFFECTIVE

Outcome	Major Interventions	Suggested Interventions	

Client Satisfaction: Access to Care Resources
 	
Definition:
Extent of positive per-
  ception of access to
  nursing staff, supplies,
  and equipment
  needed for care
	Case Management	Cost Containment
		Financial Resource
		  Assistance
		Insurance Authorization
		Referral
			Self-Care Assistance
			Support Group
			Sustenance Support

Health Beliefs: Perceived Resources
 	
Definition:
Personal conviction that
  one has adequate
  means to carry out a
  health behavior
	Financial Resource
	  Assistance
	Support System
	  Enhancement
		Energy Management
		Environmental
		  Management: Home
		  Preparation
		Family Involvement
		  Promotion
		Family Mobilization
		Health System
		  Guidance
			Insurance Authorization
			  Referral
			Self-Care Assistance
			Self-Care Assistance:
			  IADL
			Self-Efficacy
			  Enhancement
			Sustenance Support

NOC-NIC LINKAGES FOR HEALTH MAINTENANCE, INEFFECTIVE			
Outcome	**Major Interventions**	**Suggested Interventions**	
Health-Promoting Behavior			
Definition: Personal actions to sustain or increase wellness	Health Education Health Screening Risk Identification	Breast Examination Culture Brokerage Environmental Management: Safety Exercise Promotion Immunization/ Vaccination Management Nutrition Management Oral Health Promotion Self-Modification Assistance Self-Responsibility Facilitation	Sleep Enhancement Smoking Cessation Assistance Socialization Enhancement Spiritual Growth Facilitation Sports-Injury Preven- tion: Youth Substance Use Prevention Teaching: Safe Sex Weight Management
Health-Seeking Behavior			
Definition: Personal actions to promote optimal wellness, recovery, and rehabilitation	Decision-Making Support Self-Efficacy Enhancement	Counseling Culture Brokerage Exercise Promotion Health Education Health Literacy Enhancement Health Screening Health System Guidance Learning Facilitation Mutual Goal Setting Nutrition Management Patient Contracting	Self-Modification Assistance Self-Responsibility Facilitation Sexual Counseling Sleep Enhancement Smoking Cessation Assistance Substance Use Treatment Support Group Support System Enhancement Values Clarification Weight Management
Knowledge: Health Behavior			
Definition: Extent of understanding conveyed about the promotion and protection of health	Health Education	Family Planning: Contraception Learning Facilitation Learning Readiness Enhancement Nutritional Counseling Parent Education: Adolescent Parent Education: Childrearing Family Parent Education: Infant Preconception Counseling Risk Identification Risk Identification: Childbearing Family	Smoking Cessation Assistance Substance Use Prevention Teaching: Foot Care Teaching: Group Teaching: Individual Teaching: Prescribed Activity/Exercise Teaching: Prescribed Diet Teaching: Prescribed Medication Teaching: Psychomotor Skill Teaching: Safe Sex

Continued

PART II - H

NOC-NIC LINKAGES FOR HEALTH MAINTENANCE, INEFFECTIVE			
Outcome	**Major Interventions**	**Suggested Interventions**	
Knowledge: Health Promotion Definition: Extent of understanding conveyed about information needed to obtain and maintain optimal health	Health Education Risk Identification	Breast Examination Childbirth Preparation Exercise Promotion Genetic Counseling Health Literacy Enhancement Health Screening Immunization/ Vaccination Management Nutritional Counseling	Oral Health Promotion Preconception Counseling Risk Identification: Genetic Teaching: Prescribed Medication Teaching: Safe Sex Vehicle Safety Promotion Weight Management
Knowledge: Health Resources Definition: Extent of understanding conveyed about relevant health care resources	Health Literacy Enhancement Health System Guidance	Discharge Planning First Aid Teaching: Group	Teaching: Individual Telephone Consultation
Participation in Health Care Decisions Definition: Personal involvement in selecting and evaluating health care options to achieve desired outcome	Decision-Making Support Mutual Goal Setting	Anticipatory Guidance Assertiveness Training Culture Brokerage Discharge Planning Fiscal Resource Management Health System Guidance	Patient Rights Protection Referral Self-Responsibility Facilitation Telephone Consultation Values Clarification
Risk Detection Definition: Personal actions to identify personal health threats	Health Screening Risk Identification Risk Identification: Childbearing Family	Abuse Protection Support Abuse Protection Support: Child Abuse Protection Support: Domestic Partner Abuse Protection Support: Elder Breast Examination	Environmental Management: Safety Environmental Management: Violence Prevention Immunization/ Vaccination Management Smoking Cessation Assistance Substance Use Prevention
Social Support Definition: Reliable assistance from others	Family Involvement Promotion Support Group Support System Enhancement	Caregiver Support Emotional Support Family Support Financial Resource Assistance Insurance Authorization	Socialization Enhancement Spiritual Support Sustenance Support Telephone Consultation

Critical reasoning note: A number of outcomes are provided to enable selection of the one(s) that best addresses the defining characteristics and/or related factors of the diagnosis for a particular client. Learning Facilitation and Learning Readiness Facilitation are interventions that can be appropriate with any knowledge outcome and teaching intervention; therefore they are not repeated with each outcome.

NURSING DIAGNOSIS: Home Maintenance, Impaired

Definition: Inability to independently maintain a safe growth-promoting immediate environment

NICS ASSOCIATED WITH DIAGNOSIS RELATED FACTORS

Family Process Maintenance	Self-Care Assistance: IADL	Teaching: Infant Safety 7-9 Months	Teaching: Toddler Safety 19-24 Months
Family Therapy	Support System Enhancement	Teaching: Infant Safety 10-12 Months	Teaching: Toddler Safety 25-36 Months
Financial Resource Assistance	Teaching: Infant Safety 0-3 Months	Teaching: Toddler Safety 13-18 Months	
Health Education	Teaching: Infant Safety 4-6 Months		
Role Enhancement			

NOC-NIC LINKAGES FOR HOME MAINTENANCE, IMPAIRED

Outcome	Major Interventions	Suggested Interventions	
Safe Home Environment			
Definition: Physical arrangements to minimize environmental factors that might cause physical harm or injury in the home	Environmental Management Home Maintenance Assistance	Environmental Management: Home Preparation Environmental Management: Safety Environmental Management: Violence Prevention	Fall Prevention Risk Identification Surveillance: Safety
Self-Care: Instrumental Activities of Daily Living (IADL)			
Definition: Ability to perform activities needed to function in the home or community independently with or without assistive device	Self-Care Assistance: IADL	Environmental Management: Safety Health Education Health System Guidance	Home Maintenance Assistance Teaching: Prescribed Medication

NURSING DIAGNOSIS: Hope, Readiness for Enhanced

Definition: A pattern of expectations and desires that is sufficient for mobilizing energy on one's own behalf and can be strengthened

NOC-NIC LINKAGES FOR HOPE, READINESS FOR ENHANCED

Outcome	Major Interventions	Suggested Interventions	
Decision-Making			
Definition: Ability to make judgments and choose between two or more alternatives	Decision-Making Support	Hope Inspiration Mutual Goal Setting Self-Awareness Enhancement	Self-Efficacy Enhancement Self-Modification Assistance Self-Responsibility Facilitation

Continued

NOC-NIC LINKAGES FOR HOPE, READINESS FOR ENHANCED

Outcome	Major Interventions	Suggested Interventions	
Health Beliefs: Perceived Ability to Perform Definition: Personal conviction that one can carry out a given health behavior	Self-Modification Assistance	Health Education Hope Inspiration Learning Facilitation Mutual Goal Setting	Self-Efficacy Enhancement Self-Responsibility Facilitation Teaching: Individual
Hope Definition: Optimism that is personally satisfying and life-supporting	Hope Inspiration	Humor Mutual Goal Setting Self-Awareness Enhancement Self-Efficacy Enhancement	Socialization Enhancement Spiritual Growth Facilitation Values Clarification
Spiritual Health Definition: Connectedness with self, others, higher power, all life, nature, and the universe that transcends and empowers the self	Hope Inspiration Spiritual Growth Facilitation	Behavior Modification: Social Skills Forgiveness Facilitation Meditation Facilitation Religious Ritual Enhancement	Self-Awareness Enhancement Socialization Enhancement Spiritual Support Values Clarification

NURSING DIAGNOSIS: Hopelessness

Definition: Subjective state in which an individual sees limited or no alternatives or personal choices available and is unable to mobilize energy on own behalf

NICS ASSOCIATED WITH DIAGNOSIS RELATED FACTORS

Abuse Protection Support	Anxiety Reduction	Support System Enhancement
Activity Therapy	Spiritual Support	Values Clarification

NOC-NIC LINKAGES FOR HOPELESSNESS

Outcome	Major Interventions	Suggested Interventions	
Depression Level Definition: Severity of melancholic mood and loss of interest in life events	Hope Inspiration Mood Management	Activity Therapy Behavior Management: Self-Harm Cognitive Restructuring Coping Enhancement Counseling Crisis Intervention Electroconvulsive Therapy (ECT) Management Emotional Support	Grief Work Facilitation Grief Work Facilitation: Perinatal Death Phototherapy: Mood/ Sleep Regulation Self-Esteem Enhancement Spiritual Support Suicide Prevention Support Group Therapy Group

PART II - H

NOC-NIC LINKAGES FOR HOPELESSNESS		
Outcome	**Major Interventions**	**Suggested Interventions**
Depression Self-Control		

Definition:
Personal actions to
  minimize melancholy
  and maintain interest
  in life events
	Mood Management
	Resiliency Promo-
	  tion
	Self-Modification
	  Assistance
		Animal-Assisted Therapy
		Art Therapy
		Behavior Modification
		Coping Enhancement
		Emotional Support
		Energy Management
		Exercise Promotion
		Grief Work Facilitation
		Grief Work Facilitation:
		  Perinatal Death
		Guilt Work Facilitation
			Hope Inspiration
			Music Therapy
			Mutual Goal Setting
			Patient Contracting
			Presence
			Recreation Therapy
			Self-Awareness
			  Enhancement
			Socialization
			  Enhancement
			Therapeutic Play
			Therapy Group

Hope		

Definition:
Optimism that is
  personally satisfying
  and life-supporting
	Hope Inspiration	Active Listening
		Complex Relationship
		  Building
		Coping Enhancement
		Counseling
		Emotional Support
		Grief Work Facilitation
		Nutritional Monitoring
		Presence
			Reminiscence Therapy
			Resiliency Promotion
			Socialization
			  Enhancement
			Spiritual Support
			Support Group
			Support System
			  Enhancement
			Values Clarification

Mood Equilibrium		

Definition:
Appropriate adjustment
  of prevailing
  emotional tone in
  response to
  circumstances
	Hope Inspiration
	Mood Management
		Animal-Assisted Therapy
		Anxiety Reduction
		Counseling
		Emotional Support
		Energy Management
		Presence
			Sleep Enhancement
			Spiritual Support
			Suicide Prevention
			Therapeutic Play
			Therapy Group

Psychomotor Energy		

Definition:
Personal drive and
  energy to maintain
  activities of daily
  living, nutrition, and
  personal safety
	Mood Management	Activity Therapy
		Cognitive Restructuring
		Coping Enhancement
		Counseling
		Decision-Making Support
		Emotional Support
		Hope Inspiration
			Nutritional Monitoring
			Self-Awareness
			  Enhancement
			Self-Esteem
			  Enhancement
			Socialization
			  Enhancement
			Support Group
			Therapy Group

Quality of Life		

Definition:
Extent of positive
  perception of current
  life circumstances
	Hope Inspiration
	Values Clarification
		Coping Enhancement
		Emotional Support
		Family Support
		Mood Management
		Reminiscence Therapy
		Resiliency Promotion
		Role Enhancement
			Self-Awareness
			  Enhancement
			Socialization
			  Enhancement
			Spiritual Support
			Support Group
			Support System
			  Enhancement
			Sustenance Support

Continued

NOC-NIC LINKAGES FOR HOPELESSNESS

Outcome	Major Interventions	Suggested Interventions	
Will to Live Definition: Desire, determination, and effort to survive	Coping Enhancement Hope Inspiration	Active Listening Bibliotherapy Cognitive Restructuring Counseling Emotional Support Journaling Self-Awareness Enhancement	Self-Esteem Enhancement Self-Modification Assistance Socialization Enhancement Spiritual Support Suicide Prevention Support Group Values Clarification

NURSING DIAGNOSIS: Hyperthermia

Definition: Body temperature elevated above normal range

NICS ASSOCIATED WITH DIAGNOSIS RELATED FACTORS

Environmental Management Fluid Management Malignant Hyperthermia Precautions	Medication Management Postanesthesia Care	Risk Identification Teaching: Disease Process	Teaching: Prescribed Activity/Exercise Teaching: Procedure/ Treatment

NOC-NIC LINKAGES FOR HYPERTHERMIA

Outcome	Major Interventions	Suggested Interventions	
Thermoregulation Definition: Balance among heat production, heat gain, and heat loss	Fever Treatment Temperature Regulation	Environmental Management Fluid Management Heat/Cold Application Heat Exposure Treatment Hypothermia Induction Therapy Infection Control Malignant Hyperthermia Precautions Medication Administration Medication Management	Medication Prescribing Pain Management Seizure Management Seizure Precautions Shock Prevention Skin Surveillance Temperature Regulation: Intraoperative Vital Signs Monitoring
Thermoregulation: Newborn Definition: Balance among heat production, heat gain, and heat loss during the first 28 days of life	Newborn Monitoring Temperature Regulation	Environmental Management Fever Treatment Fluid Management Heat Exposure Treatment Infection Control Medication Administration	Newborn Care Parent Education: Infant Seizure Management Seizure Precautions Skin Surveillance Vital Signs Monitoring
Vital Signs Definition: Extent to which temperature, pulse, respiration, and blood pressure are within normal range	Temperature Regulation Vital Signs Monitoring	Fever Treatment Heat Exposure Treatment Heat/Cold Application Hemodynamic Regulation Medication Administration	Medication Management Shock Management Shock Prevention Temperature Regulation: Intraoperative

NURSING DIAGNOSIS: Hypothermia

Definition: Body temperature below normal range

NICS ASSOCIATED WITH DIAGNOSIS RELATED FACTORS		
Environmental Management	Medication Management	Teaching: Disease Process
Exercise Promotion	Nutrition Therapy	Teaching: Procedure/ Treatment

NOC-NIC LINKAGES FOR HYPOTHERMIA			
Outcome	**Major Interventions**	**Suggested Interventions**	
Thermoregulation Definition: Balance among heat production, heat gain, and heat loss	Hypothermia Treatment Temperature Regulation	Circulatory Care: Arterial Insufficiency Circulatory Care: Venous Insufficiency Circulatory Precautions Environmental Management Heat/Cold Application	Hemodynamic Regulation Shock Prevention Temperature Regulation: Intraoperative Vital Signs Monitoring
Thermoregulation: Newborn Definition: Balance among heat production, heat gain, and heat loss during the first 28 days of life	Hypothermia Treatment Newborn Monitoring	Acid-Base Management Circulatory Precautions Environmental Management Heat/Cold Application Newborn Care Parent Education: Infant	Respiratory Monitoring Shock Prevention Technology Management Temperature Regulation Vital Signs Monitoring
Vital Signs Definition: Extent to which temperature, pulse, respiration, and blood pressure are within normal range	Hypothermia Treatment Vital Signs Monitoring	Circulatory Precautions Environmental Management Heat/Cold Application Hemodynamic Regulation Newborn Monitoring	Respiratory Monitoring Shock Prevention Skin Surveillance Temperature Regulation

PART II - I

NURSING DIAGNOSIS: Immunization Status, Readiness for Enhanced

Definition: A pattern of conforming to local, national, and/or international standards of immunization to pre-vent infectious disease(s) that is sufficient to protect a person, family, or community and can be strengthened

NOC-NIC LINKAGES FOR IMMUNIZATION STATUS, READINESS FOR ENHANCED			
Outcome	**Major Interventions**	**Suggested Interventions**	
Immunization Behavior Definition: Personal actions to obtain immunization to prevent a communicable disease	Immunization/ Vaccination Management	Health Education	Teaching: Individual
Risk Control Definition: Personal actions to prevent, eliminate, or reduce modifiable health threats	Immunization/ Vaccination Management	Health Education Risk Identification	Teaching: Individual

NURSING DIAGNOSIS: Infant Behavior, Disorganized

Definition: Disintegrated physiological and neurobehavioral responses of infant to the environment

NICS ASSOCIATED WITH DIAGNOSIS RELATED FACTORS

Environmental Management	Pain Management	Prenatal Care	Teaching: Infant Stimulation 0-4 Months
Genetic Counseling	Parent Education: Infant	Teaching: Infant Nutrition 0-3 Months	

NOC-NIC LINKAGES FOR INFANT BEHAVIOR, DISORGANIZED

Outcome	Major Interventions	Suggested Interventions	
Child Development: 1 Month Definition: Milestones of physical, cognitive, and psychosocial progression by 1 month of age **Child Development: 2 Months** Definition: Milestones of physical, cognitive, and psychosocial progression by 2 months of age	Infant Care Neurological Monitoring	Attachment Promotion Bottle Feeding Breastfeeding Assistance Calming Technique Environmental Management: Attachment Process Environmental Management: Comfort Kangaroo Care Newborn Care Nonnutritive Sucking	Nutritional Monitoring Parent Education: Infant Parenting Promotion Respiratory Monitoring Sleep Enhancement Teaching: Infant Safety 0-3 Months Teaching: Infant Stimulation 0-4 Months Touch Vital Signs Monitoring
Neurological Status Definition: Ability of the peripheral and central nervous systems to receive, process, and respond to internal and external stimuli	Developmental Care Neurological Monitoring	Laboratory Data Interpretation Newborn Monitoring Positioning Respiratory Monitoring	Sleep Enhancement Surveillance Temperature Regulation Vital Signs Monitoring
Preterm Infant Organization Definition: Extrauterine integration of physiological and behavioral function by the infant born 24 to 37 (term) weeks gestation	Developmental Care Newborn Monitoring	Attachment Promotion Bottle Feeding Breastfeeding Assistance Cutaneous Stimulation Environmental Management Environmental Management: Attachment Process Kangaroo Care Lactation Counseling Newborn Care	Nonnutritive Sucking Pain Management Parent Education: Infant Positioning Respiratory Monitoring Surveillance Teaching: Infant Stimulation 0-4 Months Temperature Regulation Tube Care: Umbilical Line Vital Signs Monitoring
Sleep Definition: Natural periodic suspension of consciousness during which the body is restored	Developmental Care	Calming Technique Environmental Management Environmental Management: Comfort	Nonnutritive Sucking Pain Management Touch

NOC-NIC LINKAGES FOR INFANT BEHAVIOR, DISORGANIZED		
Outcome	**Major Interventions**	**Suggested Interventions**
Thermoregulation: Newborn Definition: Balance among heat production, heat gain, and heat loss during the first 28 days of life	Newborn Care Temperature Regulation	Developmental Care Environmental Management Newborn Monitoring	Parent Education: Infant Vital Signs Monitoring

Critical reasoning note: Although disorganization of infant behavior is commonly associated with a preterm infant, the diagnosis is not limited to preterm infants; therefore child development outcomes for the first 2 months have been included.

NURSING DIAGNOSIS: Infant Behavior: Organized, Readiness for Enhanced

Definition: A pattern of modulation of the physiological and behavioral systems of functioning (i.e., autonomic, motor, state-organization, self-regulatory, and attentional-interactional systems) in an infant who is satisfactory but can be improved

NOC-NIC LINKAGES FOR INFANT BEHAVIOR, ORGANIZED, READINESS FOR ENHANCED		
Outcome	**Major Interventions**	**Suggested Interventions**
Child Development: 1 Month Definition: Milestones of physical, cognitive, and psychosocial progression by 1 month of age **Child Development: 2 Months** Definition: Milestones of physical, cognitive, and psycho-social progression by 2 months of age	Newborn Care Infant Care	Attachment Promotion Bottle Feeding Breastfeeding Assistance Circumcision Care Environmental Management Environmental Management: Attachment Process Kangaroo Care	Nonnutritive Sucking Parent Education: Infant Surveillance Teaching: Infant Safety 0-3 Months Teaching: Infant Stimulation 0-4 Months Touch
Child Development: 4 Months Definition: Milestones of physical, cognitive, and psychosocial progression by 4 months of age **Child Development: 6 Months** Definition: Milestones of physical, cognitive, and psychosocial progression by 6 months of age	Infant Care Parent Education: Infant	Anticipatory Guidance Bottle Feeding Environmental Management Environmental Management: Safety Health Screening Nonnutritive Sucking	Parenting Promotion Sleep Enhancement Surveillance Teaching: Infant Nutrition 4-6 Months Teaching: Infant Safety 4-6 Months Teaching: Infant Stimulation 0-4 Months Teaching: Infant Stimulation 5-8 Months

Continued

PART II - I

NOC-NIC LINKAGES FOR INFANT BEHAVIOR, ORGANIZED, READINESS FOR ENHANCED

Outcome	Major Interventions	Suggested Interventions	
Child Development: 12 Months Definition: Milestones of physical, cognitive, and psychosocial progression by 12 months of age	Infant Care Parent Education: Infant	Anticipatory Guidance Bottle Feeding Environmental Management Environmental Management: Safety Health Screening Nutrition Management Parenting Promotion Security Enhancement	Sleep Enhancement Surveillance Teaching: Infant Nutrition 10-12 Months Teaching: Infant Safety 10-12 Months Teaching: Infant Stimulation 9-12 Months
Newborn Adaptation Definition: Adaptive response to the extrauterine environment by a physiologically mature newborn during the first 28 days	Newborn Care Newborn Monitoring	Attachment Promotion Bottle Feeding Breastfeeding Assistance Environmental Management: Attachment Process Infant Care Kangaroo Care Laboratory Data Interpretation Lactation Counseling Nonnutritive Sucking	Parent Education: Infant Parenting Promotion Phototherapy: Neonate Respiratory Monitoring Sleep Enhancement Teaching: Infant Stimulation 0-4 Months Touch Vital Signs Monitoring
Sleep Definition: Natural periodic suspension of consciousness during which the body is restored	Sleep Enhancement	Calming Technique Environmental Management Environmental Management: Comfort	Infant Care Parent Education: Infant Touch

NURSING DIAGNOSIS: Infant Feeding Pattern, Ineffective

Definition: Impaired ability of an infant to suck or coordinate the suck/swallow response, resulting in inadequate oral nutrition for metabolic needs

NICS ASSOCIATED WITH DIAGNOSIS RELATED FACTORS

Developmental Care	Nonnutritive Sucking	Swallowing Therapy

NOC-NIC LINKAGES FOR INFANT FEEDING PATTERN, INEFFECTIVE

Outcome	Major Interventions	Suggested Interventions	
Breastfeeding Establishment: Infant Definition: Infant attachment to and sucking from the mother's breast for nourishment during the first 3 weeks of breastfeeding	Breastfeeding Assistance	Nonnutritive Sucking Nutritional Monitoring	Parent Education: Infant

NOC-NIC LINKAGES FOR INFANT FEEDING PATTERN, INEFFECTIVE

Outcome	Major Interventions	Suggested Interventions	
Breastfeeding Maintenance Definition: Continuation of breastfeeding from establishment to weaning for nourishment of an infant/toddler	Breastfeeding Assistance Lactation Counseling	Bottle Feeding Nonnutritive Sucking Nutrition Management	Nutritional Monitoring Parent Education: Infant Weight Management
Swallowing Status: Oral Phase Definition: Preparation, containment, and posterior movement of fluids and/or solids in the mouth	Nonnutritive Sucking	Aspiration Precautions Bottle Feeding	Breastfeeding Assistance Calming Technique

NURSING DIAGNOSIS: Insomnia

Definition: A disruption in amount and quality of sleep that impairs functioning

NICS ASSOCIATED WITH DIAGNOSIS RELATED FACTORS

Anxiety Reduction Environmental Management Grief Work Facilitation	Medication Management Mood Management Nausea Management	Pain Management Premenstrual Syndrome (PMS) Management	Urinary Elimination Management Urinary Incontinence Care

NOC-NIC LINKAGES FOR INSOMNIA

Outcome	Major Interventions	Suggested Interventions	
Fatigue Level Definition: Severity of observed or reported prolonged generalized fatigue	Mood Management Sleep Enhancement	Energy Management Massage	Medication Management Pain Management
Personal Well-Being Definition: Extent of positive perception of one's health status	Energy Management Sleep Enhancement	Coping Enhancement Medication Management Mood Management	Phototherapy: Mood/Sleep Regulation Relaxation Therapy Socialization Enhancement
Sleep Definition: Natural periodic suspension of consciousness during which the body is restored	Sleep Enhancement	Environmental Management Medication Management	Phototherapy: Mood/Sleep Regulation

PART II - I

NURSING DIAGNOSIS: Intracranial Adaptive Capacity, Decreased

Definition: Intracranial fluid dynamic mechanisms that normally compensate for increases in intracranial volumes are compromised, resulting in repeated disproportionate increases in intracranial pressure (ICP) in response to a variety of noxious and non-noxious stimuli

NICS ASSOCIATED WITH DIAGNOSIS RELATED FACTORS

Bleeding Precautions	Cerebral Perfusion Promotion	Subarachnoid Hemorrhage Precautions
Cerebral Edema Management	Intracranial Pressure (ICP) Monitoring	Vital Signs Monitoring

NOC-NIC LINKAGES FOR INTRACRANIAL ADAPTIVE CAPACITY, DECREASED

Outcome	Major Interventions	Suggested Interventions	
Neurological Status Definition: Ability of the peripheral and central nervous systems to receive, process, and respond to internal and external stimuli	Cerebral Edema Management Intracranial Pressure (ICP) Monitoring Neurological Monitoring	Cerebral Perfusion Promotion Code Management Fluid Management Fluid Monitoring Intravenous (IV) Insertion Intravenous (IV) Therapy Laboratory Data Interpretation Medication Administration	Medication Management Positioning: Neurological Respiratory Monitoring Seizure Management Seizure Precautions Surveillance: Safety Vital Signs Monitoring
Neurological Status: Consciousness Definition: Arousal, orientation, and attention to the environment	Cerebral Edema Management Intracranial Pressure (ICP) Monitoring Neurological Monitoring	Airway Management Aspiration Precautions Cerebral Perfusion Promotion Environmental Management: Safety Intravenous (IV) Insertion Intravenous (IV) Therapy Laboratory Data Interpretation Medication Administration	Medication Management Patient Rights Protection Reality Orientation Respiratory Monitoring Seizure Management Seizure Precautions Vital Signs Monitoring
Seizure Control Definition: Personal actions to reduce or minimize the occurrence of seizure episodes	Seizure Management Seizure Precautions	Airway Management Aspiration Precautions Counseling Environmental Management: Safety Health Education	Teaching: Disease Process Teaching: Individual Teaching: Prescribed Medication Teaching: Procedure/Treatment
Tissue Perfusion: Cerebral Definition: Adequacy of blood flow through the cerebral vasculature to maintain brain function	Cerebral Edema Management Cerebral Perfusion Promotion	Anxiety Reduction Intracranial Pressure (ICP) Monitoring Neurological Monitoring Pain Management Positioning: Neurological	Reality Orientation Respiratory Monitoring Thrombolytic Therapy Management Vital Signs Monitoring Vomiting Management

NURSING DIAGNOSIS: Knowledge, Deficient

Definition: Absence or deficiency of cognitive information related to a specific topic

NICS ASSOCIATED WITH DIAGNOSIS RELATED FACTORS			
Cognitive Stimulation Dementia Management	Health Literacy Enhancement Learning Facilitation	Learning Readiness Enhancement Memory Training	Teaching: Individual Teaching: Group

NOC-NIC LINKAGES FOR KNOWLEDGE, DEFICIENT		
Outcome	**Major Interventions**	**Suggested Interventions**
Client Satisfaction: Teaching Definition: Extent of positive perception of instruction provided by nursing staff to improve knowledge, understanding, and participation in care	Teaching: Disease Process Teaching: Prescribed Medication Teaching: Procedure/ Treatment	Health Education Learning Readiness Enhancement Preparatory Sensory Information Teaching: Foot Care Teaching: Individual Teaching: Prescribed Activity/Exercise Teaching: Prescribed Diet Teaching: Psychomotor Skill
Knowledge: Arthritis Management Definition: Extent of understanding conveyed about arthritis, its treatment, and the prevention of complications	Teaching: Disease Process Teaching: Prescribed Activity/Exercise	Energy Management Environmental Management: Safety Exercise Promotion Exercise Therapy: Joint Mobility Health System Guidance Pain Management Support Group Teaching: Individual Teaching: Prescribed Diet Teaching: Prescribed Medication Weight Management Weight Reduction Assistance
Knowledge: Asthma Management Definition: Extent of understanding conveyed about asthma, its treatment, and the prevention of complications	Asthma Management Teaching: Disease Process Teaching: Prescribed Medication	Anticipatory Guidance Energy Management Environmental Management: Safety Health System Guidance Immunization/ Vaccination Management Medication Administration: Inhalation Risk Identification Support Group Teaching: Individual Teaching: Prescribed Activity/Exercise Teaching: Procedure/ Treatment
Knowledge: Body Mechanics Definition: Extent of understanding conveyed about proper body alignment, balance, and coordinated movement	Body Mechanics Promotion	Exercise Promotion: Strength Training Exercise Promotion: Stretching Exercise Therapy: Ambulation Exercise Therapy: Balance Exercise Therapy: Joint Mobility Exercise Therapy: Muscle Control Risk Identification Teaching: Prescribed Activity/Exercise

Continued

PART II - K

NOC-NIC LINKAGES FOR KNOWLEDGE, DEFICIENT		
Outcome	**Major Interventions**	**Suggested Interventions**
Knowledge: Breastfeeding Definition: Extent of understanding conveyed about lactation and nourishment of an infant through breastfeeding	Breastfeeding Assistance Lactation Counseling	Health System Guidance Nonnutritive Sucking	Skin Surveillance Support Group
Knowledge: Cancer Management Definition: Extent of understanding conveyed about cause, type, progress, symptoms, and treatment of cancer	Teaching: Disease Process Teaching: Procedure/ Treatment	Anticipatory Guidance Chemotherapy Management Coping Enhancement Energy Management Financial Resource Assistance Health System Guidance Medication Management	Nausea Management Pain Management Radiation Therapy Management Risk Identification Support Group Teaching: Individual Vomiting Management
Knowledge: Cancer Threat Reduction Definition: Extent of understanding conveyed about causes, prevention, and early detection of cancer	Health Screening Risk Identification	Breast Examination Genetic Counseling Nutritional Counseling Oral Health Maintenance	Skin Surveillance Smoking Cessation Assistance Teaching: Disease Process Teaching: Safe Sex
Knowledge: Cardiac Disease Management Definition: Extent of understanding conveyed about heart disease, its treatment, and the prevention of complications	Cardiac Precautions Teaching: Disease Process	Anxiety Reduction Energy Management Cardiac Care: Rehabilitative Culture Brokerage Family Involvement Promotion Health System Guidance Nutritional Counseling Relaxation Therapy Resiliency Promotion Risk Identification	Sexual Counseling Smoking Cessation Assistance Support Group Teaching: Prescribed Activity/Exercise Teaching: Prescribed Diet Teaching: Prescribed Medication Teaching: Procedure/ Treatment Weight Management Weight Reduction Assistance

NOC-NIC LINKAGES FOR KNOWLEDGE, DEFICIENT

Outcome	Major Interventions	Suggested Interventions	
Knowledge: Child Physical Safety Definition: Extent of understanding conveyed about safely caring for a child from 1 year through 17 years of age	Teaching: Toddler Safety 13-18 Months Teaching: Toddler Safety 19-24 Months Teaching: Toddler Safety 25-36 Months	Abuse Protection Support: Child Parent Education: Adolescent Parent Education: Childrearing Family Risk Identification Risk Identification: Childbearing Family	Substance Use Prevention Surveillance: Safety Teaching: Group Vehicle Safety Promotion
Knowledge: Conception Prevention Definition: Extent of understanding conveyed about prevention of unintended pregnancy	Family Planning: Contraception	Parent Education: Adolescent	Teaching: Safe Sex
Knowledge: Congestive Heart Failure Management Definition: Extent of understanding conveyed about heart failure, its treatment, and the prevention of exacerbations	Circulatory Care: Venous Insufficiency Hypervolemia Management Teaching: Disease Process	Circulatory Care: Arterial Insufficiency Energy Management Fluid Management Fluid Monitoring Health System Guidance Medication Management Respiratory Monitoring	Support Group Teaching: Prescribed Activity/Exercise Teaching: Prescribed Diet Teaching: Prescribed Medication Teaching: Procedure/ Treatment Weight Management
Knowledge: Depression Management Definition: Extent of understanding conveyed about depression and interrelationships among causes, effects, and treatments	Teaching: Prescribed Medication Teaching: Procedure/ Treatment	Health System Guidance Journaling Medication Management Medication Reconciliation Mood Management	Self-Awareness Enhancement Self-Esteem Enhancement Substance Use Prevention Support Group Teaching: Disease Process
Knowledge: Diabetes Management Definition: Extent of understanding conveyed about diabetes mellitus, its treatment, and the prevention of complications	Teaching: Disease Process Teaching: Prescribed Diet Teaching: Prescribed Medication	Hyperglycemia Management Hypoglycemia Management Medication Administration: Subcutaneous Medication Management	Nutrition Management Teaching: Foot Care Teaching: Prescribed Activity/Exercise Teaching: Psychomotor Skill

Continued

NOC-NIC LINKAGES FOR KNOWLEDGE, DEFICIENT

Outcome	Major Interventions	Suggested Interventions	
Knowledge: Diet Definition: Extent of understanding conveyed about recommended diet	Nutritional Counseling Teaching: Prescribed Diet	Chemotherapy Management Eating Disorders Management Self-Modification Assistance	Teaching: Group Weight Management
Knowledge: Disease Process Definition: Extent of understanding conveyed about a specific disease process and prevention of complications	Teaching: Disease Process	Allergy Management Asthma Management Chemotherapy Management Discharge Planning Health System Guidance	Risk Identification Teaching: Group Teaching: Individual Teaching: Procedure/ Treatment
Knowledge: Energy Conservation Definition: Extent of understanding conveyed about energy conservation techniques	Energy Management Teaching: Prescribed Activity/Exercise	Body Mechanics Promotion Cardiac Care: Rehabilitative	Health Education Teaching: Group
Knowledge: Fall Prevention Definition: Extent of understanding conveyed about prevention of falls	Environmental Management: Safety Fall Prevention	Teaching: Individual Teaching: Toddler Safety 13-18 Months Teaching: Toddler Safety 19-24 Months	Teaching: Toddler Safety 25-36 Months
Knowledge: Fertility Promotion Definition: Extent of understanding conveyed about fertility testing and the conditions that affect conception	Family Planning: Infertility Fertility Preservation	Preconception Counseling Reproductive Technology Management Specimen Management	Teaching: Procedure/ Treatment Teaching: Safe Sex
Knowledge: Health Behavior Definition: Extent of understanding conveyed about the promotion and protection of health	Health Education Health Screening	Breast Examination Environmental Management: Safety Environmental Management: Worker Safety Exercise Promotion Genetic Counseling Health System Guidance Nutritional Counseling Oral Health Promotion Parent Education: Adolescent	Parent Education: Childrearing Family Parent Education: Infant Preconception Counseling Relaxation Therapy Risk Identification Substance Use Prevention Teaching: Group Teaching: Safe Sex Vehicle Safety Promotion

NOC-NIC LINKAGES FOR KNOWLEDGE, DEFICIENT		
Outcome	**Major Interventions**	**Suggested Interventions**

Knowledge: Health Promotion

Definition:
Extent of understanding conveyed about information needed to obtain and maintain optimal health

	Major Interventions	Suggested Interventions	

	Health Education
	Health System Guidance
		Allergy Management
		Breast Examination
		Exercise Promotion
		Health Screening
		Immunization/
		  Vaccination
		  Management
		Infection Protection
		Medication Management
			Nutritional
			  Counseling
			Relaxation Therapy
			Substance Use
			  Prevention
			Teaching: Foot Care
			Teaching: Prescribed
			  Medication
			Teaching: Safe Sex
			Weight Management

Knowledge: Health Resources

Definition:
Extent of understanding conveyed about relevant health care resources

	Health Education
	Health System Guidance
		Case Management
		Discharge Planning
			Financial Resource
			  Assistance
			Telephone
			  Consultation

Knowledge: Hypertension Management

Definition:
Extent of understanding conveyed about high blood pressure, its treatment, and the prevention of complications

	Teaching: Disease
	  Process
	Teaching: Prescribed
	  Medication
		Exercise Promotion
		Health System Guidance
		Medication Management
		Nutritional Counseling
			Smoking Cessation
			  Assistance
			Teaching: Prescribed
			  Diet
			Teaching: Procedure/
			  Treatment
			Vital Signs Monitoring

Knowledge: Illness Care

Definition:
Extent of understanding conveyed about illness-related information needed to achieve and maintain optimal health

	Teaching: Disease
	  Process
	Teaching:
	  Procedure/
	  Treatment
		Anticipatory Guidance
		Energy Management
		Health System Guidance
			Teaching: Prescribed
			  Activity/Exercise
			Teaching: Prescribed
			  Diet
			Teaching: Prescribed
			  Medication

Knowledge: Infant Care

Definition:
Extent of understanding conveyed about caring for a baby from birth to first birthday

	Parent Education:
	  Infant
		Circumcision Care
		Infant Care
		Lactation Counseling
		Parenting Promotion
		Teaching: Infant Nutrition
		  0-3 Months
		Teaching: Infant Nutrition
		  4-6 Months
		Teaching: Infant Nutrition
		  7-9 Months
		Teaching: Infant Nutrition
		  10-12 Months
		Teaching: Infant Safety
		  0-3 Months
			Teaching: Infant
			  Safety 4-6 Months
			Teaching: Infant
			  Safety 7-9 Months
			Teaching: Infant Safety
			  10-12 Months
			Teaching: Infant
			  Stimulation
			  0-4 Months
			Teaching: Infant
			  Stimulation
			  5-8 Months
			Teaching: Infant
			  Stimulation
			  9-12 Months

PART II - K

Continued

NOC-NIC LINKAGES FOR KNOWLEDGE, DEFICIENT		
Outcome	**Major Interventions**	**Suggested Interventions**
Knowledge: Infection Management Definition: Extent of understanding conveyed about infection, its treatment, and the prevention of complications	Infection Control Risk Identification	Health System Guidance Incision Site Care Medication Management Teaching: Disease Process Teaching: Prescribed Medication Teaching: Procedure/ Treatment Wound Care
Knowledge: Labor & Delivery Definition: Extent of understanding conveyed about labor and vaginal delivery	Childbirth Preparation	Anticipatory Guidance Labor Suppression Teaching: Group
Knowledge: Medication Definition: Extent of understanding conveyed about the safe use of medication	Teaching: Prescribed Medication	Allergy Management Analgesic Administration Asthma Management Hyperglycemia Management Hypoglycemia Management Immunization/ Vaccination Management Patient-Controlled Analgesia (PCA) Assistance
Knowledge: Multiple Sclerosis Management Definition: Extent of understanding conveyed about multiple sclerosis, its treatment, and the prevention of relapses or exacerbations	Energy Management Teaching: Disease Process	Case Management Health System Guidance Support Group Teaching: Prescribed Activity/Exercise Teaching: Prescribed Diet Teaching: Prescribed Medication Teaching: Procedure/ Treatment Teaching: Psychomotor Skill
Knowledge: Ostomy Care Definition: Extent of understanding conveyed about maintenance of an ostomy for elimination	Ostomy Care	Medication Administration: Skin Skin Care: Topical Treatments Skin Surveillance Teaching: Prescribed Diet Teaching: Procedure/ Treatment Teaching: Psychomotor Skill
Knowledge: Pain Management Definition: Extent of understanding conveyed about causes, symptoms, and treatment of pain	Pain Management Teaching: Prescribed Medication	Analgesic Administration Aromatherapy Health System Guidance Heat/Cold Application Medication Reconciliation Patient-Controlled Analgesia (PCA) Assistance Progressive Muscle Relaxation Relaxation Therapy Self-Hypnosis Facilitation Support Group Teaching: Prescribed Activity/Exercise Transcutaneous Electrical Nerve Stimulation (TENS)

NOC-NIC LINKAGES FOR KNOWLEDGE, DEFICIENT		
Outcome	**Major Interventions**	**Suggested Interventions**

Knowledge: Parenting

Definition:
Extent of understanding conveyed about provision of a nurturing and constructive environment for a child from 1 year through 17 years of age

Parent Education: Adolescent
Parent Education: Childrearing Family

Developmental Enhancement: Adolescent
Developmental Enhancement: Child
Teaching: Toddler Nutrition 13-18 Months
Teaching: Toddler Nutrition 19-24 Months
Teaching: Toddler Nutrition 25-36 Months

Teaching: Toddler Safety 13-18 Months
Teaching: Toddler Safety 19-24 Months
Teaching: Toddler Safety 25-36 Months
Teaching: Toilet Training

Knowledge: Personal Safety

Definition:
Extent of understanding conveyed about prevention of unintentional injuries

Environmental Management: Safety
Risk Identification

Environmental Management: Community
Environmental Management: Worker Safety
Fall Prevention
Substance Use Prevention
Teaching: Infant Safety 0-3 Months
Teaching: Infant Safety 4-6 Months
Teaching: Infant Safety 7-9 Months

Teaching: Infant Safety 10-12 Months
Teaching: Toddler Safety 13-18 Months
Teaching: Toddler Safety 19-24 Months
Teaching: Toddler Safety 25-36 Months
Vehicle Safety Promotion

Knowledge: Postpartum Maternal Health

Definition:
Extent of understanding conveyed about maternal health in the period following the birth of an infant

Lactation Counseling
Postpartal Care

Energy Management
Exercise Promotion
Health System Guidance
Mood Management

Nutritional Counseling
Teaching: Prescribed Activity/Exercise
Weight Reduction Assistance

Knowledge: Preconception Maternal Health

Definition:
Extent of understanding conveyed about maternal health prior to conception to ensure a healthy pregnancy

Preconception Counseling

Environmental Management: Safety
Genetic Counseling

Substance Use Prevention

Knowledge: Pregnancy

Definition:
Extent of understanding conveyed about promotion of a healthy pregnancy and prevention of complications

Childbirth Preparation
Prenatal Care

Body Mechanics Promotion
Environmental Management: Safety
Health System Guidance
High-Risk Pregnancy Care
Nutritional Counseling

Substance Use Prevention
Teaching: Prescribed Activity/Exercise
Teaching: Prescribed Diet
Teaching: Prescribed Medication

PART II - K

Continued

	NOC-NIC LINKAGES FOR KNOWLEDGE, DEFICIENT		
Outcome	**Major Interventions**	**Suggested Interventions**	
Knowledge: Pregnancy & Postpartum Sexual Functioning Definition: Extent of understanding conveyed about sexual function during pregnancy and postpartum	Sexual Counseling	Family Planning: Contraception Postpartal Care	Prenatal Care
Knowledge: Prescribed Activity Definition: Extent of understanding conveyed about prescribed activity and exercise	Teaching: Prescribed Activity/Exercise	Energy Management Exercise Promotion Exercise Therapy: Ambulation	Exercise Therapy: Muscle Control Teaching: Group
Knowledge: Preterm Infant Care Definition: Extent of understanding conveyed about the care of a premature infant born 24 to 37 weeks (term) gestation	Developmental Care	Attachment Promotion Financial Resource Assistance Health System Guidance	Parent Education: Infant Teaching: Infant Stimulation 0-4 Months
Knowledge: Sexual Functioning Definition: Extent of understanding conveyed about sexual development and responsible sexual practices	Teaching: Safe Sex Teaching: Sexuality	Family Planning: Contraception Parent Education: Adolescent	Parent Education: Childrearing Family Sexual Counseling
Knowledge: Substance Use Control Definition: Extent of understanding conveyed about controlling the use of addictive drugs, toxic chemicals, tobacco, or alcohol	Substance Use Prevention Substance Use Treatment	Health Education Health System Guidance Preconception Counseling	Smoking Cessation Assistance Teaching: Group
Knowledge: Treatment Procedure Definition: Extent of understanding conveyed about a procedure required as part of a treatment regimen	Teaching: Procedure/ Treatment Teaching: Psychomotor Skill	Asthma Management Culture Brokerage Decision-Making Support	Preparatory Sensory Information Prosthesis Care Teaching: Disease Process

NOC-NIC LINKAGES FOR KNOWLEDGE, DEFICIENT		
Outcome	**Major Interventions**	**Suggested Interventions**
Knowledge: Treatment Regimen Definition: Extent of understanding conveyed about a specific treatment regimen	Teaching: Disease Process Teaching: Procedure/ Treatment	Allergy Management Asthma Management Chemotherapy Management Health System Guidance Medication Management Nutritional Counseling	Radiation Therapy Management Teaching: Group Teaching: Prescribed Activity/Exercise Teaching: Prescribed Diet Teaching: Prescribed Medication
Knowledge: Weight Management Definition: Extent of understanding conveyed about the promotion and maintenance of optimal body weight and fat percentage congruent with height, frame, gender, and age	Nutritional Counseling Weight Management	Behavior Modification Eating Disorders Management Exercise Promotion Health System Guidance	Medication Management Teaching: Group Weight Gain Assistance Weight Reduction Assistance

Critical reasoning note: If the condition or problem about which the patient is to be taught is not listed, the generic outcomes related to health or disease process can be selected and any of the teaching interventions or generic education interventions that fit the problem can be selected.

NURSING DIAGNOSIS: Knowledge, Readiness for Enhanced

Definition: The presence or acquisition of cognitive information related to a specific topic is sufficient for meeting health-related goals and can be strengthened

NOC-NIC LINKAGES FOR KNOWLEDGE, READINESS FOR ENHANCED		
Outcome	**Major Interventions**	**Suggested Interventions**
Knowledge: Health Behavior Definition: Extent of understanding conveyed about the promotion and protection of health	Health Education Learning Facilitation Learning Readiness Enhancement	Health System Guidance Immunization/ Vaccination Management Self-Modification Assistance Self-Responsibility Facilitation Smoking Cessation Assistance	Sports-Injury Prevention: Youth Substance Use Prevention Teaching: Safe Sex Vehicle Safety Promotion

Continued

PART II - K

NOC-NIC LINKAGES FOR KNOWLEDGE, READINESS FOR ENHANCED			
Outcome	**Major Interventions**	**Suggested Interventions**	
Knowledge: Health Promotion			
Definition: Extent of understanding conveyed about information needed to obtain and maintain optimal health	Health Education Learning Facilitation Learning Readiness Enhancement	Breast Examination Smoking Cessation Assistance Substance Use Prevention Teaching: Individual Teaching: Prescribed Activity/Exercise	Teaching: Prescribed Diet Teaching: Prescribed Medication Teaching: Procedure/ Treatment Teaching: Safe Sex Weight Management
Knowledge: Health Resources			
Definition: Extent of understanding conveyed about relevant health care resources	Health System Guidance Learning Facilitation Learning Readiness Enhancement	Culture Brokerage Discharge Planning Financial Resource Assistance	Health Education Teaching: Individual

Critical reasoning note: If outcomes and interventions are needed for a specific problem, see specific areas under the diagnosis Knowledge, Deficient.

NURSING DIAGNOSIS: Latex Allergy Response

Definition: A hypersensitive response to natural latex rubber products

NICS ASSOCIATED WITH DIAGNOSIS RELATED FACTORS	
Environmental Management: Safety	Latex Precautions

NOC-NIC LINKAGES FOR LATEX ALLERGY RESPONSE			
Outcome	**Major Interventions**	**Suggested Interventions**	
Allergic Response: Localized			
Definition: Severity of localized hypersensitive immune response to a specific environmental (exogenous) antigen	Allergy Management Latex Precautions	Environmental Management Medication Administration Medication Administration: Nasal Medication Administration: Skin Pruritus Management	Respiratory Monitoring Risk Identification Skin Care: Topical Treatments Skin Surveillance Teaching: Individual

NOC-NIC LINKAGES FOR LATEX ALLERGY RESPONSE

Outcome	Major Interventions	Suggested Interventions	
Allergic Response: Systemic Definition: Severity of systemic hypersensitive immune response to a specific environmental (exogenous) antigen	Anaphylaxis Management Emergency Care Respiratory Monitoring	Airway Insertion and Stabilization Airway Management Airway Suctioning Artificial Airway Management Code Management Fluid Management Intravenous (IV) Insertion Intravenous (IV) Therapy Latex Precautions	Medication Administration Medication Administration: Intravenous (IV) Medication Management Oxygen Therapy Risk Identification Shock Prevention Vital Signs Monitoring
Tissue Integrity: Skin & Mucous Membranes Definition: Structural intactness and normal physiological function of skin and mucous membranes	Latex Precautions Skin Surveillance	Medication Administration Medication Administration: Skin Medication Management Pruritus Management	Skin Care: Topical Treatments Teaching: Individual Wound Care

NURSING DIAGNOSIS: Lifestyle, Sedentary

Definition: Reports a habit of life that is characterized by a low physical activity level

NICS ASSOCIATED WITH DIAGNOSIS RELATED FACTORS

Health Education	Teaching: Prescribed Activity/Exercise

NOC-NIC LINKAGES FOR LIFESTYLE, SEDENTARY

Outcome	Major Interventions	Suggested Interventions	
Motivation Definition: Inner urge that moves or prompts an individual to positive action(s)	Self-Modification Assistance Self-Responsibility Facilitation	Decision-Making Support Self-Awareness Enhancement	Self-Efficacy Enhancement Self-Esteem Enhancement
Physical Fitness Definition: Performance of physical activities with vigor	Exercise Promotion	Activity Therapy Exercise Promotion: Strength Training Exercise Promotion: Stretching Exercise Therapy: Joint Mobility	Teaching: Prescribed Activity/Exercise Vital Signs Monitoring Weight Management

Critical reasoning note: Motivation is provided as a potential outcome because it is often an intermediary outcome that must be addressed in some situations to change behaviors necessary to increase physical activity.

NURSING DIAGNOSIS: Memory, Impaired

Definition: Inability to remember or recall bits of information or behavioral skills

NICS ASSOCIATED WITH DIAGNOSIS RELATED FACTORS			

Cardiac Care
Cardiac Care: Acute
Cardiac Precautions
	Cerebral Edema
	  Management
	Cerebral Perfusion
	  Protection
		Environmental
		  Management
		Fluid/Electrolyte
		  Management
			Oxygen Therapy
			Ventilation Assistance

NOC-NIC LINKAGES FOR MEMORY, IMPAIRED		
Outcome	**Major Interventions**	**Suggested Interventions**

Cognitive Orientation
Definition:
Ability to identify
  person, place, and
  time accurately
	Delirium Management
	Dementia
	  Management
	Reality Orientation
		Cognitive Stimulation Patient Rights Protection
		Memory Training Reminiscence Therapy
		Neurological Substance Use
		  Monitoring Treatment

Memory
Definition:
Ability to cognitively
  retrieve and report
  previously stored
  information
	Dementia
	  Management
	Memory Training
		Active Listening Medication
		Anxiety Reduction Management
		Cognitive Stimulation Patient Rights Protection
		Emotional Support Reality Orientation
		Family Support Reminiscence Therapy

Neurological Status
Definition:
Ability of the peripheral
  and central nervous
  systems to receive,
  process, and respond
  to internal and
  external stimuli
	Cerebral Perfusion
	  Promotion
	Neurological
	  Monitoring
		Electrolyte Medication
		  Management Management
		Electrolyte Monitoring Oxygen Therapy
		Fluid/Electrolyte Respiratory Monitoring
		  Management Substance Use
		Fluid Management Treatment
		Fluid Monitoring Surveillance
		Medication Vital Signs Monitoring
		  Administration

NURSING DIAGNOSIS: Mobility: Bed, Impaired

Definition: Limitation of independent movement from one bed position to another

NICS ASSOCIATED WITH DIAGNOSIS RELATED FACTORS			

Cognitive Stimulation
Environmental
  Management
	Exercise Promotion
	Exercise Promotion:
	  Strength Training
		Exercise Promotion:
		  Stretching
		Pain Management
			Sedation Management
			Weight Reduction
			  Assistance

PART II - M

NOC-NIC LINKAGES FOR MOBILITY: BED, IMPAIRED		
Outcome	**Major Interventions**	**Suggested Interventions**
Body Positioning: Self-Initiated Definition: Ability to change own body position independently with or without assistive device	Exercise Promotion: Strength Training Exercise Therapy: Muscle Control	Body Mechanics Promotion Energy Management Exercise Promotion: Stretching Exercise Therapy: Joint Mobility Fall Prevention	Positioning Self-Care Assistance Self-Care Assistance: Transfer Teaching: Prescribed Activity/Exercise Traction/Immobilization Care
Coordinated Movement Definition: Ability of muscles to work together voluntarily for purposeful movement	Exercise Promotion: Strength Training Exercise Therapy: Muscle Control	Body Mechanics Promotion Exercise Promotion: Stretching Exercise Therapy: Balance Exercise Therapy: Joint Mobility Massage	Pain Management Progressive Muscle Relaxation Relaxation Therapy Teaching: Prescribed Activity/Exercise
Mobility Definition: Ability to move purposefully in own environment independently with or without assistive device	Exercise Promotion: Strength Training	Bed Rest Care Exercise Promotion Exercise Promotion: Stretching Exercise Therapy: Joint Mobility Exercise Therapy: Muscle Control Medication Management Pain Management	Self-Care Assistance Self-Care Assistance: Bathing/Hygiene Self-Care Assistance: Dressing/Grooming Self-Care Assistance: Toileting Self-Care Assistance: Transfer

PART II - M

NURSING DIAGNOSIS: Mobility: Physical, Impaired

Definition: Limitation in independent, purposeful physical movement of the body or of one or more extremities

NICS ASSOCIATED WITH DIAGNOSIS RELATED FACTORS			
Anxiety Reduction Behavior Modification Cognitive Stimulation Culture Brokerage	Energy Management Environmental Management Exercise Promotion Exercise Promotion: Strength Training	Exercise Therapy: Joint Mobility Medication Management Mood Management Nutrition Therapy	Pain Management Teaching: Prescribed Activity/Exercise Weight Management Weight Reduction Assistance

Continued

NOC-NIC LINKAGES FOR MOBILITY: PHYSICAL, IMPAIRED

Outcome	Major Interventions	Suggested Interventions	
Ambulation Definition: Ability to walk from place to place independently with or without assistive device	Exercise Promotion: Strength Training Exercise Therapy: Ambulation	Activity Therapy Body Mechanics Promotion Energy Management Environmental Management: Safety Exercise Promotion Exercise Promotion: Stretching	Exercise Therapy: Balance Exercise Therapy: Joint Mobility Exercise Therapy: Muscle Control Fall Prevention Surveillance: Safety Teaching: Prescribed Activity/Exercise
Balance Definition: Ability to maintain body equilibrium	Exercise Promotion: Strength Training Exercise Therapy: Balance	Activity Therapy Body Mechanics Promotion Energy Management Environmental Management: Safety	Exercise Promotion Exercise Therapy: Joint Mobility Exercise Therapy: Muscle Control Fall Prevention
Body Mechanics Performance Definition: Personal actions to maintain proper body alignment and to prevent muscular skeletal strain	Body Mechanics Promotion Exercise Therapy: Ambulation	Exercise Promotion: Strength Training Exercise Promotion: Stretching Exercise Therapy: Balance Exercise Therapy: Joint Mobility Exercise Therapy: Muscle Control	Self-Care Assistance Self-Care Assistance: IADL Self-Care Assistance: Toileting Self-Care Assistance: Transfer Teaching: Individual
Client Satisfaction: Functional Assistance Definition: Extent of positive perception of nursing assistance to achieve mobility and self-care	Body Mechanics Promotion Exercise Promotion	Environmental Management Exercise Therapy: Ambulation Fall Prevention Mutual Goal Setting	Self-Care Assistance Self-Care Assistance: Toileting Teaching: Prescribed Medication Transfer
Coordinated Movement Definition: Ability of muscles to work together voluntarily for purposeful movement	Exercise Promotion: Strength Training Exercise Therapy: Muscle Control	Body Mechanics Promotion Energy Management Exercise Promotion: Stretching Exercise Therapy: Ambulation	Exercise Therapy: Balance Exercise Therapy: Joint Mobility Teaching: Prescribed Activity/Exercise

NOC-NIC LINKAGES FOR MOBILITY: PHYSICAL, IMPAIRED		
Outcome	**Major Interventions**	**Suggested Interventions**
Joint Movement: (Specify joint) Definition: Active range of motion of _____ (specify joint) with self-initiated movement	Exercise Therapy: Joint Mobility	Analgesic Administration Body Mechanics Promotion Energy Management Exercise Promotion Exercise Promotion: Strength Training / Exercise Promotion: Stretching Exercise Therapy: Ambulation Exercise Therapy: Balance Exercise Therapy: Muscle Control Teaching: Prescribed Activity/Exercise
Joint Movement: Passive Definition: Joint movement with assistance	Exercise Therapy: Joint Mobility	Energy Management Pain Management / Skin Surveillance
Mobility Definition: Ability to move purposefully in own environment independently with or without assistive device	Exercise Therapy: Ambulation Exercise Therapy: Balance Exercise Therapy: Joint Mobility Exercise Therapy: Muscle Control	Activity Therapy Body Mechanics Promotion Cast Care: Maintenance Cast Care: Wet Circulatory Precautions Energy Management Environmental Management: Safety Exercise Promotion Exercise Promotion: Strength Training Exercise Promotion: Stretching Fall Prevention Neurological Monitoring / Pain Management Peripheral Sensation Management Positioning Positioning: Intraoperative Positioning: Neurological Positioning: Wheelchair Pressure Management Skin Surveillance Surveillance: Safety Teaching: Prescribed Activity/Exercise Traction/Immobilization Care
Neurological Status: Central Motor Control Definition: Ability of the central nervous system to coordinate skeletal muscle activity for body movement	Body Mechanics Promotion	Exercise Therapy: Ambulation Exercise Therapy: Balance Exercise Therapy: Joint Mobility Exercise Therapy: Muscle Control / Neurological Monitoring Seizure Precautions Seizure Management

Continued

PART II - M

NOC-NIC LINKAGES FOR MOBILITY: PHYSICAL, IMPAIRED		
Outcome	**Major Interventions**	**Suggested Interventions**
Skeletal Function Definition: Ability of the bones to support the body and facilitate movement	Body Mechanics Promotion Exercise Therapy: Ambulation	Energy Management Exercise Promotion Exercise Promotion: Strength Training Exercise Promotion: Stretching Exercise Therapy: Balance Exercise Therapy: Joint Mobility Exercise Therapy: Muscle Control	Medication Administration: Intraosseous Positioning Self-Care Assistance: Transfer Traction/Immobilization Care Weight Management
Transfer Performance Definition: Ability to change body location independently with or without assistive device	Exercise Promotion: Strength Training Exercise Therapy: Muscle Control Self-Care Assistance: Transfer	Anxiety Reduction Body Mechanics Promotion Energy Management Environmental Management: Safety Exercise Promotion Exercise Promotion: Stretching Exercise Therapy: Balance Exercise Therapy: Joint Mobility	Fall Prevention Positioning Positioning: Wheelchair Self-Care Assistance Surveillance: Safety Teaching: Prescribed Activity/Exercise Teaching: Psychomotor Skill

NURSING DIAGNOSIS: Mobility: Wheelchair, Impaired

Definition: Limitation of independent operation of wheelchair within environment

NICS ASSOCIATED WITH DIAGNOSIS RELATED FACTORS			
Cognitive Stimulation Energy Management Environmental Management	Exercise Promotion Exercise Promotion: Strength Training	Mood Management Pain Management	Teaching: Prescribed Activity/Exercise Weight Reduction Assistance

NOC-NIC LINKAGES FOR MOBILITY: WHEELCHAIR, IMPAIRED		
Outcome	**Major Interventions**	**Suggested Interventions**
Ambulation: Wheelchair Definition: Ability to move from place to place in a wheelchair	Exercise Promotion: Strength Training Positioning: Wheelchair	Body Mechanics Promotion Energy Management Environmental Management: Safety Exercise Promotion Exercise Promotion: Stretching Exercise Therapy: Balance	Exercise Therapy: Muscle Control Fall Prevention Medication Management Positioning: Neurological Self-Care Assistance: Transfer Teaching: Prescribed Activity/Exercise

NOC-NIC LINKAGES FOR MOBILITY: WHEELCHAIR, IMPAIRED		
Outcome	**Major Interventions**	**Suggested Interventions**

Balance

Definition:
Ability to maintain body equilibrium

Exercise Promotion: Strength Training
Exercise Therapy: Balance

Energy Management
Environmental Management: Safety
Exercise Promotion
Exercise Therapy: Ambulation
Exercise Therapy: Joint Mobility

Exercise Therapy: Muscle Control
Fall Prevention
Positioning: Wheelchair
Weight Management

Coordinated Movement

Definition:
Ability of muscles to work together voluntarily for purposeful movement

Exercise Promotion: Strength Training
Exercise Therapy: Muscle Control

Body Mechanics Promotion
Energy Management
Exercise Promotion: Stretching

Exercise Therapy: Joint Mobility
Positioning: Wheelchair
Teaching: Prescribed Activity/Exercise

Mobility

Definition:
Ability to move purposefully in own environment independently with or without assistive device

Exercise Promotion: Strength Training
Positioning: Wheelchair

Body Mechanics Promotion
Energy Management
Environmental Management: Safety
Exercise Promotion
Exercise Promotion: Stretching
Exercise Therapy: Balance

Exercise Therapy: Muscle Control
Fall Prevention
Mutual Goal Setting
Pain Management
Positioning
Teaching: Prescribed Activity/Exercise

Transfer Performance

Definition:
Ability to change body location independently with or without assistive device

Self-Care Assistance: Transfer

Energy Management
Exercise Promotion: Strength Training
Exercise Promotion: Stretching
Exercise Therapy: Balance
Exercise Therapy: Joint Mobility

Exercise Therapy: Muscle Control
Nutrition Management
Positioning: Wheelchair
Teaching: Prescribed Activity/Exercise

PART II - M

NURSING DIAGNOSIS: Moral Distress

Definition: Response to the inability to carry out one's chosen ethical/moral decision/action

NICS ASSOCIATED WITH DIAGNOSIS RELATED FACTORS		

Conflict Mediation
Culture Brokerage
	Decision-Making
	  Support
	Patient Rights
	  Protection
		Truth Telling
		Values Clarification

NOC-NIC LINKAGES FOR MORAL DISTRESS			
Outcome	**Major Interventions**	**Suggested Interventions**	

Anxiety Level
Definition:
Severity of manifested
  apprehension, tension, or
  uneasiness arising from
  an unidentifiable source
Fear Level
Definition:
Severity of manifested
  apprehension, tension, or
  uneasiness arising from
  an identifiable source
	Anxiety Reduction	Active Listening
		Anger Control
		  Assistance
		Calming Technique
		Counseling
		Crisis Intervention
		Decision-Making
		  Support
		Emotional Support
		Guilt Work Facilitation
			Music Therapy
			Patient Rights
			  Protection
			Relaxation Therapy
			Sleep Enhancement
			Spiritual Support
			Values Clarification
			Vital Signs Monitoring

Comfort Status:
Psychospiritual
Definition:
Psychospiritual ease related
  to self-concept, emotional
  well-being, source of
  inspiration, and meaning
  and purpose in one's life
	Anxiety Reduction
	Spiritual Support
		Calming Technique
		Emotional Support
		Guilt Work Facilitation
		Mood Management
		Music Therapy
		Self-Awareness
		  Enhancement
			Self-Esteem
			  Enhancement
			Spiritual Growth
			  Facilitation
			Suicide Prevention
			Truth Telling
			Values Clarification

Dignified Life Closure
Definition:
Personal actions to
  maintain control while
  approaching end of life
	Decision-Making
	  Support
	Patient Rights
	  Protection
		Anxiety Reduction
		Dying Care
		Grief Work Facilitation
		Guilt Work Facilitation
		Hope Inspiration
		Music Therapy
			Mutual Goal Setting
			Reminiscence Therapy
			Spiritual Growth
			  Facilitation
			Spiritual Support
			Values Clarification

Personal Autonomy
Definition:
Personal actions of a
  competent individual to
  exercise governance in
  life decisions
	Decision-Making
	  Support
	Patient Rights
	  Protection
		Anxiety Reduction
		Conflict Mediation
		Emotional Support
		Health System
		  Guidance
			Mutual Goal Setting
			Self-Awareness
			  Enhancement
			Values Clarification

Spiritual Health
Definition:
Connectedness with self,
  others, higher power, all
  life, nature, and the uni-
  verse that transcends and
  empowers the self
	Spiritual Growth
	  Facilitation
	Spiritual Support
		Active Listening
		Art Therapy
		Forgiveness
		  Facilitation
		Guilt Work Facilitation
		Hope Inspiration
			Meditation Facilitation
			Music Therapy
			Self-Awareness
			  Enhancement
			Values Clarification

Critical reasoning note: The outcomes Anxiety Level and Fear Level have been consolidated because the same interventions can be used for this diagnosis.

NURSING DIAGNOSIS: Nausea

Definition: A subjective unpleasant, wave-like sensation in the back of the throat, epigastrium, or abdomen that may lead to the urge or need to vomit

NICS ASSOCIATED WITH DIAGNOSIS RELATED FACTORS			
Anxiety Reduction	Environmental	Medication	Teaching: Disease
Cerebral Edema	Management	Management	Process
Management	Gastrointestinal	Pain Management	
Chemotherapy	Intubation	Prenatal Care	
Management	Intracranial Pressure		
	(ICP) Monitoring		

NOC-NIC LINKAGES FOR NAUSEA			
Outcome	**Major Interventions**	**Suggested Interventions**	
Appetite			
Definition:	Nausea	Calming Technique	Pain Management
Desire to eat when ill or receiving treatment	Management	Medication Management Oral Health Maintenance	Vomiting Management
Nausea & Vomiting Control			
Definition:	Nausea	Biofeedback	Oral Health Promotion
Personal actions to control nausea, retching, and vomiting symptoms	Management	Distraction Guided Imagery Medication Administration Oral Health Maintenance	Pain Management Relaxation Therapy Self-Hypnosis Facilitation Vomiting Management
Nausea & Vomiting: Disruptive Effect			
Definition:	Nausea	Anxiety Reduction	Nutritional Monitoring
Severity of observed or reported disruptive effects of nausea, retching, and vomiting on daily functioning	Management	Chemotherapy Management Emotional Support Fluid/Electrolyte Monitoring Fluid Monitoring Mood Management	Relaxation Therapy Role Enhancement Sleep Enhancement Vomiting Management
Nausea & Vomiting Severity			
Definition:	Nausea	Acid-Base Monitoring	Fluid Management
Severity of nausea, retching, and vomiting symptoms	Management	Aspiration Precautions Calming Technique Electrolyte Monitoring Fluid/Electrolyte Management	Fluid Monitoring Vital Signs Monitoring Vomiting Management

Critical reasoning note: Although the diagnosis does not include vomiting, the outcomes include both nausea and vomiting. The interventions have been limited to the control of nausea as much as possible, with some interventions addressing vomiting.

PART II - N

NURSING DIAGNOSIS: Neonatal Jaundice

Definition: The yellow orange tint of the neonate's skin and mucous membranes that occurs after 24 hours of life as a result of unconjugated bilirubin in the circulation

NICS ASSOCIATED WITH DIAGNOSIS RELATED FACTORS			
Bottle Feeding Breastfeeding Assistance	Developmental Care	Newborn Care	Newborn Monitoring

NOC-NIC LINKAGES FOR NEONATAL JAUNDICE

Outcome	Major Interventions	Suggested Interventions
Newborn Adaptation Definition: Adaptive response to the extrauterine environment by a physiologically mature newborn during the first 28 days	Phototherapy: Neonate	Newborn Monitoring

NURSING DIAGNOSIS: Noncompliance

Definition: Behavior of person and/or caregiver that fails to coincide with a health-promoting or therapeutic plan agreed on by the person (and/or family and/or community) and healthcare professional. In the presence of an agreed-on, health-promoting or therapeutic plan, person's or caregiver's behavior is fully or partially nonadherent and may lead to clinically ineffective or partially ineffective outcomes

NICS ASSOCIATED WITH DIAGNOSIS RELATED FACTORS			

Case Management
Complex Relationship
  Building
Culture Brokerage
	Discharge Planning
	Financial Resource
	  Assistance
	Health System
	  Guidance
		Insurance
		  Authorization
		Learning Facilitation
		Teaching: Individual
			Teaching: Procedure/
			  Treatment
			Truth Telling
			Values Clarification

NOC-NIC LINKAGES FOR NONCOMPLIANCE

Outcome	Major Interventions	Suggested Interventions	

Caregiver Performance: Direct Care
Definition:
Provision by family care provider of appropriate personal and health care for a family member
	Caregiver Support
	Learning Facilitation
		Anticipatory Guidance
		Coping Enhancement
		Discharge Planning
		Family Involvement
		  Promotion
		Home Maintenance
		  Assistance
		Referral
		Respite Care
			Support System
			  Enhancement
			Teaching: Disease Process
			Teaching: Prescribed
			  Activity/Exercise
			Teaching: Prescribed Diet
			Teaching: Prescribed
			  Medication
			Teaching: Procedure/
			  Treatment
			Teaching: Psychomotor
			  Skill

NOC-NIC LINKAGES FOR NONCOMPLIANCE		
Outcome	**Major Interventions**	**Suggested Interventions**

Caregiver Performance: Indirect Care

Definition: Arrangement and oversight by family care provider of appropriate care for a family member

Caregiver Support
Health System Guidance

Case Management
Coping Enhancement
Culture Brokerage
Decision-Making Support
Family Involvement Promotion
Financial Resource Assistance

Home Maintenance Assistance
Insurance Authorization
Patient Rights Protection
Referral
Support System Enhancement

Compliance Behavior

Definition: Personal actions to promote wellness, recovery, and rehabilitation recommended by a health professional

Health System Guidance
Mutual Goal Setting

Behavior Modification
Case Management
Culture Brokerage
Decision-Making Support
Discharge Planning
Family Involvement Promotion
Financial Resource Assistance
Health Education
Health Literacy Enhancement
Learning Facilitation
Learning Readiness Enhancement
Parent Education: Adolescent
Parent Education: Childrearing Family
Parent Education: Infant
Patient Contracting

Self-Modification Assistance
Self-Responsibility Facilitation
Smoking Cessation Assistance
Substance Use Prevention
Support Group
Support System Enhancement
Surveillance
Teaching: Prescribed Activity/Exercise
Teaching: Prescribed Diet
Teaching: Prescribed Medication
Teaching: Procedure/Treatment
Teaching: Psychomotor Skill
Teaching: Safe Sex
Telephone Consultation

Compliance Behavior: Prescribed Diet

Definition: Personal actions to follow food and fluid intake recommended by a health professional for a specific health condition

Nutritional Counseling
Teaching: Prescribed Diet

Behavior Modification
Culture Brokerage
Diet Staging
Discharge Planning
Fluid Monitoring
Mutual Goal Setting
Nutritional Monitoring
Self-Efficacy Enhancement

Self-Responsibility Facilitation
Teaching: Toddler Nutrition 13-18 Months
Teaching: Toddler Nutrition 19-24 Months
Teaching: Toddler Nutrition 25-36 Months

Continued

PART II - N

NOC-NIC LINKAGES FOR NONCOMPLIANCE		
Outcome	**Major Interventions**	**Suggested Interventions**
Compliance: Prescribed Medication Definition: Personal actions to administer medication safely to meet therapeutic goals as recommended by a health professional	Medication Management Teaching: Prescribed Medication	Behavior Modification Chemotherapy Management Culture Brokerage Discharge Planning Hormone Replacement Therapy Medication Reconciliation	Mutual Goal Setting Self-Efficacy Enhancement Self-Responsibility Facilitation Skin Care: Topical Treatments Thrombolytic Therapy Management
Motivation Definition: Inner urge that moves or prompts an individual to positive action(s)	Self-Efficacy Enhancement Self-Responsibility Facilitation	Coping Enhancement Decision-Making Support Family Involvement Promotion Financial Resource Assistance Mutual Goal Setting Resiliency Promotion	Self-Esteem Enhancement Self-Modification Assistance Support Group Teaching: Individual Values Clarification
Treatment Behavior: Illness or Injury Definition: Personal actions to palliate or eliminate pathology	Self-Responsibility Facilitation Teaching: Procedure/ Treatment	Allergy Management Asthma Management Behavior Modification Chemotherapy Management Energy Management Family Involvement Promotion Health System Guidance Learning Facilitation Learning Readiness Enhancement Mutual Goal Setting Patient Contracting Radiation Therapy Management Self-Care Assistance Self-Efficacy Enhancement Self-Modification Assistance	Smoking Cessation Assistance Substance Use Treatment Support Group Support System Enhancement Surveillance Teaching: Disease Process Teaching: Individual Teaching: Prescribed Activity/Exercise Teaching: Prescribed Diet Teaching: Prescribed Medication Teaching: Psychomotor Skill Telephone Consultation Weight Gain Assistance Weight Reduction Assistance

NURSING DIAGNOSIS: Nutrition: Imbalanced, Less than Body Requirements

Definition: Intake of nutrients insufficient to meet metabolic needs

NICS ASSOCIATED WITH DIAGNOSIS RELATED FACTORS

Chemotherapy Management	Financial Resource Assistance	Nausea Management	Sustenance Support
Diarrhea Management	Mood Management	Radiation Therapy Management	Swallowing Therapy
Eating Disorders Management			

NOC-NIC LINKAGES FOR NUTRITION: IMBALANCED, LESS THAN BODY REQUIREMENTS

Outcome	Major Interventions	Suggested Interventions	
Appetite			
Definition: Desire to eat when ill or receiving treatment	Nutrition Therapy Nutritional Monitoring	Diet Staging Energy Management Environmental Management Fluid Management	Nutrition Management Oral Health Maintenance Oral Health Promotion
Compliance Behavior: Prescribed Diet			
Definition: Personal actions to follow food and fluid intake recommended by a health professional for a specific health condition	Nutritional Counseling Teaching: Prescribed Diet	Culture Brokerage Eating Disorders Management Fluid Management Nutrition Management	Nutritional Monitoring Self-Efficacy Enhancement Self-Responsibility Facilitation
Gastrointestinal Function			
Definition: Extent to which foods (ingested or tube-fed) are moved from ingestion to excretion	Diarrhea Management	Bowel Management Cutaneous Stimulation Feeding	Medication Management Nutrition Therapy Pain Management
Nutritional Status			
Definition: Extent to which nutrients are available to meet metabolic needs	Nutrition Therapy Nutritional Monitoring	Diet Staging Eating Disorders Management Energy Management Enteral Tube Feeding Gastrointestinal Intubation Nutrition Management	Nutritional Counseling Teaching: Prescribed Diet Total Parenteral Nutrition (TPN) Administration Vital Signs Monitoring Weight Gain Assistance
Nutritional Status: Biochemical Measures			
Definition: Body fluid components and chemical indices of nutritional status	Laboratory Data Interpretation Nutrition Therapy	Eating Disorders Management Nutrition Management Nutritional Counseling Teaching: Prescribed Diet	Total Parenteral Nutrition (TPN) Administration Weight Gain Assistance

PART II - N

Continued

NOC-NIC LINKAGES FOR NUTRITION: IMBALANCED, LESS THAN BODY REQUIREMENTS

Outcome	Major Interventions	Suggested Interventions	
Nutritional Status: Nutrient Intake Definition: Nutrient intake to meet metabolic needs	Nutrition Therapy Nutritional Monitoring	Enteral Tube Feeding Feeding Laboratory Data Interpretation Nutrition Management Nutritional Counseling Self-Care Assistance: Feeding	Sustenance Support Teaching: Prescribed Diet Total Parenteral Nutrition (TPN) Administration Weight Gain Assistance
Weight: Body Mass Definition: Extent to which body weight, muscle, and fat are congruent to height, frame, gender, and age	Weight Gain Assistance Weight Management	Behavior Modification Eating Disorders Management	Exercise Promotion Nutrition Therapy
Weight Gain Behavior Definition: Personal actions to gain weight following voluntary or involuntary significant weight loss	Nutritional Counseling Weight Gain Assistance	Eating Disorders Management Enteral Tube Feeding Fluid/Electrolyte Management Medication Management Nutrition Management Nutrition Therapy Nutritional Monitoring Oral Health Maintenance Oral Health Promotion	Support Group Support System Enhancement Sustenance Support Teaching: Prescribed Activity/Exercise Teaching: Prescribed Diet Teaching: Prescribed Medication Total Parenteral Nutrition (TPN) Administration

NURSING DIAGNOSIS: Nutrition: Imbalanced, More than Body Requirements

Definition: Intake of nutrients that exceeds metabolic needs

NICS ASSOCIATED WITH DIAGNOSIS RELATED FACTORS

Behavior Modification Nutritional Counseling	Nutritional Monitoring Self-Responsibility Facilitation	Self-Modification Assistance Teaching: Prescribed Diet

NOC-NIC LINKAGES FOR NUTRITION: IMBALANCED, MORE THAN BODY REQUIREMENTS

Outcome	Major Interventions	Suggested Interventions	
Nutritional Status: Food & Fluid Intake Definition: Amount of food and fluid taken into the body over a 24-hour period	Behavior Modification Nutritional Counseling	Fluid Monitoring Nutritional Monitoring Self-Responsibility Facilitation	Teaching: Prescribed Diet Weight Reduction Assistance

NOC-NIC LINKAGES FOR NUTRITION: IMBALANCED, MORE THAN BODY REQUIREMENTS		
Outcome	**Major Interventions**	**Suggested Interventions**

Weight Loss Behavior
 	
Definition:
Personal actions to lose weight through diet, exercise, and behavior modification
	Nutrition Management
	Nutritional Monitoring
	Weight Reduction
	   Assistance
		Eating Disorders
		   Management
		Exercise Promotion
		Mutual Goal Setting
		Nutritional Counseling
			Self-Awareness
			   Enhancement
			Self-Modification
			   Assistance
			Support Group

Critical reasoning note: The outcome Weight Loss Behavior is included because it addresses both the weight gain and the eating pattern behaviors in the defining characteristics.

NURSING DIAGNOSIS: Nutrition, Readiness for Enhanced

Definition: A pattern of nutrient intake that is sufficient for meeting metabolic needs and can be strengthened

NOC-NIC LINKAGES FOR NUTRITION, READINESS FOR ENHANCED		
Outcome	**Major Interventions**	**Suggested Interventions**

Adherence Behavior: Healthy Diet
 	
Definition:
Personal actions to monitor and optimize a healthy and nutritional dietary regimen
	Health Education
	Nutritional Monitoring
		Culture Brokerage
		Mutual Goal Setting
		Nutritional Counseling
			Self-Modification
			   Assistance
			Self-Responsibility
			   Facilitation
			Weight Management

Knowledge: Diet
 	
Definition:
Extent of understanding conveyed about recommended diet
	Teaching: Individual
	Teaching: Prescribed
	   Diet
		Health Education
		Learning Facilitation
		Learning Readiness
		   Enhancement
		Nutritional Counseling
			Parent Education:
			   Childrearing Family
			Prenatal Care
			Teaching: Group

Nutritional Status
 	
Definition:
Extent to which nutrients are available to meet metabolic needs
	Nutrition Management
	Nutritional Counseling
		Nutritional Monitoring
		Prenatal Care
		Teaching: Prescribed
		   Diet
			Weight Gain Assistance
			Weight Management
			Weight Reduction
			   Assistance

Nutritional Status: Nutrient Intake Definition: Nutrient intake to meet metabolic needs	Nutritional Monitoring	Nutrition Management Nutritional Counseling	Weight Management
Weight Maintenance Behavior Definition: Personal actions to maintain optimum body weight	Nutritional Monitoring Weight Management	Fluid Management Nutrition Management Nutritional Counseling	Self-Awareness Enhancement Sleep Enhancement Teaching: Individual

NURSING DIAGNOSIS: Oral Mucous Membrane, Impaired

Definition: Disruption of the lips and/or soft tissue of the oral cavity

NICS ASSOCIATED WITH DIAGNOSIS RELATED FACTORS			
Bleeding Precautions	Insurance	Referral	Substance Use
Chemotherapy	Authorization	Self-Care Assistance	Treatment
Management	Oral Health		Teaching: Individual
Financial Resource	Maintenance		
Assistance			

NOC-NIC LINKAGES FOR ORAL MUCOUS MEMBRANE, IMPAIRED		
Outcome	**Major Interventions**	**Suggested Interventions**
Oral Hygiene Definition: Condition of the mouth, teeth, gums, and tongue	Oral Health Restoration	Bleeding Precautions Bleeding Reduction Chemotherapy Management Infection Control Infection Protection / Medication Management Nutrition Management Oral Health Maintenance Oral Health Promotion Pain Management
Tissue Integrity: Skin & Mucous Membranes Definition: Structural intactness and normal physiological function of skin and mucous membranes	Oral Health Restoration	Bleeding Precautions Chemotherapy Management Fluid Management Infection Control Infection Protection Medication Management / Nutrition Management Oral Health Maintenance Oral Health Promotion Radiation Therapy Management Wound Care

NURSING DIAGNOSIS: Pain, Acute

Definition: Unpleasant sensory and emotional experience arising from actual or potential tissue damage or described in terms of such damage (International Association for the Study of Pain); sudden or slow onset of any intensity from mild to severe with an anticipated or predictable end and a duration of <6 months

NICS ASSOCIATED WITH DIAGNOSIS RELATED FACTORS			
Grief Work Facilitation	Premenstrual	Rape-Trauma Treatment	Wound Care: Burns
Incision Site Care	Syndrome (PMS)	Trauma Therapy: Child	
	Management		

NOC-NIC LINKAGES FOR PAIN, ACUTE

Outcome	Major Interventions	Suggested Interventions	
Client Satisfaction: Pain Management Definition: Extent of positive perception of nursing care to relieve pain	Pain Management	Analgesic Administration Aromatherapy Cutaneous Stimulation Distraction Heat/Cold Application Massage Medication Administration: Intraspinal Medication Administration: Intravenous (IV)	Patient-Controlled Analgesia (PCA) Assistance Positioning Splinting Teaching: Prescribed Medication Transcutaneous Electrical Nerve Stimulation (TENS)
Discomfort Level Definition: Severity of observed or reported mental or physical discomfort	Medication Management Pain Management	Acupressure Analgesic Administration Anxiety Reduction Bathing Biofeedback Bowel Management Calming Technique Coping Enhancement Cutaneous Stimulation Distraction Dying Care Emotional Support Energy Management Environmental Management: Comfort Flatulence Reduction Guided Imagery Heat/Cold Application Humor Hypnosis Massage Medication Administration	Medication Administration: Intramuscular (IM) Medication Administration: Intravenous (IV) Medication Administration: Oral Medication Prescribing Meditation Facilitation Music Therapy Nausea Management Oxygen Therapy Positioning Presence Relaxation Therapy Sedation Management Sleep Enhancement Splinting Therapeutic Touch Transcutaneous Electrical Nerve Stimulation (TENS) Vomiting Management
Pain Control Definition: Personal actions to control pain	Medication Administration Pain Management Patient-Controlled Analgesia (PCA) Assistance	Acupressure Cutaneous Stimulation Distraction Guided Imagery Heat/Cold Application Medication Administration: Intramuscular (IM) Medication Administration: Intraspinal Medication Administration: Intravenous (IV) Medication Administration: Oral Medication Prescribing Music Therapy Positioning	Preparatory Sensory Information Relaxation Therapy Self-Hypnosis Facilitation Sleep Enhancement Splinting Teaching: Individual Teaching: Prescribed Medication Teaching: Procedure/ Treatment Therapeutic Touch

PART II - N

Continued

NOC-NIC LINKAGES FOR PAIN, ACUTE

Outcome	Major Interventions	Suggested Interventions	
Pain Level Definition: Severity of observed or reported pain	Pain Management Surveillance	Active Listening Analgesic Administration Anxiety Reduction Emotional Support	Positioning Splinting Therapeutic Touch Vital Signs Monitoring

Critical reasoning note: The related factors include any agents that can cause pain, including psychological agents. Depending on the causative agent, a number of other NIC interventions could be selected.

NURSING DIAGNOSIS: Pain, Chronic

Definition: Unpleasant sensory and emotional experience arising from actual or potential tissue damage or described in terms of such damage (International Association for the Study of Pain); sudden or slow onset of any intensity from mild to severe, constant or recurring without an anticipated or predictable end and a duration of >6 months

NICS ASSOCIATED WITH DIAGNOSIS RELATED FACTORS

Teaching: Disease
  Process
	Teaching: Prescribed
	  Medication
		Teaching: Procedure/
		  Treatment

NOC-NIC LINKAGES FOR PAIN, CHRONIC

Outcome	Major Interventions	Suggested Interventions	

Client Satisfaction:
Pain Management
 	
Definition:
Extent of positive
  perception of
  nursing care to
  relieve pain
	Pain Management	Acupressure
		Analgesic
		  Administration
		Aromatherapy
		Cutaneous Stimulation
		Distraction
		Environmental
		  Management: Comfort
		Heat/Cold Application
		Massage
		Medication
		  Administration:
		  Intravenous (IV)
		Multidisciplinary Care
		  Conference
		Music Therapy
			Patient-Controlled
			  Analgesia (PCA)
			  Assistance
			Positioning
			Progressive Muscle
			  Relaxation
			Referral
			Splinting
			Support Group
			Teaching: Individual
			Teaching: Prescribed
			  Medication
			Transcutaneous Electrical
			  Nerve Stimulation
			  (TENS)

NOC-NIC LINKAGES FOR PAIN, CHRONIC

Outcome	Major Interventions	Suggested Interventions	
Pain: Adverse Psychological Response			
Definition: Severity of observed or reported adverse cognitive and emotional responses to physical pain	Mood Management Pain Management	Active Listening Activity Therapy Anger Control Assistance Animal-Assisted Therapy Anxiety Reduction Coping Enhancement Emotional Support Guided Imagery Hope Inspiration Humor Journaling	Medication Management Music Therapy Presence Self-Esteem Enhancement Sleep Enhancement Spiritual Support Substance Use Prevention Suicide Prevention Support Group Support System Enhancement Touch
Pain Control			
Definition: Personal actions to control pain	Medication Management Pain Management	Acupressure Analgesic Administration Biofeedback Cutaneous Stimulation Distraction Environmental Management: Comfort Family Involvement Promotion Guided Imagery Heat/Cold Application Massage Medication Administration Medication Administration: Intramuscular (IM) Medication Administration: Intravenous (IV) Medication Administration: Oral Medication Prescribing Patient-Controlled Analgesia (PCA) Assistance	Positioning Progressive Muscle Relaxation Relaxation Therapy Self-Hypnosis Facilitation Self-Modification Assistance Self-Responsibility Facilitation Sleep Enhancement Splinting Support Group Support System Enhancement Surveillance Teaching: Individual Teaching: Prescribed Medication Teaching: Procedure/ Treatment Telephone Consultation Therapeutic Touch Transcutaneous Electrical Nerve Stimulation (TENS)

Continued

PART II - P

NOC-NIC LINKAGES FOR PAIN, CHRONIC

Outcome	Major Interventions	Suggested Interventions	
Pain: Disruptive Effects			
Definition: Severity of observed or reported disruptive effects of chronic pain on daily functioning	Coping Enhancement Pain Management	Activity Therapy Anxiety Reduction Behavior Modification Body Mechanics Promotion Bowel Management Consultation Decision-Making Support Energy Management Environmental Management: Comfort Exercise Promotion Exercise Promotion: Stretching Exercise Therapy: Ambulation Exercise Therapy: Joint Mobility	Family Process Maintenance Hope Inspiration Massage Medication Management Nutritional Counseling Nutritional Monitoring Progressive Muscle Relaxation Role Enhancement Self-Care Assistance Sleep Enhancement Socialization Enhancement
Pain Level			
Definition: Severity of observed or reported pain	Pain Management	Active Listening Anxiety Reduction Emotional Support Positioning	Splinting Surveillance Therapeutic Touch Vital Signs Monitoring

Critical reasoning note: Three teaching interventions that can address chronic physical or psychosocial disability are identified for the related factors. Depending on the type of disability, the care provider can consider outcomes and interventions specific for the disability.

NURSING DIAGNOSIS: Parental Role Conflict

Definition: Parent experience of role confusion and conflict in response to crisis

NICS ASSOCIATED WITH DIAGNOSIS RELATED FACTORS

Coping Enhancement Family Process Maintenance	Family Therapy	Respite Care	Teaching: Procedure/ Treatment

NOC-NIC LINKAGES FOR PARENTAL ROLE CONFLICT

Outcome	Major Interventions	Suggested Interventions	
Caregiver Home Care Readiness			
Definition: Preparedness of a caregiver to assume responsibility for the health care of a family member in the home	Decision-Making Support Discharge Planning	Anticipatory Guidance Anxiety Reduction Caregiver Support Family Involvement Promotion Financial Resource Assistance Health System Guidance Support System Enhancement	Teaching: Disease Process Teaching: Individual Teaching: Prescribed Activity/Exercise Teaching: Prescribed Diet Teaching: Prescribed Medication Teaching: Procedure/ Treatment

NOC-NIC LINKAGES FOR PARENTAL ROLE CONFLICT

Outcome	Major Interventions	Suggested Interventions	
Caregiver Lifestyle Disruption Definition: Severity of disturbances in the lifestyle of a family member due to caregiving	Caregiver Support Role Enhancement	Coping Enhancement Emotional Support Family Integrity Promotion Family Involvement Promotion Family Process Maintenance Financial Resource Assistance Health System Guidance	Insurance Authorization Respite Care Sleep Enhancement Socialization Enhancement Support Group Support System Enhancement
Knowledge: Parenting Definition: Extent of understanding conveyed about provision of a nurturing and constructive environment for a child from 1 year through 17 years of age	Parent Education: Adolescent Parent Education: Childrearing Family	Parenting Promotion Risk Identification Teaching: Safe Sex Teaching: Sexuality Teaching: Toddler Nutrition 13-18 Months Teaching: Toddler Nutrition 19-24 Months	Teaching: Toddler Nutrition 25-36 Months Teaching: Toddler Safety 13-18 Months Teaching: Toddler Safety 19-24 Months Teaching: Toddler Safety 25-36 Months Teaching: Toilet Training Vehicle Safety Promotion
Parenting Performance Definition: Parental actions to provide a child a nurturing and constructive physical, emotional, and social environment	Developmental Enhancement: Adolescent Developmental Enhancement: Child Parenting Promotion	Abuse Protection Support: Child Anxiety Reduction Coping Enhancement Counseling Crisis Intervention Decision-Making Support Emotional Support Family Integrity Promotion: Childbearing Family Family Process Maintenance	Guilt Work Facilitation Health System Guidance Home Maintenance Assistance Normalization Promotion Parent Education: Adolescent Parent Education: Childrearing Family Role Enhancement Self-Esteem Enhancement Socialization Enhancement Support System Enhancement
Role Performance Definition: Congruence of an individual's role behavior with role expectations	Parenting Promotion Role Enhancement	Attachment Promotion Behavior Modification Caregiver Support Childbirth Preparation Counseling Decision-Making Support Emotional Support	Family Integrity Promotion Family Therapy Self-Awareness Enhancement Self-Esteem Enhancement Support Group Support System Enhancement Values Clarification

NURSING DIAGNOSIS: Parenting, Impaired

Definition: Inability of the primary caretaker to create, maintain, or regain an environment that promotes the optimum growth and development of the child

NICS ASSOCIATED WITH DIAGNOSIS RELATED FACTORS

Anxiety Reduction
Behavior Management:
  Overactivity/
  Inattention
Behavior Management:
  Sexual
Behavior Modification:
  Social Skills
Conflict Mediation
Coping Enhancement

Decision-Making
  Support
Environmental
  Management: Safety
Family Involvement
  Promotion
Family Planning:
  Unintended
  Pregnancy
Family Support

Financial Resource
  Assistance
Mood Management
Parent Education:
  Adolescent
Parent Education:
  Childrearing Family
Parent Education:
  Infant
Prenatal Care

Self-Esteem
  Enhancement
Sleep Enhancement
Substance Use
  Prevention
Substance Use
  Treatment
Support System
  Enhancement
Values Clarification

NOC-NIC LINKAGES FOR PARENTING, IMPAIRED

Outcome	Major Interventions	Suggested Interventions	
Child Development: 1 Month Definition: Milestones of physical, cognitive, and psychosocial progression by 1 month of age **Child Development: 2 Months** Definition: Milestones of physical, cognitive, and psychosocial progression by 2 months of age	Attachment Promotion Parent Education: Infant	Abuse Protection Support: Child Anticipatory Guidance Bottle Feeding Breastfeeding Assistance Environmental Management: Attachment Process Family Integrity Promotion: Childbearing Family Family Involvement Promotion	Family Support Home Maintenance Assistance Infant Care Lactation Counseling Newborn Care Teaching: Infant Nutrition 0-3 Months Teaching: Infant Safety 0-3 Months Teaching: Infant Stimulation 0-4 Months
Child Development: 4 Months Definition: Milestones of physical, cognitive, and psycho-social progression by 4 months of age **Child Development: 6 Months** Definition: Milestones of physical, cognitive, and psycho-social progression by 6 months of age	Family Integrity Promotion: Childbearing Family Parent Education: Infant Parenting Promotion	Abuse Protection Support: Child Anticipatory Guidance Bottle Feeding Environmental Management: Safety Family Involvement Promotion Family Process Maintenance Health System Guidance Infant Care Lactation Counseling	Sibling Support Surveillance Sustenance Support Teaching: Infant Nutrition 4-6 Months Teaching: Infant Safety 4-6 Months Teaching: Infant Stimulation 0-4 Months Teaching: Infant Stimulation 5-8 Months

NOC-NIC LINKAGES FOR PARENTING, IMPAIRED		
Outcome	**Major Interventions**	**Suggested Interventions**
Child Development: 12 Months Definition: Milestones of physical, cognitive, and psychosocial progression by 12 months of age	Family Integrity Promotion: Childbearing Family Parenting Promotion	Abuse Protection Support: Child Anticipatory Guidance Developmental Enhancement: Child Environmental Management: Safety Family Process Maintenance Nutrition Management Parent Education: Childrearing Family Security Enhancement Sibling Support	Surveillance Sustenance Support Teaching: Infant Nutrition 10-12 Months Teaching: Infant Safety 10-12 Months Teaching: Toddler Nutrition 13-18 Months Teaching: Toddler Safety 13-18 Months Therapeutic Play
Child Development: 2 Years Definition: Milestones of physical, cognitive, and psychosocial progression by 2 years of age	Developmental Enhancement: Child Parenting Promotion	Abuse Protection Support: Child Bowel Training Environmental Management: Safety Family Integrity Promotion: Childbearing Family Family Process Maintenance Family Therapy Parent Education: Childrearing Family Security Enhancement Sibling Support	Surveillance Sustenance Support Teaching: Toddler Nutrition 19-24 Months Teaching: Toddler Nutrition 25-36 Months Teaching: Toddler Safety 19-24 Months Teaching: Toddler Safety 25-36 Months Teaching: Toilet Training
Child Development: 3 Years Definition: Milestones of physical, cognitive, and psychosocial progression by 3 years of age	Developmental Enhancement: Child Environmental Management: Safety Parenting Promotion	Abuse Protection Support: Child Behavior Management: Overactivity/ Inattention Family Integrity Promotion Family Process Maintenance Family Therapy Parent Education: Childrearing Family Security Enhancement	Sibling Support Surveillance Sustenance Support Teaching: Toddler Nutrition 25-36 Months Teaching: Toddler Safety 25-36 Months Teaching: Toilet Training

Continued

PART II - P

	NOC-NIC LINKAGES FOR PARENTING, IMPAIRED	
Outcome	**Major Interventions**	**Suggested Interventions**
Child Development: 4 Years Definition: Milestones of physical, cognitive, and psychosocial progression by 4 years of age	Developmental Enhancement: Child Parenting Promotion	Abuse Protection Support: Child Behavior Management: Overactivity/ Inattention Bowel Incontinence Care: Encopresis Environmental Management: Safety Family Integrity Promotion	Family Therapy Parent Education: Childrearing Family Security Enhancement Sibling Support Sustenance Support Therapeutic Play
Child Development: 5 Years Definition: Milestones of physical, cognitive, and psychosocial progression by 5 years of age	Developmental Enhancement: Child Parent Education: Childrearing Family Parenting Promotion	Abuse Protection Support: Child Behavior Management: Overactivity/ Inattention Bowel Incontinence Care: Encopresis Environmental Management: Safety Family Integrity Promotion	Family Therapy Security Enhancement Sibling Support Sustenance Support Therapeutic Play Urinary Incontinence Care: Enuresis
Child Development: Middle Childhood Definition: Milestones of physical, cognitive, and psychosocial progression from 6 years through 11 years of age	Developmental Enhancement: Child Parent Education: Childrearing Family Parenting Promotion	Abuse Protection Support: Child Family Integrity Promotion Family Therapy Mutual Goal Setting Sibling Support Spiritual Support	Sports-Injury Prevention: Youth Substance Use Prevention Sustenance Support Teaching: Individual Values Clarification
Child Development: Adolescence Definition: Milestones of physical, cognitive, and psychosocial progression from 12 years through 17 years of age	Developmental Enhancement: Adolescent Parent Education: Adolescent Parenting Promotion	Abuse Protection Support Family Integrity Promotion Family Involvement Promotion Family Process Maintenance Family Support Family Therapy Health System Guidance Mutual Goal Setting	Role Enhancement Spiritual Support Sports-Injury Prevention: Youth Substance Use Prevention Support System Enhancement Teaching: Individual Values Clarification

NOC-NIC LINKAGES FOR PARENTING, IMPAIRED			
Outcome	**Major Interventions**	**Suggested Interventions**	
Parent-Infant Attachment			
Definition: Parent and infant behaviors that demonstrate an enduring affectionate bond	Attachment Promotion Environmental Management: Attachment Process Kangaroo Care	Anticipatory Guidance Breastfeeding Assistance Emotional Support Family Integrity Promotion	Infant Care Intrapartal Care Lactation Counseling Parent Education: Infant
Parenting Performance			
Definition: Parental actions to provide a child with a nurturing and constructive physical, emotional, and social environment	Parenting Promotion Role Enhancement	Abuse Protection Support: Child Anticipatory Guidance Anxiety Reduction Breastfeeding Assistance Caregiver Support Coping Enhancement Counseling Developmental Enhancement: Adolescent Developmental Enhancement: Child Family Integrity Promotion Family Integrity Promotion: Childbearing Family Family Involvement Promotion	Family Process Maintenance Family Support Family Therapy Health System Guidance Home Maintenance Assistance Parent Education: Adolescent Parent Education: Childrearing Family Parent Education: Infant Prenatal Care Self-Esteem Enhancement Support Group Support System Enhancement Values Clarification
Parenting: Psychosocial Safety			
Definition: Parental actions to protect a child from social contacts that might cause harm or injury	Abuse Protection Support: Child Parenting Promotion Risk Identification: Childbearing Family	Counseling Developmental Enhancement: Adolescent Developmental Enhancement: Child Family Therapy Parent Education: Adolescent Parent Education: Childrearing Family Parent Education: Infant	Risk Identification Self-Modification Assistance Self-Responsibility Facilitation Substance Use Prevention Support Group Surveillance: Safety Trauma Therapy: Child

Continued

PART II - P

NOC-NIC LINKAGES FOR PARENTING, IMPAIRED		
Outcome	**Major Interventions**	**Suggested Interventions**

Role Performance
 	
Definition:
Congruence of an individual's role behavior with role expectations
	Parent Education:
	  Adolescent
	Parent Education:
	  Childrearing Family
	Parent Education:
	  Infant
	Role Enhancement
		Caregiver Support
		Childbirth Preparation
		Counseling
		Decision-Making
		  Support
		Emotional Support
		Family Integrity
		  Promotion
		Family Therapy
			Health Education
			Self-Awareness
			  Enhancement
			Self-Esteem
			  Enhancement
			Self-Modification
			  Assistance
			Self-Responsibility
			  Facilitation
			Support Group
			Support System
			  Enhancement

Safe Home Environment
 	
Definition:
Physical arrangements to minimize environmental factors that might cause physical harm or injury in the home
	Environmental
	  Management:
	  Safety
	Surveillance:
	  Safety
		Environmental
		  Management:
		  Violence Prevention
		Home Maintenance
		  Assistance
		Teaching: Infant Safety
		  0-3 Months
		Teaching: Infant Safety
		  4-6 Months
		Teaching: Infant Safety
		  7-9 Months
		Teaching: Infant Safety
		  10-12 Months
			Teaching: Toddler Safety
			  13-18 Months
			Teaching: Toddler Safety
			  19-24 Months
			Teaching: Toddler Safety
			  25-36 Months

Social Support
 	
Definition:
Reliable assistance from others
	Support Group
	Support System
	  Enhancement
		Caregiver Support
		Emotional Support
		Family Involvement
		  Promotion
		Family Support
			Financial Resource
			  Assistance
			Referral
			Spiritual Support
			Sustenance Support

NURSING DIAGNOSIS: Parenting, Readiness for Enhanced

Definition: A pattern of providing an environment for children or other dependent person(s) that is sufficient to nurture growth and development, and can be strengthened

NOC-NIC LINKAGES FOR PARENTING, READINESS FOR ENHANCED		
Outcome	**Major Interventions**	**Suggested Interventions**

Family Functioning
 	
Definition:
Capacity of the family system to meet the needs of its members during developmental transitions
	Family Integrity
	  Promotion
	Family Integrity
	  Promotion:
	  Childbearing Family
		Developmental
		  Enhancement:
		  Adolescent
		Developmental
		  Enhancement: Child
		Family Support
		Parent Education:
		  Adolescent
			Parent Education:
			  Childrearing Family
			Parenting Promotion
			Resiliency Promotion
			Support System
			  Enhancement

NOC-NIC LINKAGES FOR PARENTING, READINESS FOR ENHANCED		
Outcome	**Major Interventions**	**Suggested Interventions**
Knowledge: Child Physical Safety		
Definition: Extent of understanding conveyed about safely caring for a child from 1 year through 17 years of age	Teaching: Toddler Safety 13-18 Months Teaching: Toddler Safety 19-24 Months Teaching: Toddler Safety 25-36 Months	Environmental Management: Safety Learning Readiness Enhancement Parent Education: Childrearing Family / Sports-Injury Prevention: Youth Vehicle Safety Promotion
Knowledge: Infant Care		
Definition: Extent of understanding conveyed about caring for a baby from birth to first birthday	Parent Education: Infant	Anticipatory Guidance Childbirth Preparation Circumcision Care Lactation Counseling Environmental Management: Attachment Process Teaching: Infant Nutrition 0-3 Months Teaching: Infant Nutrition 4-6 Months Teaching: Infant Nutrition 7-9 Months Teaching: Infant Nutrition 10-12 Months Teaching: Infant Safety 0-3 Months / Teaching: Infant Safety 4-6 Months Teaching: Infant Safety 7-9 Months Teaching: Infant Safety 10-12 Months Teaching: Infant Stimulation 0-4 Months Teaching: Infant Stimulation 5-8 Months Teaching: Infant Stimulation 9-12 Months
Knowledge: Parenting		
Definition: Extent of understanding conveyed about provision of a nurturing and constructive environment for a child from 1 year through 17 years of age	Parent Education: Adolescent Parent Education: Childrearing Family	Abuse Protection Support: Child Environmental Management: Safety Nutritional Counseling Teaching: Group Teaching: Individual Teaching: Toddler Nutrition 13-18 Months Teaching: Toddler Nutrition 19-24 Months / Teaching: Toddler Nutrition 25-36 Months Teaching: Toddler Safety 13-18 Months Teaching: Toddler Safety 19-24 Months Teaching: Toddler Safety 25-36 Months Teaching: Toilet Training
Parenting: Adolescent Physical Safety		
Definition: Parental actions to prevent physical injury in an adolescent from 12 years through 17 years of age	Parent Education: Adolescent Parenting Promotion	Abuse Protection Support: Religious Environmental Management: Safety Sports-Injury Prevention: Youth / Substance Use Prevention Suicide Prevention Vehicle Safety Promotion

PART II - P

Continued

NOC-NIC LINKAGES FOR PARENTING, READINESS FOR ENHANCED		
Outcome	**Major Interventions**	**Suggested Interventions**
Parenting: Early/ Middle Childhood Physical Safety Definition: Parental actions to avoid physical injury of a child from 3 years through 11 years of age	Parent Education: 　Childrearing Family Parenting Promotion	Abuse Protection 　Support: Child Environmental 　Management: Safety Risk Identification	Sports-Injury Prevention: 　Youth Substance Use Prevention
Parenting: Infant/ Toddler Physical Safety Definition: Parental actions to avoid physical injury of a child from birth through 2 years of age	Parent Education: 　Infant Parenting Promotion	Abuse Protection 　Support: Child Environmental 　Management: Safety Teaching: Infant Safety 　0-3 Months Teaching: Infant Safety 　4-6 Months Teaching: Infant Safety 　7-9 Months Teaching: Infant Safety 　10-12 Months	Teaching: Toddler Safety 　13-18 Months Teaching: Toddler Safety 　19-24 Months
Parenting Performance Definition: Parental actions to provide a child with a nurturing and constructive physical, emotional, and social environment	Developmental 　Enhancement: 　Adolescent Development 　Enhancement: Child Parenting Promotion	Attachment Promotion Environmental 　Management: Safety Family Integrity 　Promotion Family Integrity 　Promotion: 　Childbearing Family	Resiliency Promotion Role Enhancement
Parenting: Psychosocial Safety Definition: Parental actions to protect a child from social contacts that might cause harm or injury	Parent Education: 　Adolescent Parent Education: 　Childrearing Family	Developmental 　Enhancement: 　Adolescent Developmental 　Enhancement: Child	Environmental 　Management: Safety Parenting Promotion Role Enhancement

NURSING DIAGNOSIS: Personal Identity, Disturbed

Definition: Inability to maintain an integrated and complete perception of self

NICS ASSOCIATED WITH DIAGNOSIS RELATED FACTORS			
Crisis Intervention	Developmental	Religious Addiction	Self-Esteem
Culture Brokerage	Enhancement:	Prevention	Enhancement
Dementia Management	Child	Relocation Stress	Substance Use
Developmental	Family Therapy	Reduction	Prevention
Enhancement:	Mood Management	Role Enhancement	Substance Use
Adolescent			Treatment

NOC-NIC LINKAGES FOR PERSONAL IDENTITY, DISTURBED			
Outcome	**Major Interventions**	**Suggested Interventions**	
Distorted Thought Self-Control			
Definition: Self-restraint of disruptions in perception, thought processes, and thought content	Delusion Management Hallucination Management	Anxiety Reduction Cognitive Restructuring Delirium Management Dementia Management	Environmental Management Medication Management Mood Management Reality Orientation
Identity			
Definition: Distinguishes between self and non-self and characterizes one's essence	Self-Awareness Enhancement Self-Esteem Enhancement	Behavior Modification: Social Skills Body Image Enhancement Cognitive Restructuring Complex Relationship Building Coping Enhancement Counseling Developmental Enhancement: Adolescent	Developmental Enhancement: Child Reality Orientation Sexual Counseling Socialization Enhancement Support Group Therapy Group Values Clarification
Sexual Identity			
Definition: Acknowledgement and acceptance of own sexual identity	Self-Awareness Enhancement Teaching: Sexuality	Cognitive Restructuring Complex Relationship Building Coping Enhancement Counseling Developmental Enhancement: Adolescent	Developmental Enhancement: Child Guilt Work Facilitation Sexual Counseling Socialization Enhancement Support System Enhancement Values Clarification

PART II - P

NURSING DIAGNOSIS: Post-Trauma Syndrome

Definition: Sustained maladaptive response to a traumatic, overwhelming event

NICS ASSOCIATED WITH DIAGNOSIS RELATED FACTORS

Abuse Protection
  Support
Abuse Protection
  Support: Child
Abuse Protection
  Support: Domestic
  Partner
Abuse Protection
  Support: Elder

Communicable
  Disease
  Management
Environmental
  Management: Safety
Environmental
  Management:
  Violence Prevention

Environmental
  Management: Worker
  Safety
Fall Prevention

Sports-Injury
  Prevention: Youth
Vehicle Safety
  Promotion

NOC-NIC LINKAGES FOR POST-TRAUMA SYNDROME

Outcome	Major Interventions	Suggested Interventions	
Abuse Recovery: Emotional			
Definition: Extent of healing of psychological injuries due to abuse	Counseling Support System Enhancement Therapy Group	Anger Control Assistance Anxiety Reduction Assertiveness Training Behavior Management: Self-Harm Coping Enhancement Emotional Support Family Support Forgiveness Facilitation Grief Work Facilitation Guilt Work Facilitation Impulse Control Training	Mood Management Security Enhancement Self-Esteem Enhancement Socialization Enhancement Spiritual Support Substance Use Prevention Suicide Prevention Support Group Trauma Therapy: Child Urinary Incontinence Care: Enuresis
Abuse Recovery: Financial			
Definition: Extent of control of monetary and legal matters following financial exploitation	Coping Enhancement Counseling Financial Resource Assistance	Assertiveness Training Decision-Making Support Patient Rights Protection Security Enhancement	Self-Efficacy Enhancement Self-Esteem Enhancement Support System Enhancement
Abuse Recovery: Sexual			
Definition: Extent of healing of physical and psychological injuries due to sexual abuse or exploitation	Counseling Rape-Trauma Treatment Therapy Group	Active Listening Anger Control Assistance Anxiety Reduction Assertiveness Training Behavior Management: Self-Harm Behavior Management: Sexual Emotional Support Family Support Forgiveness Facilitation Grief Work Facilitation Guilt Work Facilitation Hope Inspiration	Impulse Control Training Mood Management Self-Efficacy Enhancement Self-Esteem Enhancement Sexual Counseling Socialization Enhancement Spiritual Support Substance Use Prevention Suicide Prevention Support Group Support System Enhancement Trauma Therapy: Child

NOC-NIC LINKAGES FOR POST-TRAUMA SYNDROME		
Outcome	**Major Interventions**	**Suggested Interventions**
Anxiety Level Definition: Severity of manifested apprehension, tension, or uneasiness arising from an unidentifiable source	Anxiety Reduction	Abuse Protection Support Animal-Assisted Therapy Exercise Promotion Medication Management	Music Therapy Progressive Muscle Relaxation Relaxation Therapy Security Enhancement
Coping Definition: Personal actions to manage stressors that tax an individual's resources	Coping Enhancement Counseling	Anxiety Reduction Behavior Management: Self-Harm Emotional Support Grief Work Facilitation Hope Inspiration Mood Management	Sibling Support Socialization Enhancement Spiritual Support Support Group Support System Enhancement Trauma Therapy: Child
Depression Level Definition: Severity of melancholic mood and loss of interest in life events	Mood Management Suicide Prevention	Anger Control Assistance Animal-Assisted Therapy Anxiety Reduction Counseling Exercise Promotion Forgiveness Facilitation Grief Work Facilitation Guilt Work Facilitation Hope Inspiration	Medication Administration Milieu Therapy Patient Contracting Self-Esteem Enhancement Sleep Enhancement Socialization Enhancement Substance Use Prevention Weight Management
Fear Level Definition: Severity of manifested apprehension, tension, or uneasiness arising from an identifiable source	Anxiety Reduction Coping Enhancement	Calming Technique Crisis Intervention Emotional Support Environmental Management: Safety	Medication Management Security Enhancement Truth Telling Vital Signs Monitoring
Fear Level: Child Definition: Severity of manifested apprehension, tension, or uneasiness arising from an identifiable source in a child from 1 year through 17 years of age	Anxiety Reduction Trauma Therapy: Child	Abuse Protection Support: Child Animal-Assisted Therapy Art Therapy Calming Technique Distraction Emotional Support Environmental Management: Safety	Medication Administration Music Therapy Security Enhancement Therapeutic Play Truth Telling Vital Signs Monitoring

Continued

PART II - P

NOC-NIC LINKAGES FOR POST-TRAUMA SYNDROME			
Outcome	**Major Interventions**	**Suggested Interventions**	
Impulse Self-Control			
Definition: Self-restraint of compulsive or impulsive behaviors	Coping Enhancement Impulse Control Training	Behavior Management: Self-Harm Environmental Management: Safety Mutual Goal Setting Patient Contracting Risk Identification	Self-Awareness Enhancement Substance Use Prevention Suicide Prevention Support Group Support System Enhancement
Self-Mutilation Restraint			
Definition: Personal actions to refrain from intentional self-inflicted injury (nonlethal)	Behavior Management: Self-Harm Coping Enhancement	Anxiety Reduction Behavior Modification Cognitive Restructuring Counseling Environmental Management: Safety	Impulse Control Training Mutual Goal Setting Patient Contracting Self-Awareness Enhancement Surveillance: Safety

NURSING DIAGNOSIS: Power, Readiness for Enhanced

Definition: A pattern of participating knowingly in change that is sufficient for well-being and can be strengthened

NOC-NIC LINKAGES FOR POWER, READINESS FOR ENHANCED			
Outcome	**Major Interventions**	**Suggested Interventions**	
Health Beliefs: Perceived Control			
Definition: Personal conviction that one can influence a health outcome	Self-Efficacy Enhancement	Decision-Making Support Self-Esteem Enhancement	Self-Modification Assistance Self-Responsibility Facilitation
Health Promoting Behavior			
Definition: Personal actions to sustain or increase wellness	Self-Modification Assistance	Anxiety Reduction Energy Management Exercise Promotion Financial Resource Assistance Health Screening Immunization/ Vaccination Management Infection Protection Nutrition Management	Risk Identification Self-Efficacy Enhancement Self-Responsibility Facilitation Sleep Enhancement Socialization Enhancement Substance Use Prevention Support System Enhancement Weight Management

NOC-NIC LINKAGES FOR POWER, READINESS FOR ENHANCED			
Outcome	**Major Interventions**	**Suggested Interventions**	
Knowledge: Health Promotion Definition: Extent of understanding conveyed about information needed to obtain and maintain optimal health	Health Education	Exercise Promotion Genetic Counseling Health Literacy Enhancement Health Screening Learning Facilitation	Nutritional Counseling Risk Identification Substance Use Prevention Teaching: Individual Teaching: Prescribed Medication
Participation in Health Care Decisions Definition: Personal involvement in selecting and evaluating health care options to achieve desired outcome	Decision-Making Support Self-Responsibility Facilitation	Assertiveness Training Fiscal Resource Management Health Literacy Enhancement	Health System Guidance Mutual Goal Setting Self-Efficacy Enhancement
Personal Autonomy Definition: Personal actions of a competent individual to exercise governance in life decisions	Decision-Making Support	Abuse Protection Support Assertiveness Training	Conflict Mediation Self-Modification Assistance
Personal Resiliency Definition: Positive adaptation and function of an individual following significant adversity or crisis	Coping Enhancement Resiliency Promotion	Abuse Protection Support Anger Control Assistance Conflict Mediation Decision-Making Support Emotional Support Mood Management Risk Identification	Role Enhancement Self-Efficacy Enhancement Self-Esteem Enhancement Self-Responsibility Facilitation Substance Use Prevention Support Group Teaching: Safe Sex

PART II - P

NURSING DIAGNOSIS: Powerlessness

Definition: Perception that one's own action will not significantly affect an outcome; a perceived lack of control over a current situation or immediate happening

NICS ASSOCIATED WITH DIAGNOSIS RELATED FACTORS		
Assertiveness Training Behavior Modification	Behavior Modification: Social Skills Case Management	Health System Guidance Teaching: Procedure/Treatment

Continued

NOC-NIC LINKAGES FOR POWERLESSNESS		
Outcome	**Major Interventions**	**Suggested Interventions**
Depression Self-Control Definition: Personal actions to minimize melancholy and maintain interest in life events	Mood Management Self-Efficacy Enhancement	Activity Therapy Cognitive Restructuring Coping Enhancement Emotional Support Exercise Promotion Grief Work Facilitation Guilt Work Facilitation: Perinatal Death Health System Guidance Hope Inspiration Journaling Medication Management — Presence Risk Identification Self-Awareness Enhancement Self-Esteem Enhancement Sleep Enhancement Substance Use Prevention Support Group Teaching: Procedure/ Treatment Therapy Group Weight Management
Health Beliefs: Perceived Ability to Perform Definition: Personal conviction that one can carry out a given health behavior	Mutual Goal Setting Self-Efficacy Enhancement	Coping Enhancement Health System Guidance Hope Inspiration Patient Contracting Self-Awareness Enhancement — Self-Esteem Enhancement Self-Modification Assistance Teaching: Individual Values Clarification
Health Beliefs: Perceived Control Definition: Personal conviction that one can influence a health outcome	Decision-Making Support Self-Responsibility Facilitation	Assertiveness Training Culture Brokerage Patient Rights Protection Self-Esteem Enhancement — Self-Modification Assistance Teaching: Individual Values Clarification
Health Beliefs: Perceived Resources Definition: Personal conviction that one has adequate means to carry out a health behavior	Financial Resource Assistance Support System Enhancement	Culture Brokerage Health System Guidance Insurance Authorization — Patient Rights Protection Referral Sustenance Support
Participation in Health Care Decisions Definition: Personal involvement in selecting and evaluating health care options to achieve desired outcome	Decision-Making Support Health System Guidance Self-Responsibility Facilitation	Active Listening Admission Care Assertiveness Training Culture Brokerage — Discharge Planning Patient Rights Protection Values Clarification

NOC-NIC LINKAGES FOR POWERLESSNESS		
Outcome	**Major Interventions**	**Suggested Interventions**
Personal Autonomy Definition: Personal actions of a competent individual to exercise governance in life decisions	Decision-Making Support Patient Rights Protection	Assertiveness Training Culture Brokerage Health System Guidance Hope Inspiration	Mutual Goal Setting Self-Esteem Enhancement Self-Responsibility Facilitation

NURSING DIAGNOSIS: Protection, Ineffective

Definition: Decrease in the ability to guard the self from internal or external threats such as illness or injury

NICS ASSOCIATED WITH DIAGNOSIS RELATED FACTORS		
Infection Control Infection Control: Intraoperative	Infection Protection Nutrition Therapy	Nutritional Monitoring Substance Use Treatment

NOC-NIC LINKAGES FOR PROTECTION, INEFFECTIVE		
Outcome	**Major Interventions**	**Suggested Interventions**
Blood Coagulation Definition: Extent to which blood clots within normal period of time	Bleeding Precautions	Bleeding Reduction Blood Products Administration	Emergency Care Hemorrhage Control
Cognitive Orientation Definition: Ability to identify person, place, and time accurately	Reality Orientation	Anxiety Reduction Delirium Management Dementia Management	Dementia Management: Bathing Reminiscence Therapy
Fatigue Level Definition: Severity of observed or reported prolonged generalized fatigue	Energy Management	Mood Management Nutrition Management Pain Management	Self-Care Assistance Sleep Enhancement Teaching: Prescribed Activity/Exercise
Immune Status Definition: Natural and acquired appropriately targeted resistance to internal and external antigens	Infection Protection	Chemotherapy Management Energy Management Health Screening Immunization/Vaccination Management Infection Control Medication Management Pruritus Management	Radiation Therapy Management Respiratory Monitoring Risk Identification Skin Surveillance Teaching: Individual Teaching: Prescribed Medication Weight Management
Immunization Behavior Definition: Personal actions to obtain immunization to prevent a communicable disease	Immunization/ Vaccination Management Risk Identification	Health Education Health System Guidance	Parent Education: Infant Teaching: Individual

Continued

NOC-NIC LINKAGES FOR PROTECTION, INEFFECTIVE

Outcome	Major Interventions	Suggested Interventions	
Mobility Definition: Ability to move purposefully in own environment independently with or without assistive device	Exercise Therapy: Ambulation Exercise Therapy: Balance	Body Mechanics Promotion Exercise Promotion Exercise Promotion: Strength Training Exercise Promotion: Stretching	Exercise Therapy: Joint Mobility Exercise Therapy: Muscle Control Teaching: Prescribed Activity/Exercise
Neurological Status: Peripheral Definition: Ability of the peripheral nervous system to transmit impulses to and from the central nervous system	Peripheral Sensation Management	Exercise Promotion: Strength Training Exercise Therapy: Muscle Control Lower Extremity Monitoring	Pain Management Unilateral Neglect Management
Nutritional Status Definition: Extent to which nutrients are available to meet metabolic needs	Eating Disorders Management Nutritional Counseling	Diet Staging Enteral Tube Feeding Gastrointestinal Intubation Nutrition Management Nutrition Therapy Nutritional Monitoring	Prenatal Care Teaching: Prescribed Diet Total Parenteral Nutrition (TPN) Administration Weight Management
Respiratory Status Definition: Movement of air in and out of the lungs and exchange of carbon dioxide and oxygen at the alveolar level	Respiratory Monitoring Ventilation Assistance	Airway Management Anxiety Reduction Aspiration Precautions Chest Physiotherapy Cough Enhancement	Energy Management Mechanical Ventilation Management: Noninvasive Oxygen Therapy
Symptom Control Definition: Personal actions to minimize perceived adverse changes in physical and emotional functioning	Energy Management Infection Protection	Anxiety Reduction Bleeding Precautions Bleeding Reduction Diet Staging Exercise Promotion: Strength Training Exercise Therapy: Ambulation Fever Treatment Infection Control Nutritional Monitoring	Peripheral Sensation Management Pressure Ulcer Care Pressure Ulcer Prevention Pruritus Management Reality Orientation Respiratory Monitoring Temperature Regulation Ventilation Assistance Wound Care
Tissue Integrity: Skin & Mucous Membranes Definition: Structural intactness and normal physiological function of skin and mucous membranes	Pressure Management	Amputation Care Incision Site Care Lower Extremity Monitoring Pressure Ulcer Care Pressure Ulcer Prevention	Pruritus Management Skin Care: Donor Site Skin Care: Graft Site Skin Care: Topical Treatments Skin Surveillance

NOC-NIC LINKAGES FOR PROTECTION, INEFFECTIVE

Outcome	Major Interventions	Suggested Interventions
Wound Healing: Primary Intention Definition: Extent of regeneration of cells and tissues following intentional closure	Incision Site Care Wound Care	Amputation Care Infection Control: Intraoperative Skin Care: Donor Site Skin Care: Graft Site	Skin Surveillance Suturing Wound Care: Closed Drainage

---

NURSING DIAGNOSIS: Rape-Trauma Syndrome

Definition: Sustained maladaptive response to a forced, violent sexual penetration against the victim's will and consent

NICS ASSOCIATED WITH DIAGNOSIS RELATED FACTORS

Abuse Protection Support

Abuse Protection Support: Child

Abuse Protection Support: Domestic Partner

Abuse Protection Support: Elder

NOC-NIC LINKAGES FOR RAPE-TRAUMA SYNDROME

Outcome	Major Interventions	Suggested Interventions
Abuse Protection Definition: Protection of self and/or dependent others from abuse	Abuse Protection Support Abuse Protection Support: Child Abuse Protection Support: Domestic Partner Abuse Protection Support: Elder	Counseling Decision-Making Support Environmental Management: Safety Environmental Management: Violence Prevention Family Support	Risk Identification Security Enhancement Self-Efficacy Enhancement Support System Enhancement Surveillance: Safety
Abuse Recovery: Emotional Definition: Extent of healing of psychological injuries due to abuse	Counseling Therapy Group Trauma Therapy: Child	Anger Control Assistance Anxiety Reduction Assertiveness Training Behavior Management: Self-Harm Coping Enhancement Emotional Support Forgiveness Facilitation Grief Work Facilitation Impulse Control Training	Mood Management Security Enhancement Self-Esteem Enhancement Socialization Enhancement Substance Use Prevention Suicide Prevention Support Group Support System Enhancement
Abuse Recovery: Physical Definition: Extent of healing of physical injuries due to abuse	Health Screening Risk Identification	Body Image Enhancement Health Education Infection Control Medication Administration	Nutritional Monitoring Rape-Trauma Treatment Wound Care

Continued

NOC-NIC LINKAGES FOR RAPE-TRAUMA SYNDROME		
Outcome	**Major Interventions**	**Suggested Interventions**

Abuse Recovery: Sexual
 	
Definition:
Extent of healing of physical and psychological injuries due to sexual abuse or exploitation
	Therapy Group
	Trauma Therapy: Child
		Abuse Protection Support
		Active Listening
		Anger Control Assistance
		Anxiety Reduction
		Assertiveness Training
		Behavior Management:
		  Self-Harm
		Behavior Management: Sexual
		Decision-Making Support
		Eating Disorders Management
		Emotional Support
		Forgiveness Facilitation
		Grief Work Facilitation
		Guilt Work Facilitation
			Hope Inspiration
			Mood Management
			Relaxation Therapy
			Security Enhancement
			Self-Efficacy Enhancement
			Self-Esteem Enhancement
			Sexual Counseling
			Sleep Enhancement
			Substance Use Prevention
			Suicide Prevention
			Support Group
			Support System
			  Enhancement
			Therapeutic Play

Sexual Functioning
 	
Definition:
Integration of physical, socioemotional, and intellectual aspects of sexual expression and performance
	Behavior
	  Management:
	  Sexual
	Sexual Counseling
		Anxiety Reduction
		Forgiveness Facilitation
		Grief Work Facilitation
		Guilt Work Facilitation
		Impulse Control Training
			Self-Awareness
			  Enhancement
			Self-Esteem Enhancement
			Self-Modification
			  Assistance
			Self-Responsibility
			  Facilitation
			Substance Use Prevention

NURSING DIAGNOSIS: Relationship, Readiness for Enhanced

Definition: A pattern of mutual partnership that is sufficient to provide each other's needs and can be strengthened

NOC-NIC LINKAGES FOR RELATIONSHIP, READINESS FOR ENHANCED		
Outcome	**Major Interventions**	**Suggested Interventions**
Development: Late Adulthood Definition: Cognitive, psychosocial, and moral progression from 65 years of age and older	Role Enhancement	Anger Control Assistance Anxiety Reduction Conflict Mediation Counseling Grief Work Facilitation Humor Mood Management	Reminiscence Therapy Self-Modification Assistance Sexual Counseling Substance Use Prevention Teaching: Safe Sex Truth Telling Values Clarification
Development: Middle Adulthood Definition: Cognitive, psychosocial, and moral progression from 40 through 64 years of age	Role Enhancement	Conflict Mediation Counseling Family Support Forgiveness Facilitation Grief Work Facilitation Humor	Self-Modification Assistance Substance Use Prevention Sexual Counseling Truth Telling Values Clarification

NOC-NIC LINKAGES FOR RELATIONSHIP, READINESS FOR ENHANCED

Outcome	Major Interventions	Suggested Interventions	
Development: Young Adulthood			
Definition: Cognitive, psychosocial, and moral progression from 18 through 39 years of age	Role Enhancement	Conflict Mediation Counseling Family Support Forgiveness Facilitation Guilt Work Facilitation Self-Awareness Enhancement Self-Esteem Enhancement	Self-Modification Assistance Self-Responsibility Facilitation Substance Use Prevention Teaching: Sexuality Truth Telling Values Clarification
Role Performance			
Definition: Congruence of an individual's role behavior with role expectations	Role Enhancement	Conflict Mediation Counseling Family Integrity Promotion	Family Support Resiliency Promotion

Clinical reasoning note: The defining characteristics of the diagnosis indicate the relationship is between partners in a marital or intimate relationship. The outcomes are broader than the marital/intimate relationship, but the interventions have been selected, as much as possible, to suggest those most helpful in the marital relationship.

NURSING DIAGNOSIS: Religiosity, Impaired

Definition: Impaired ability to exercise reliance on beliefs and/or participate in rituals of a particular faith tradition

NICS ASSOCIATED WITH DIAGNOSIS RELATED FACTORS

Anxiety Reduction Coping Enhancement Crisis Intervention	Culture Brokerage Pain Management	Religious Ritual Enhancement Security Enhancement	Socialization Enhancement Support System Enhancement

NOC-NIC LINKAGES FOR RELIGIOSITY, IMPAIRED

Outcome	Major Interventions	Suggested Interventions	
Comfort Status: Psychospiritual			
Definition: Psychospiritual ease related to self-concept, emotional well-being, source of inspiration, and meaning and purpose in one's life	Anxiety Reduction Spiritual Support	Emotional Support Guilt Work Facilitation Religious Ritual Enhancement	Self-Awareness Enhancement Spiritual Growth Facilitation Values Clarification
Hope			
Definition: Optimism that is personally satisfying and life-supporting	Hope Inspiration Spiritual Support	Emotional Support Religious Ritual Enhancement Self-Awareness Enhancement Self-Efficacy Enhancement	Self-Esteem Enhancement Spiritual Growth Facilitation Values Clarification

Continued

PART II - R

NOC-NIC LINKAGES FOR RELIGIOSITY, IMPAIRED		
Outcome	**Major Interventions**	**Suggested Interventions**
Spiritual Health Definition: Connectedness with self, others, higher power, all life, nature, and the universe that transcends and empowers the self	Religious Ritual Enhancement Spiritual Support	Active Listening Decision-Making Support Guilt Work Facilitation Hope Inspiration　　　Meditation Facilitation 　　　Self-Awareness Enhancement 　　　Values Clarification

NURSING DIAGNOSIS: Religiosity, Readiness for Enhanced

Definition: Ability to increase reliance on religious beliefs and/or participate in rituals of a particular faith tradition

NOC-NIC LINKAGES FOR RELIGIOSITY, READINESS FOR ENHANCED		
Outcome	**Major Interventions**	**Suggested Interventions**
Hope Definition: Optimism that is personally satisfying and life-supporting	Hope Inspiration Spiritual Growth Facilitation	Religious Ritual Enhancement Self-Awareness Enhancement Self-Efficacy Enhancement　　　Self-Esteem Enhancement 　　　Spiritual Support 　　　Values Clarification
Spiritual Health Definition: Connectedness with self, others, higher power, all life, nature, and the universe that transcends and empowers the self	Religious Ritual Enhancement Spiritual Growth Facilitation	Decision-Making Support Forgiveness Facilitation Hope Inspiration Meditation Facilitation　　　Religious Addiction Prevention 　　　Spiritual Support 　　　Values Clarification

NURSING DIAGNOSIS: Relocation Stress Syndrome

Definition: Physiological and/or psychosocial disturbance following transfer from one environment to another

NICS ASSOCIATED WITH DIAGNOSIS RELATED FACTORS			
Coping Enhancement Counseling	Discharge Planning Grief Work Facilitation	Risk Identification Self-Efficacy Enhancement	Socialization Enhancement Support System Enhancement

NOC-NIC LINKAGES FOR RELOCATION STRESS SYNDROME		
Outcome	**Major Interventions**	**Suggested Interventions**
Anxiety Level Definition: Severity of manifested apprehension, tension, or uneasiness arising from an unidentifiable source	Anxiety Reduction Relocation Stress Reduction	Active Listening Anger Control Assistance Behavior Management Calming Technique Coping Enhancement Decision-Making Support Massage Mood Management Relaxation Therapy Security Enhancement Sleep Enhancement Spiritual Support Support Group Support System Enhancement Visitation Facilitation Vital Signs Monitoring
Child Adaptation to Hospitalization Definition: Adaptive response of a child from 3 years through 17 years of age to hospitalization	Security Enhancement Trauma Therapy: Child	Admission Care Anger Control Assistance Anticipatory Guidance Anxiety Reduction Calming Technique Coping Enhancement Emotional Support Environmental Management Family Involvement Promotion Patient Rights Protection Preparatory Sensory Information Presence Sibling Support Sleep Enhancement Support System Enhancement Teaching: Individual Therapeutic Play Truth Telling Visitation Facilitation
Coping Definition: Personal actions to manage stressors that tax an individual's resources	Coping Enhancement Relocation Stress Reduction	Active Listening Anger Control Assistance Anticipatory Guidance Anxiety Reduction Calming Technique Emotional Support Hope Inspiration Mood Management Music Therapy Relaxation Therapy Reminiscence Therapy Resiliency Promotion Self-Esteem Enhancement Sleep Enhancement Support Group Support System Enhancement Visitation Facilitation
Depression Level Definition: Severity of melancholic mood and loss of interest in life events	Hope Inspiration Mood Management	Activity Therapy Anger Control Assistance Animal-Assisted Therapy Counseling Emotional Support Exercise Promotion Guilt Work Facilitation Medication Management Nutritional Monitoring Self-Esteem Enhancement Sleep Enhancement Spiritual Support Support System Enhancement Weight Management

PART II - R

Continued

NOC-NIC LINKAGES FOR RELOCATION STRESS SYNDROME

Outcome	Major Interventions	Suggested Interventions	
Loneliness Severity			
Definition: Severity of emotional, social, or existential isolation response	Family Involvement Promotion Socialization Enhancement	Active Listening Activity Therapy Animal-Assisted Therapy Assertiveness Training Emotional Support Hope Inspiration Mood Management	Presence Recreation Therapy Sleep Enhancement Spiritual Support Support System Enhancement Visitation Facilitation
Psychosocial Adjustment: Life Change			
Definition: Adaptive psychosocial response of an individual to a significant life change	Coping Enhancement Relocation Stress Reduction	Active Listening Activity Therapy Anger Control Assistance Decision-Making Support Emotional Support Hope Inspiration	Mutual Goal Setting Resiliency Promotion Role Enhancement Self-Esteem Enhancement Socialization Enhancement Spiritual Support
Quality of Life			
Definition: Extent of positive perception of current life circumstances	Relocation Stress Reduction Values Clarification	Coping Enhancement Decision-Making Support Family Involvement Promotion Family Support Hope Inspiration Patient Rights Protection	Role Enhancement Security Enhancement Self-Esteem Enhancement Socialization Enhancement Spiritual Support Support System Enhancement
Stress Level			
Definition: Severity of manifested physical or mental tension resulting from factors that alter an existing equilibrium	Coping Enhancement Relocation Stress Reduction	Anger Control Assistance Anxiety Reduction Decision-Making Support Emotional Support Massage Mood Management Nausea Management	Relaxation Therapy Security Enhancement Sleep Enhancement Spiritual Support Substance Use Prevention Support System Enhancement

NURSING DIAGNOSIS: Resilience, Impaired Individual

Definition: Decreased ability to sustain a pattern of positive responses to an adverse situation or crisis

NICS ASSOCIATED WITH DIAGNOSIS RELATED FACTORS

Delusion Management Environmental Management: Violence Prevention	Family Planning: Contraception Hallucination Management Impulse Control Training	Parent Education: Adolescent Parent Education: Childrearing Family	Parenting Promotion Substance Use Prevention

NOC-NIC LINKAGES FOR RESILIENCE, IMPAIRED INDIVIDUAL		
Outcome	**Major Interventions**	**Suggested Interventions**
Coping		

Definition:
Personal actions to
  manage stressors that
  tax an individual's
  resources
	Coping Enhancement
	Resiliency Promotion
		Anxiety Reduction
		Crisis Intervention
		Mood Management
		Role Enhancement
			Self-Esteem
			  Enhancement
			Self-Modification
			  Assistance
			Substance Use
			  Prevention
			Support System
			  Enhancement

Depression Level		

Definition:
Severity of melancholic
  mood and loss of
  interest in life events
	Mood Management
	Resiliency Promotion
		Activity Therapy
		Anger Control
		  Assistance
		Guilt Work Facilitation
		Medication
		  Management
		Role Enhancement
			Self-Esteem
			  Enhancement
			Socialization
			  Enhancement
			Substance Use
			  Prevention
			Support System
			  Enhancement

Personal Resiliency		

Definition:
Positive adaptation and
  function of an
  individual following
  significant adversity
  or crisis
	Resiliency Promotion	Conflict Mediation
		Coping Enhancement
		Decision-Making
		  Support
		Emotional Support
		Mood Management
		Risk Identification
			Role Enhancement
			Self-Efficacy
			  Enhancement
			Self-Esteem
			  Enhancement
			Self-Responsibility
			  Facilitation
			Substance Use
			  Prevention
			Support Group

PART II - R

NURSING DIAGNOSIS: Resilience, Readiness for Enhanced

Definition: A pattern of positive responses to an adverse situation or crisis that can be strengthened to optimize human potential

NICS ASSOCIATED WITH DIAGNOSIS RELATED FACTORS			

Delusion Management
Environmental
  Management:
  Violence Prevention
	Family Planning:
	  Contraception
	Hallucination
	  Management
	Impulse Control
	  Training
		Parent Education:
		  Adolescent
		Parent Education:
		  Childrearing Family
			Parenting Promotion
			Substance Use
			  Prevention

Continued

NOC-NIC LINKAGES FOR RESILIENCE, READINESS FOR ENHANCED

Outcome	Major Interventions	Suggested Interventions	
Coping			
Definition: Personal actions to manage stressors that tax an individual's resources	Coping Enhancement Resiliency Promotion	Conflict Mediation Crisis Intervention Health System Guidance Role Enhancement	Self-Esteem Enhancement Self-Modification Assistance Socialization Enhancement Support System Enhancement
Personal Resiliency			
Definition: Positive adaptation and function of an individual following significant adversity or crisis	Resiliency Promotion	Conflict Mediation Coping Enhancement Decision-Making Support Risk Identification Role Enhancement	Self-Efficacy Enhancement Self-Esteem Enhancement Self-Responsibility Facilitation Support Group

NURSING DIAGNOSIS: Role Performance, Ineffective

Definition: Patterns of behavior and self-expression that do not match the environmental context, norms, and expectations

NICS ASSOCIATED WITH DIAGNOSIS RELATED FACTORS

Abuse Protection Support	Conflict Mediation	Health System Guidance	Self-Esteem Enhancement
Anxiety Reduction	Delusion Management	Mood Management	Support System Enhancement
Body Image Enhancement	Energy Management	Pain Management	Substance Use Treatment
Cognitive Stimulation			

NOC-NIC LINKAGES FOR ROLE PERFORMANCE, INEFFECTIVE

Outcome	Major Interventions	Suggested Interventions	
Caregiver Performance: Direct Care			
Definition: Provision by family care provider of appropriate personal and health care for a family member	Self-Efficacy Enhancement	Abuse Protection Support Chemotherapy Management Environmental Management: Safety Surveillance Teaching: Disease Process	Teaching: Prescribed Activity/Exercise Teaching: Prescribed Diet Teaching: Prescribed Medication Teaching: Procedure/ Treatment Teaching: Psychomotor Skill
Caregiver Performance: Indirect Care			
Definition: Arrangement and oversight by family care provider of appropriate care for a family member	Self-Efficacy Enhancement	Decision-Making Support Environmental Management: Safety Financial Resource Assistance Health Education	Health System Guidance Patient Rights Protection Supply Management Telephone Consultation

NOC-NIC LINKAGES FOR ROLE PERFORMANCE, INEFFECTIVE		
Outcome	**Major Interventions**	**Suggested Interventions**
Coping		
Definition: Personal actions to manage stressors that tax an individual's resources	Coping Enhancement Role Enhancement	Anticipatory Guidance Anxiety Reduction Counseling Decision-Making Support Mood Management	Spiritual Support Support Group Support System Enhancement Values Clarification
Depression Level		
Definition: Severity of melancholic mood and loss of interest in life events	Hope Inspiration Mood Management	Activity Therapy Animal-Assisted Therapy Cognitive Restructuring Counseling Energy Management Guilt Work Facilitation Medication Management Nutritional Monitoring Self-Awareness Enhancement Self-Esteem Enhancement	Sleep Enhancement Spiritual Support Substance Use Prevention Substance Use Treatment Suicide Prevention Support Group Support System Enhancement Therapy Group Weight Management
Parenting Performance		
Definition: Parental actions to provide a child with a nurturing and constructive physical, emotional, and social environment	Parenting Promotion Role Enhancement	Abuse Protection Support: Domestic Partner Coping Enhancement Environmental Management: Attachment Process Family Planning: Contraception	Health System Guidance Parent Education: Adolescent Parent Education: Childrearing Family Parent Education: Infant Support System Enhancement
Psychosocial Adjustment: Life Change		
Definition: Adaptive psychosocial response of an individual to a significant life change	Anticipatory Guidance Coping Enhancement	Abuse Protection Support Anxiety Reduction Counseling Decision-Making Support Emotional Support Mood Management	Mutual Goal Setting Role Enhancement Self-Esteem Enhancement Self-Responsibility Facilitation Socialization Enhancement Spiritual Support
Role Performance		
Definition: Congruence of an individual's role behavior with role expectations	Role Enhancement	Abuse Protection Support Anticipatory Guidance Anxiety Reduction Counseling Mood Management Resiliency Promotion	Self-Awareness Enhancement Self-Esteem Enhancement Support Group Support System Enhancement Teaching: Sexuality Values Clarification

PART II - R

NURSING DIAGNOSIS: Self-Care Deficit: Bathing

Definition: Impaired ability to perform or complete bathing/hygiene activities for self

NICS ASSOCIATED WITH DIAGNOSIS RELATED FACTORS			

Anxiety Reduction
Cognitive Stimulation
	Dementia Management
	Environmental
	  Management
		Exercise Promotion:
		  Strength Training
		Pain Management
			Self-Responsibility
			  Facilitation
			Unilateral Neglect
			  Management

NOC-NIC LINKAGES FOR SELF-CARE DEFICIT: BATHING		
Outcome	**Major Interventions**	**Suggested Interventions**

Self-Care: Bathing
Definition:
Ability to cleanse own
  body independently
  with or without
  assistive device
	Self-Care Assistance:
	  Bathing/Hygiene
		Bathing
		Dementia Management:
		  Bathing
		Ear Care
		Energy Management
		Environmental
		  Management: Comfort
		Environmental
		  Management: Safety
		Exercise Promotion
			Fall Prevention
			Foot Care
			Hair Care
			Nail Care
			Perineal Care
			Teaching: Individual

Self-Care: Hygiene
Definition:
Ability to maintain own
  personal cleanliness
  and kempt appear-
  ance independently
  with or without as-
  sistive device
	Self-Care Assistance:
	  Bathing/Hygiene
		Bathing
		Contact Lens Care
		Ear Care
		Energy Management
		Foot Care
		Hair Care
			Nail Care
			Oral Health Maintenance
			Oral Health Promotion
			Oral Health Restoration
			Perineal Care
			Teaching: Individual

Critical reasoning note: Self-Care: Hygiene has been included as an outcome because the NANDA-I definition for the diagnosis includes bathing/hygiene activities although they are not included in the defining characteristics. Self-Care Status could be an appropriate outcome to select when the patient has multiple self-care deficits. Any of the interventions suggested for the specific self-care deficits can be selected as appropriate for the particular patient problem.

NURSING DIAGNOSIS: Self-Care Deficit: Dressing

Definition: An impaired ability to perform or complete dressing and grooming activities for self

NICS ASSOCIATED WITH DIAGNOSIS RELATED FACTORS

Anxiety Reduction
Cognitive Stimulation
	Dementia Management
	Environmental
	  Management
		Exercise Promotion:
		  Strength Training
		Pain Management
			Self-Responsibility
			  Facilitation
			Sleep Enhancement

NOC-NIC LINKAGES FOR SELF-CARE DEFICIT: DRESSING

Outcome	Major Interventions	Suggested Interventions	

Self-Care: Dressing
Definition:
Ability to dress self
  independently
  with or without
  assistive device
	Self-Care Assistance:
	  Dressing/Grooming
		Communication
		  Enhancement:
		  Visual Deficit
		Energy Management
		Environmental
		  Management
		Environmental
		  Management: Comfort
			Environmental
			  Management: Safety
			Exercise Promotion
			Fall Prevention
			Self-Care Assistance
			Teaching: Individual

Clinical reasoning note: Self-Care Status could be an appropriate outcome to select when the patient has multiple self-care deficits. Any of the interventions suggested for the specific self-care deficits can be selected as appropriate for the particular patient problem.

NURSING DIAGNOSIS: Self-Care Deficit: Feeding

Definition: Impaired ability to perform or complete self-feeding activities

NICS ASSOCIATED WITH DIAGNOSIS RELATED FACTORS

Anxiety Reduction
Cognitive Stimulation
	Environmental
	  Management
	Exercise Promotion:
	  Strength Training
		Pain Management
		Self-Responsibility
		  Facilitation
			Sleep Enhancement
			Swallowing Therapy

NOC-NIC LINKAGES FOR SELF-CARE DEFICIT: FEEDING

Outcome	Major Interventions	Suggested Interventions	

Nutritional Status:
Food & Fluid Intake
Definition:
Amount of food and
  fluid taken into the
  body over a 24-hour
  period
	Nutritional
	  Monitoring
	Self-Care Assistance:
	  Feeding
		Enteral Tube Feeding
		Environmental
		  Management
		Feeding
		Fluid Management
		Fluid Monitoring
		Intravenous (IV)
		  Therapy
			Nutrition Management
			Oral Health Maintenance
			Swallowing Therapy
			Teaching: Individual
			Teaching: Prescribed Diet
			Total Parenteral
			  Nutrition (TPN)
			  Administration

Self-Care: Eating
Definition:
Ability to prepare and
  ingest food and fluid
  independently
  with or without
  assistive device
	Self-Care Assistance:
	  Feeding
		Aspiration Precautions
		Environmental
		  Management
		Family Involvement
		  Promotion
		Feeding
		Nutrition Management
			Nutritional Monitoring
			Oral Health Maintenance
			Positioning
			Swallowing Therapy

Continued

PART II - S

NOC-NIC LINKAGES FOR SELF-CARE DEFICIT: FEEDING		
Outcome	**Major Interventions**	**Suggested Interventions**
Swallowing Status Definition: Safe passage of fluids and/or solids from the mouth to the stomach	Self-Care Assistance: Feeding Swallowing Therapy	Aspiration Precautions Feeding Nutrition Management	Positioning Referral Teaching: Individual

Critical reasoning note: Swallowing Therapy is a possible intervention for the related factors neuromuscular and musculoskeletal impairment and is an intervention for the defining characteristic impaired ability to swallow food. Self-Care Status could be an appropriate outcome to select when the patient has multiple self-care deficits. Any of the interventions suggested for the specific self-care deficits can be selected as appropriate for the particular patient problem.

NURSING DIAGNOSIS: Self-Care Deficit: Toileting

Definition: Impaired ability to perform or complete toileting activities for self

NICS ASSOCIATED WITH DIAGNOSIS RELATED FACTORS			
Anxiety Reduction Cognitive Stimulation	Dementia Management Environmental Management	Exercise Promotion: Strength Training Pain Management	Self-Care Assistance: Transfer Self-Responsibility Facilitation

NOC-NIC LINKAGES FOR SELF-CARE DEFICIT: TOILETING		
Outcome	**Major Interventions**	**Suggested Interventions**
Ostomy Self-Care Definition: Personal actions to maintain ostomy for elimination	Ostomy Care	Bowel Irrigation Bowel Management Diarrhea Management Flatulence Reduction Incision Site Care Nutritional Counseling	Self-Care Assistance: Bathing/Hygiene Skin Care: Topical Treatments Skin Surveillance Teaching: Individual Teaching: Prescribed Diet Wound Care
Self-Care: Toileting Definition: Ability to toilet self independently with or without assistive device	Bowel Management Self-Care Assistance: Toileting	Bowel Incontinence Care: Encopresis Bowel Training Constipation/Impaction Management Exercise Promotion Medication Management	Perineal Care Prompted Voiding Skin Surveillance Urinary Elimination Management Urinary Incontinence Care

Clinical reasoning note: Self-Care Status could be an appropriate outcome to select when the patient has multiple self-care deficits. Any of the interventions suggested for the specific self-care deficits can be selected as appropriate for the particular patient problem.

NURSING DIAGNOSIS: Self-Care, Readiness for Enhanced

Definition: A pattern of performing activities for oneself that helps to meet health-related goals and can be strengthened

NOC-NIC LINKAGES FOR SELF-CARE, READINESS FOR ENHANCED		
Outcome	**Major Interventions**	**Suggested Interventions**
Discharge Readiness: Independent Living Definition: Readiness of a patient to relocate from a health care institution to living independently	Discharge Planning	Financial Resource Assistance Health Education Self-Care Assistance Self-Care Assistance: IADL	Support System Enhancement Teaching: Disease Process Teaching: Prescribed Medication Teaching: Procedure/ Treatment
Self-Care Status Definition: Ability to perform personal care activities and instrumental activities of daily living	Self-Efficacy Enhancement Teaching: Individual	Self-Care Assistance Self-Care Assistance: IADL Teaching: Prescribed Activity/Exercise	Teaching: Prescribed Diet Teaching: Prescribed Medication Teaching: Procedure/ Treatment
Self-Care: Activities of Daily Living (ADL) Definition: Ability to perform the most basic physical tasks and personal care activities independently with or without assistive device	Self-Efficacy Enhancement Teaching: Individual	Self-Care Assistance	Teaching: Prescribed Activity/Exercise
Self-Care: Instrumental Activities of Daily Living (IADL) Definition: Ability to perform activities needed to function in the home or community independently with or without assistive device	Environmental Management: Home Preparation Self-Efficacy Enhancement	Exercise Promotion Health Literacy Enhancement Home Maintenance Assistance Self-Care Assistance: IADL	Teaching: Individual Teaching: Prescribed Diet Teaching: Prescribed Medication Teaching: Psychomotor Skill
Self-Care: Non-Parenteral Medication Definition: Ability to administer oral and topical medications to meet therapeutic goals independently with or without assistive device	Self-Efficacy Enhancement Teaching: Prescribed Medication	Medication Administration: Ear Medication Administration: Eye Medication Administration: Nasal	Medication Administration: Oral Medication Administration: Skin Medication Administration: Vaginal

Continued

PART II - S

NOC-NIC LINKAGES FOR SELF-CARE, READINESS FOR ENHANCED

Outcome	Major Interventions	Suggested Interventions	
Self-Care: Parenteral Medication Definition: Ability to administer parenteral medications to meet therapeutic goals independently with or without assistive device	Self-Efficacy Enhancement Teaching: Prescribed Medication	Medication Administration: Intradermal Medication Administration: Intramuscular (IM) Medication Administration: Intravenous (IV)	Medication Administration: Subcutaneous

NURSING DIAGNOSIS: Self-Concept, Readiness for Enhanced

Definition: A pattern of perceptions or ideas about the self that is sufficient for well-being and can be strengthened

NOC-NIC LINKAGES FOR SELF-CONCEPT, READINESS FOR ENHANCED

Outcome	Major Interventions	Suggested Interventions	
Body Image Definition: Perception of own appearance and body functions	Body Image Enhancement	Coping Enhancement Developmental Enhancement: Adolescent Developmental Enhancement: Child	Ostomy Care Self-Awareness Enhancement Self-Esteem Enhancement Weight Management
Personal Well-Being Definition: Extent of positive perception of one's health status	Self-Awareness Enhancement Self-Esteem Enhancement	Coping Enhancement Decision-Making Support Exercise Promotion Hope Inspiration Learning Facilitation Meditation Facilitation Progressive Muscle Relaxation	Recreation Therapy Role Enhancement Self-Modification Assistance Self-Responsibility Facilitation Socialization Enhancement Spiritual Growth Facilitation
Self-Esteem Definition: Personal judgment of self-worth	Self-Awareness Enhancement Self-Esteem Enhancement	Assertive Training Body Image Enhancement Body Mechanics Promotion Developmental Enhancement: Adolescent	Developmental Enhancement: Child Role Enhancement Weight Management

NURSING DIAGNOSIS: Self-Esteem: Chronic Low

Definition: Long-standing negative self-evaluating/feelings about self or self-capabilities

NICS ASSOCIATED WITH DIAGNOSIS RELATED FACTORS

Abuse Protection Support	Parent Education: Adolescent	Recreation Therapy	Socialization Enhancement
Culture Brokerage	Parent Education: Childrearing Family	Religious Addiction Prevention	Support System Enhancement
Grief Work Facilitation	Parenting Promotion	Self-Awareness Enhancement	Trauma Therapy: Child
Grief Work Facilitation: Perinatal Death			

NOC-NIC LINKAGES FOR SELF-ESTEEM: CHRONIC LOW

Outcome	Major Interventions	Suggested Interventions	
Depression Level Definition: Severity of melancholic mood and loss of interest in life events	Hope Inspiration Mood Management	Behavior Management: Self-Harm Counseling Crisis Intervention Emotional Support Grief Work Facilitation Guilt Work Facilitation Milieu Therapy Self-Awareness Enhancement Self-Esteem Enhancement	Self-Modification Assistance Spiritual Support Substance Use Prevention Suicide Prevention Support Group Support System Enhancement Therapeutic Play Therapy Group
Self-Esteem Definition: Personal judgment of self-worth	Self-Esteem Enhancement	Activity Therapy Assertiveness Training Body Image Enhancement Cognitive Restructuring Complex Relationship Building Coping Enhancement Counseling Developmental Enhancement: Adolescent Developmental Enhancement: Child	Emotional Support Guilt Work Facilitation Resiliency Promotion Role Enhancement Self-Awareness Enhancement Self-Efficacy Enhancement Socialization Enhancement Spiritual Support Support System Enhancement

PART II - S

NURSING DIAGNOSIS: Self-Esteem: Situational Low

Definition: Development of a negative perception of self-worth in response to a current situation (specify)

NICS ASSOCIATED WITH DIAGNOSIS RELATED FACTORS			
Body Image Enhancement Developmental Enhancement: Adolescent	Developmental Enhancement: Child Grief Work Facilitation	Grief Work Facilitation: Perinatal Death Relocation Stress Reduction	Role Enhancement Values Clarification

NOC-NIC LINKAGES FOR SELF-ESTEEM: SITUATIONAL LOW		
Outcome	**Major Interventions**	**Suggested Interventions**
Adaptation to Physical Disability Definition: Adaptive response to a significant functional challenge due to a physical disability	Body Image Enhancement Self-Esteem Enhancement	Amputation Care Anxiety Reduction Coping Enhancement Counseling Emotional Support Grief Work Facilitation — Resiliency Promotion Risk Identification Role Enhancement Self-Efficacy Enhancement Support System Enhancement
Grief Resolution Definition: Adjustment to actual or impending loss	Grief Work Facilitation Grief Work Facilitation: Perinatal Death	Active Listening Coping Enhancement Counseling Emotional Support — Hope Inspiration Spiritual Support Support Group
Personal Resiliency Definition: Positive adaptation and function of an individual following significant adversity or crisis	Resiliency Promotion Self-Esteem Enhancement	Abuse Protection Support Behavior Modification Coping Enhancement Crisis Intervention Decision-Making Support — Mood Management Self-Awareness Enhancement Self-Efficacy Enhancement Support Group
Psychosocial Adjustment: Life Change Definition: Adaptive psychosocial response of an individual to a significant life change	Anticipatory Guidance Coping Enhancement	Counseling Decision-Making Support Emotional Support Mutual Goal Setting Recreation Therapy — Resiliency Promotion Role Enhancement Self-Esteem Enhancement Support System Enhancement
Self-Esteem Definition: Personal judgment of self-worth	Coping Enhancement Self-Esteem Enhancement	Active Listening Assertiveness Training Cognitive Restructuring Counseling Crisis Intervention Emotional Support Grief Work Facilitation — Guilt Work Facilitation Resiliency Promotion Self-Awareness Enhancement Socialization Enhancement Spiritual Support Support Group

NURSING DIAGNOSIS: Self-Health Management, Ineffective

Definition: Pattern of regulating and integrating into daily living a therapeutic regimen for treatment of illness and the sequelae of illness that is unsatisfactory for meeting specific health goals

NICS ASSOCIATED WITH DIAGNOSIS RELATED FACTORS			
Childbirth Preparation Developmental Care	Family Involvement Promotion	Lactation Counseling	Parent Education: Infant

NOC-NIC LINKAGES FOR SELF-HEALTH MANAGEMENT, INEFFECTIVE		
Outcome	**Major Interventions**	**Suggested Interventions**
Alcohol Abuse Cessation Behavior Definition: Personal actions to eliminate alcohol use that pose a threat to health	Self-Modification Assistance Substance Use Treatment	Behavior Modification Coping Enhancement Counseling Family Involvement Promotion Health Screening Medication Management Self-Awareness Enhancement · · · Self-Efficacy Enhancement Self-Responsibility Facilitation Substance Use Treatment: Alcohol Withdrawal Support Group Teaching: Disease Process
Asthma Self-Management Definition: Personal actions to prevent or reverse inflammatory condition resulting in bronchial constriction of the airways	Asthma Management Teaching: Disease Process	Energy Management Environmental Management: Safety Infection Protection Medication Administration: Inhalation Medication Administration: Oral Medication Management Self-Efficacy Enhancement · · · Self-Modification Assistance Support Group Teaching: Prescribed Activity/Exercise Teaching: Prescribed Diet Teaching: Prescribed Medication
Blood Glucose Level Definition: Extent to which glucose levels in plasma and urine are maintained in normal range	Bedside Laboratory Testing Laboratory Data Interpretation	Capillary Blood Sample · · · Teaching: Psychomotor Skill
Cardiac Disease Self-Management Definition: Personal actions to manage heart disease, its treatment, and prevent disease progression	Teaching: Disease Process Teaching: Prescribed Activity/Exercise Teaching: Prescribed Diet Teaching: Prescribed Medication	Cardiac Care: Rehabilitative Cardiac Precautions Energy Management Exercise Promotion Immunization/Vaccination Management Medication Management Nutrition Management · · · Self-Efficacy Enhancement Self-Modification Assistance Sexual Counseling Smoking Cessation Assistance Vital Signs Monitoring Weight Management

Continued

PART II - S

NOC-NIC LINKAGES FOR SELF-HEALTH MANAGEMENT, INEFFECTIVE

Outcome	Major Interventions	Suggested Interventions	
Compliance Behavior Definition: Personal actions to promote wellness, recovery, and rehabilitation recommended by a health professional	Self-Efficacy Enhancement Self-Responsibility Facilitation Teaching: Procedure/ Treatment	Behavior Modification Bibliotherapy Coping Enhancement Counseling Culture Brokerage Emotional Support Family Involvement Promotion Family Mobilization Financial Resource Assistance Health Literacy Enhancement Health System Guidance Learning Facilitation Learning Readiness Enhancement	Mutual Goal Setting Nutritional Counseling Risk Identification Support System Enhancement Teaching: Disease Process Teaching: Prescribed Activity/Exercise Teaching: Prescribed Diet Teaching: Prescribed Medication Teaching: Psychomotor Skill Telephone Consultation Telephone Follow-up Values Clarification
Compliance Behavior: Prescribed Diet Definition: Personal actions to follow food and fluid intake recommended by a health professional for a specific health condition	Nutritional Counseling Teaching: Prescribed Diet	Behavior Modification Culture Brokerage Health System Guidance Learning Readiness Enhancement	Nutritional Monitoring Self-Efficacy Enhancement Self-Responsibility Facilitation Support System Enhancement
Compliance Behavior: Prescribed Medication Definition: Personal actions to administer medication safely to meet therapeutic goals as recommended by a health professional	Teaching: Prescribed Medication	Hormone Replacement Therapy Learning Readiness Enhancement Medication Administration Medication Administration: Intramuscular (IM) Medication Administration: Intravenous (IV)	Medication Administration: Skin Medication Administration: Subcutaneous Medication Management Self-Efficacy Enhancement Self-Responsibility Facilitation Teaching: Psychomotor Skill

NOC-NIC LINKAGES FOR SELF-HEALTH MANAGEMENT, INEFFECTIVE		
Outcome	**Major Interventions**	**Suggested Interventions**
Diabetes Self-Management Definition: Personal actions to manage diabetes mellitus, its treatment, and prevent disease progression	Teaching: Disease Process Teaching: Prescribed Diet Teaching: Prescribed Medication Teaching: Procedure/Treatment	Hyperglycemia Management Hypoglycemia Management Immunization/Vaccination Management Infection Protection Medication Administration: Intradermal Medication Administration: Oral Medication Management Nutrition Management Nutritional Counseling	Preconception Counseling Self-Efficacy Enhancement Self-Modification Assistance Self-Responsibility Facilitation Teaching: Foot Care Teaching: Group Teaching: Individual Teaching: Psychomotor Skill
Drug Abuse Cessation Behavior Definition: Personal actions to eliminate drug use that poses a threat to health	Self-Awareness Enhancement Self-Modification Assistance Substance Use Treatment	Behavior Modification Coping Enhancement Counseling Family Involvement Promotion Health Screening Medication Management	Self-Efficacy Enhancement Self-Responsibility Facilitation Substance Use Treatment: Drug Withdrawal Support Group
Health Beliefs: Perceived Control Definition: Personal conviction that one can influence a health outcome	Decision-Making Support Self-Efficacy Enhancement	Assertiveness Training Cognitive Restructuring Coping Enhancement Counseling	Journaling Learning Facilitation Self-Responsibility Facilitation
Medication Response Definition: Therapeutic and adverse effects of prescribed medication	Teaching: Individual Teaching: Prescribed Medication	Allergy Management Asthma Management Chemotherapy Management Health Education Hormone Replacement Therapy	Learning Readiness Enhancement Medication Administration Medication Management Teaching: Disease Process

Continued

NOC-NIC LINKAGES FOR SELF-HEALTH MANAGEMENT, INEFFECTIVE

Outcome	Major Interventions	Suggested Interventions	
Multiple Sclerosis Self-Management Definition: Personal actions to manage multiple sclerosis and prevent disease progression	Teaching: Disease Process Teaching: Prescribed Activity/Exercise Teaching: Prescribed Diet Teaching: Prescribed Medication	Bowel Management Decision-Making Support Energy Management Exercise Promotion Immunization/ Vaccination Management Medication Administration: Intramuscular (IM)	Medication Administration: Oral Medication Management Self-Efficacy Enhancement Self-Modification Assistance Support Group Urinary Elimination Management
Participation in Health Care Decisions Definition: Personal involvement in selecting and evaluating health care options to achieve desired outcome	Decision-Making Support Health System Guidance	Active Listening Assertiveness Training Behavior Modification Bibliotherapy Coping Enhancement Counseling Culture Brokerage Discharge Planning	Family Involvement Promotion Health Care Information Exchange Patient Rights Protection Referral Self-Responsibility Facilitation Telephone Consultation Values Clarification
Postpartum Maternal Health Behavior Definition: Personal actions to promote health of a mother in the period following birth of an infant	Postpartal Care	Anticipatory Guidance Anxiety Reduction Attachment Promotion Cesarean Section Care Energy Management Exercise Promotion Family Integrity Promotion: Childbearing Family Family Planning: Contraception Fluid Monitoring	Infection Protection Mood Management Nutritional Counseling Nutritional Monitoring Pain Management Pelvic Muscle Exercise Perineal Care Sexual Counseling Sleep Enhancement Support Group
Prenatal Health Behavior Definition: Personal actions to promote a healthy pregnancy and a healthy newborn	Prenatal Care	Abuse Protection Support: Domestic Partner Body Mechanics Promotion Environmental Management: Safety Exercise Promotion Medication Management Nutrition Management	Oral Health Promotion Sexual Counseling Substance Use Prevention Substance Use Treatment Vehicle Safety Promotion Weight Management

NOC-NIC LINKAGES FOR SELF-HEALTH MANAGEMENT, INEFFECTIVE

Outcome	Major Interventions	Suggested Interventions	
Seizure Control Definition: Personal actions to reduce or minimize the occurrence of seizure episodes	Medication Management Teaching: Prescribed Medication	Anxiety Reduction Environmental Management: Safety Risk Identification Role Enhancement	Sleep Enhancement Socialization Enhancement Teaching: Prescribed Activity/Exercise
Self-Care: Non-Parenteral Medication Definition: Ability to administer oral and topical medications to meet therapeutic goals independently with or without assistive device	Self-Care Assistance Teaching: Prescribed Medication	Learning Facilitation Medication Administration: Ear Medication Administration: Enteral Medication Administration: Eye Medication Administration: Inhalation Medication Administration: Nasal Medication Administration: Oral	Medication Administration: Rectal Medication Administration: Skin Medication Administration: Vaginal Self-Efficacy Enhancement Skin Care: Topical Treatments
Self-Care: Parenteral Medication Definition: Ability to administer parenteral medications to meet therapeutic goals independently with or without assistive device	Teaching: Prescribed Medication Teaching: Psychomotor Skill	Learning Facilitation Medication Administration: Intradermal Medication Administration: Intramuscular (IM) Medication Administration: Intravenous (IV) Medication Administration: Subcutaneous	Patient-Controlled Analgesia (PCA) Assistance Self-Efficacy Enhancement Self-Responsibility Facilitation Teaching: Disease Process
Smoking Cessation Behavior Definition: Personal actions to eliminate tobacco use	Smoking Cessation Assistance	Coping Enhancement Counseling Health Screening Medication Management Self-Awareness Enhancement	Self-Efficacy Enhancement Self-Modification Assistance Self-Responsibility Facilitation Support Group Support System Enhancement

Continued

PART II - S

NOC-NIC LINKAGES FOR SELF-HEALTH MANAGEMENT, INEFFECTIVE

Outcome	Major Interventions	Suggested Interventions	
Symptom Control Definition: Personal actions to minimize perceived adverse changes in physical and emotional functioning	Self-Modification Assistance Teaching: Disease Process	Active Listening Behavior Modification Coping Enhancement Crisis Intervention Exercise Promotion	Financial Resource Assistance Nutritional Counseling Self-Responsibility Facilitation Teaching: Prescribed Activity/Exercise Teaching: Prescribed Medication
Systemic Toxin Clearance: Dialysis Definition: Clearance of toxins from the body with peritoneal dialysis or hemodialysis	Hemodialysis Therapy Peritoneal Dialysis Therapy	Acid-Base Management Acid-Base Monitoring Electrolyte Management Electrolyte Management: Hypercalcemia Electrolyte Management: Hyperkalemia Electrolyte Management: Hypermagnesemia Electrolyte Management: Hypernatremia	Electrolyte Management: Hyperphosphatemia Electrolyte Monitoring Fluid/Electrolyte Management Laboratory Data Interpretation Teaching: Procedure/Treatment Teaching: Psychomotor Skill Vital Signs Monitoring
Treatment Behavior: Illness or Injury Definition: Personal actions to palliate or eliminate pathology	Self-Responsibility Facilitation Teaching: Disease Process Teaching: Procedure/Treatment	Behavior Modification Coping Enhancement Emotional Support Family Involvement Promotion Learning Facilitation Mutual Goal Setting Support Group Support System Enhancement	Teaching: Individual Teaching: Prescribed Activity/Exercise Teaching: Prescribed Diet Teaching: Prescribed Medication Teaching: Psychomotor Skill Telephone Consultation Telephone Follow-up

Critical reasoning note: Although the diagnosis does not address specific health conditions, we have provided both general outcomes related to health behaviors and outcomes for specific health problems.

NURSING DIAGNOSIS: Self Health Management, Readiness for Enhanced

Definition: A pattern of regulating and integrating into daily living a therapeutic regimen for treatment of illness and its sequelae that is sufficient for meeting health-related goals and can be strengthened

NOC-NIC LINKAGES FOR SELF HEALTH MANAGEMENT, READINESS FOR ENHANCED

Outcome	Major Interventions	Suggested Interventions	
Adherence Behavior Definition: Self-initiated actions to promote optimal wellness, recovery, and rehabilitation	Health Education Health System Guidance	Decision-Making Support Learning Facilitation Learning Readiness Enhancement	Self-Efficacy Enhancement Self-Modification Assistance Smoking Cessation Assistance
Compliance Behavior Definition: Personal actions to promote wellness, recovery, and rehabilitation recommended by a health professional	Mutual Goal Setting Self-Modification Assistance	Culture Brokerage Health System Guidance Learning Facilitation Learning Readiness Enhancement Nutritional Counseling Patient Rights Protection	Self-Efficacy Enhancement Teaching: Individual Teaching: Prescribed Activity/Exercise Teaching: Prescribed Diet Teaching: Prescribed Medication Telephone Consultation
Health Orientation Definition: Personal commitment to health behaviors as lifestyle priorities	Health Education	Culture Brokerage Mutual Goal Setting Risk Identification	Role Enhancement Self-Responsibility Facilitation Values Clarification
Knowledge: Treatment Regimen Definition: Extent of understanding conveyed about a specific treatment regimen	Teaching: Individual Teaching: Procedure/Treatment	Learning Facilitation Learning Readiness Enhancement Nutritional Counseling Teaching: Disease Process Teaching: Group	Teaching: Prescribed Activity/Exercise Teaching: Prescribed Diet Teaching: Prescribed Medication Teaching: Psychomotor Skill
Participation in Health Care Decisions Definition: Personal involvement in selecting and evaluating health care options to achieve desired outcome	Decision-Making Support Health System Guidance	Assertiveness Training Culture Brokerage Family Involvement Promotion	Mutual Goal Setting Self-Responsibility Facilitation

PART II - S

Continued

NOC-NIC LINKAGES FOR SELF HEALTH MANAGEMENT, READINESS FOR ENHANCED

Outcome	Major Interventions	Suggested Interventions	

Risk Control
Definition: Personal actions to prevent, eliminate, or reduce modifiable health threats
	Health Education
	Risk Identification
		Health Screening
		Immunization/
		  Vaccination
		  Management
		Infection Control
			Surveillance
			Surveillance:
			  Late Pregnancy
			Surveillance: Safety

Treatment Behavior: Illness or Injury
Definition: Personal actions to palliate or eliminate pathology
	Anticipatory Guidance
	Self-Modification
	  Assistance
		Decision-Making
		  Support
		Infection Protection
		Learning Readiness
		  Enhancement
		Nutritional Counseling
		Self-Efficacy
		  Enhancement
		Self-Responsibility
		  Facilitation
			Teaching: Disease
			  Process
			Teaching: Prescribed
			  Activity/Exercise
			Teaching: Prescribed
			  Diet
			Teaching: Prescribed
			  Medication
			Teaching: Procedure/
			  Treatment
			Teaching: Psychomotor
			  Skill

NURSING DIAGNOSIS: Self-Mutilation

Definition: Deliberate self-injurious behavior causing tissue damage with the intent of causing nonfatal injury to attain relief of tension

NICS ASSOCIATED WITH DIAGNOSIS RELATED FACTORS

Abuse Protection
  Support: Child
Anxiety Reduction
Behavior Management:
  Social Skills
Body Image
  Enhancement
	Cognitive
	  Restructuring
	Coping Enhancement
	Counseling
		Eating Disorders
		  Management
		Family Therapy
		Impulse Control
		  Training
			Self-Esteem
			  Enhancement
			Substance Use
			  Treatment
			Therapy Group

NOC-NIC LINKAGES FOR SELF-MUTILATION

Outcome	Major Interventions	Suggested Interventions	

Identity
Definition:
Distinguishes between self and non-self and characterizes one's essence
	Cognitive
	  Restructuring
	Self-Awareness
	  Enhancement
		Body Image
		  Enhancement
		Counseling
		Delusion Management
		Developmental
		  Enhancement:
		  Adolescent
			Developmental
			  Enhancement: Child
			Hallucination
			  Management
			Self-Esteem
			  Enhancement
			Socialization
			  Enhancement
			Values Clarification

NOC-NIC LINKAGES FOR SELF-MUTILATION

Outcome	Major Interventions	Suggested Interventions	
Impulse Self-Control Definition: Self-restraint of compulsive or impulsive behaviors	Impulse Control Training Limit Setting Patient Contracting	Anger Control Assistance Anxiety Reduction Area Restriction Behavior Management Behavior Management: Self-Harm Behavior Modification Environmental Management: Safety	Environmental Management: Violence Prevention Milieu Therapy Seclusion Self-Modification Assistance Self-Responsibility Facilitation
Self-Mutilation Restraint Definition: Personal actions to refrain from intentional self-inflicted injury (nonlethal)	Behavior Management: Self-Harm Impulse Control Training Wound Care	Activity Therapy Anger Control Assistance Animal-Assisted Therapy Anxiety Reduction Area Restriction Behavior Management Behavior Modification Calming Technique Chemical Restraint Counseling Environmental Management: Safety	Family Therapy Limit Setting Medication Administration Mutual Goal Setting Patient Contracting Physical Restraint Risk Identification Self-Responsibility Facilitation Surveillance: Safety Suicide Prevention Therapy Group

PART II - S

NURSING DIAGNOSIS: Self-Neglect

Definition: A constellation of culturally framed behaviors involving one or more self-care activities in which there is a failure to maintain a socially accepted standard of health and well-being

NICS ASSOCIATED WITH DIAGNOSIS RELATED FACTORS

Anxiety Reduction Behavior Management	Behavior Modification Dementia Management	Health Education Learning Facilitation	Mood Management Substance Use Treatment

NOC-NIC LINKAGES FOR SELF-NEGLECT

Outcome	Major Interventions	Suggested Interventions	
Self-Care: Activities of Daily Living (ADL) Definition: Ability to perform most basic physical tasks and personal care activities independently with or without assistive device	Self-Care Assistance	Delusion Management Dementia Management: Bathing Exercise Therapy: Ambulation Mood Management Oral Health Maintenance Oral Health Restoration Self-Care Assistance: Bathing/Hygiene	Self-Care Assistance: Dressing/Grooming Self-Care Assistance: Toileting Self-Care Assistance: Transfer Substance Use Treatment

Continued

NOC-NIC LINKAGES FOR SELF-NEGLECT

Outcome	Major Interventions	Suggested Interventions	
Self-Care: Bathing Definition: Ability to cleanse own body independently with or without assistive device **Self-Care: Hygiene** Definition: Ability to maintain own personal cleanliness and kempt appearance independently with or without assistive device	Self-Care Assistance: Bathing/Hygiene	Bathing Culture Brokerage Dementia Management: Bathing Ear Care Eye Care Foot Care Hair Care	Nail Care Oral Health Maintenance Patient Rights Protection Perineal Care Prosthesis Care Skin Surveillance
Self-Care: Dressing Definition: Ability to dress self independently with or without assistive device	Self-Care Assistance: Dressing/Grooming	Culture Brokerage Dressing Hair Care	Patient Rights Protection Prosthesis Care
Self-Care: Instrumental Activities of Daily Living (IADL) Definition: Ability to perform activities needed to function in the home or community independently with or without assistive device	Self-Care Assistance: IADL	Delusion Management Environmental Management	Mood Management Substance Use Treatment
Self-Care: Oral Hygiene Definition: Ability to care for own mouth and teeth independently with or without assistive device	Oral Health Maintenance	Oral Health Promotion	Oral Health Restoration
Self-Care: Toileting Definition: Ability to toilet self independently with or without assistive device	Self-Care Assistance: Toileting	Bowel Incontinence Care Bowel Management Constipation/Impaction Management Diarrhea Management Flatulence Reduction Ostomy Care	Rectal Prolapse Management Prompted Voiding Skin Surveillance Urinary Habit Training Urinary Incontinence Care

Critical reasoning note: The outcomes Self-Care: Bathing and Self-Care: Hygiene are combined because many of the interventions could be included with either bathing or hygiene. The user can determine if one or both of the outcomes should be selected.

NURSING DIAGNOSIS: Sensory Perception: Auditory, Disturbed

Definition: Change in the amount or patterning of incoming stimuli accompanied by a diminished, exaggerated, distorted, or impaired response to such stimuli

NICS ASSOCIATED WITH DIAGNOSIS RELATED FACTORS

Anxiety Reduction	Electrolyte Management	Environmental Management	Neurological Monitoring

NOC-NIC LINKAGES FOR SENSORY PERCEPTION: AUDITORY, DISTURBED

Outcome	Major Interventions	Suggested Interventions	
Communication: Receptive			
Definition: Reception and interpretation of verbal and/or nonverbal messages	Communication Enhancement: Hearing Deficit	Cognitive Stimulation Ear Care	Environmental Management Reality Orientation
Hearing Compensation Behavior			
Definition: Personal actions to identify, monitor, and compensate for hearing loss	Communication Enhancement: Hearing Deficit	Cognitive Stimulation Ear Care Emotional Support	Environmental Management Medication Administration: Ear
Neurological Status: Cranial Sensory/ Motor Function			
Definition: Ability of the cranial nerves to convey sensory and motor impulses	Communication Enhancement: Hearing Deficit	Cerebral Edema Management Cerebral Perfusion Promotion Ear Care Environmental Management	Medication Administration Medication Management Neurological Monitoring
Sensory Function: Hearing			
Definition: Extent to which sounds are correctly sensed	Communication Enhancement: Hearing Deficit	Ear Care Environmental Management	Medication Administration: Ear

PART II - S

NURSING DIAGNOSIS: Sensory Perception: Gustatory, Disturbed

Definition: Change in the amount or patterning of incoming stimuli accompanied by a diminished, exaggerated, distorted, or impaired response to such stimuli

NICS ASSOCIATED WITH DIAGNOSIS RELATED FACTORS			
Anxiety Reduction	Electrolyte Management	Environmental Management	Neurological Monitoring

NOC-NIC LINKAGES FOR SENSORY PERCEPTION: GUSTATORY, DISTURBED		
Outcome	**Major Interventions**	**Suggested Interventions**
Appetite Definition: Desire to eat when ill or receiving treatment	Nausea Management Nutrition Management	Fluid Management Medication Management Oral Health Maintenance · Oral Health Promotion Oral Health Restoration Vomiting Management
Nutritional Status: Food & Fluid Intake Definition: Amount of food and fluid taken into the body over a 24-hour period	Fluid Monitoring Nutritional Monitoring	Bottle Feeding Feeding Fluid Management Medication Management Nausea Management · Nutrition Management Oral Health Restoration Self-Care Assistance: Feeding Swallowing Therapy Vomiting Management
Sensory Function: Taste & Smell Definition: Extent to which chemicals inhaled or dissolved in saliva are correctly sensed	Nutritional Monitoring	Aromatherapy Fluid Management Fluid Monitoring · Nausea Management Nutrition Management Vomiting Management

NURSING DIAGNOSIS: Sensory Perception: Kinesthetic, Disturbed

Definition: Change in the amount or patterning of incoming stimuli accompanied by a diminished, exaggerated, distorted, or impaired response to such stimuli

NICS ASSOCIATED WITH DIAGNOSIS RELATED FACTORS			
Anxiety Reduction	Electrolyte Management	Environmental Management	Neurological Monitoring

NOC-NIC LINKAGES FOR SENSORY PERCEPTION: KINESTHETIC, DISTURBED		
Outcome	**Major Interventions**	**Suggested Interventions**
Balance Definition: Ability to maintain body equilibrium	Exercise Therapy: Balance Exercise Therapy: Muscle Control	Body Mechanics Promotion Exercise Therapy: Ambulation · Fall Prevention

NOC-NIC LINKAGES FOR SENSORY PERCEPTION: KINESTHETIC, DISTURBED

Outcome	Major Interventions	Suggested Interventions	
Coordinated Movement			
Definition: Ability of muscles to work together voluntarily for purposeful movement	Exercise Therapy: Muscle Control	Body Mechanics Promotion Exercise Promotion Exercise Promotion: Strength Training Exercise Promotion: Stretching	Exercise Therapy: Ambulation Exercise Therapy: Balance Exercise Therapy: Joint Mobility
Neurological Status: Spinal Sensory/ Motor Function			
Definition: Ability of the spinal nerves to convey sensory and motor impulses	Neurological Monitoring	Dysreflexia Management Peripheral Sensation Management	Surveillance Unilateral Neglect Management
Sensory Function: Proprioception			
Definition: Extent to which the position and movement of the head and body are correctly sensed	Exercise Therapy: Balance	Body Mechanics Promotion Exercise Promotion Exercise Promotion: Strength Training	Exercise Therapy: Ambulation Exercise Therapy: Muscle Control

PART II - S

NURSING DIAGNOSIS: Sensory Perception: Olfactory, Disturbed

Definition: Change in the amount or patterning of incoming stimuli accompanied by a diminished, exaggerated, distorted, or impaired response to such stimuli

NICS ASSOCIATED WITH DIAGNOSIS RELATED FACTORS

Anxiety Reduction	Electrolyte Management	Environmental Management	Neurological Monitoring

NOC-NIC LINKAGES FOR SENSORY PERCEPTION: OLFACTORY, DISTURBED

Outcome	Major Interventions	Suggested Interventions	
Appetite			
Definition: Desire to eat when ill or receiving treatment	Nausea Management Nutrition Management	Diet Staging Fluid Management Fluid Monitoring	Medication Management Vomiting Management
Neurological Status: Cranial Sensory/Motor Function			
Definition: Ability of the cranial nerves to convey sensory and motor impulses	Neurological Monitoring	Aromatherapy Cerebral Edema Management Cerebral Perfusion Promotion	Medication Management Nausea Management
Sensory Function: Taste & Smell			
Definition: Extent to which chemicals inhaled or dissolved in saliva are correctly sensed	Aromatherapy Neurological Monitoring	Nausea Management Medication Management	Vomiting Management

NURSING DIAGNOSIS: Sensory Perception: Tactile, Disturbed

Definition: Change in the amount or patterning of incoming stimuli accompanied by a diminished, exaggerated, distorted, or impaired response to such stimuli

NICS ASSOCIATED WITH DIAGNOSIS RELATED FACTORS			
Anxiety Reduction	Electrolyte Management	Environmental Management	Neurological Monitoring

NOC-NIC LINKAGES FOR SENSORY PERCEPTION: TACTILE, DISTURBED			
Outcome	Major Interventions	Suggested Interventions	
Neurological Status: Spinal Sensory/Motor Function Definition: Ability of the spinal nerves to convey sensory and motor impulses	Peripheral Sensation Management	Dysreflexia Management Neurological Monitoring	Surveillance Unilateral Neglect Management
Sensory Function: Cutaneous Definition: Extent to which stimulation of the skin is correctly sensed	Peripheral Sensation Management	Amputation Care Lower Extremity Monitoring Neurological Monitoring	Positioning Pressure Management Skin Surveillance

NURSING DIAGNOSIS: Sensory Perception: Visual, Disturbed

Definition: Change in the amount or patterning of incoming stimuli accompanied by a diminished, exaggerated, distorted, or impaired response to such stimuli

NICS ASSOCIATED WITH DIAGNOSIS RELATED FACTORS			
Anxiety Reduction	Electrolyte Management	Environmental Management	Neurological Monitoring

NOC-NIC LINKAGES FOR SENSORY PERCEPTION: VISUAL, DISTURBED			
Outcome	Major Interventions	Suggested Interventions	
Neurological Status: Cranial Sensory/Motor Function Definition: Ability of the cranial nerves to convey sensory and motor impulses	Communication Enhancement: Visual Deficit Neurological Monitoring	Cerebral Edema Management Cerebral Perfusion Promotion	Environmental Management Medication Management
Sensory Function: Vision Definition: Extent to which visual images are correctly sensed	Communication Enhancement: Visual Deficit	Eye Care Medication Administration: Eye	Medication Management Neurological Monitoring
Vision Compensation Behavior Definition: Personal actions to compensate for visual impairment	Communication Enhancement: Visual Deficit Environmental Management: Safety	Contact Lens Care Environmental Management Eye Care	Fall Prevention Medication Administration: Eye Medication Management

NURSING DIAGNOSIS: Sexual Dysfunction

Definition: The state in which an individual experiences a change in sexual function during the sexual response phases of desire, excitation, and/or orgasm, which is viewed as unsatisfying, unrewarding, or inadequate

NICS ASSOCIATED WITH DIAGNOSIS RELATED FACTORS			
Abuse Protection Support	Postpartal Care	Prenatal Care	Teaching: Sexuality

NOC-NIC LINKAGES FOR SEXUAL DYSFUNCTION		
Outcome	**Major Interventions**	**Suggested Interventions**
Abuse Recovery: Sexual		
Definition: Extent of healing of physical and psychological injuries due to sexual abuse or exploitation	Abuse Protection Support Counseling Sexual Counseling	Abuse Protection Support: Child Abuse Protection Support: Domestic Partner Abuse Protection Support: Elder Active Listening Anger Control Assistance Assertiveness Training Behavior Management: Self-Harm Emotional Support Guilt Work Facilitation Hope Inspiration Mood Management — Resiliency Promotion Self-Awareness Enhancement Self-Esteem Enhancement Sleep Enhancement Spiritual Support Substance Use Prevention Suicide Prevention Support Group Support System Enhancement Teaching: Sexuality Therapy Group Values Clarification
Knowledge: Pregnancy & Postpartum Sexual Functioning		
Definition: Extent of understanding conveyed about sexual function during pregnancy and postpartum	Postpartal Care Prenatal Care	Family Planning: Contraception Mood Management Sexual Counseling — Teaching: Individual Teaching: Safe Sex
Physical Aging		
Definition: Normal physical changes that occur with the natural aging process	Sexual Counseling	Anxiety Reduction Body Image Enhancement Emotional Support Hormone Replacement Therapy — Medication Management Self-Esteem Enhancement Self-Modification Assistance
Risk Control: Sexually Transmitted Diseases (STD)		
Definition: Personal actions to prevent, eliminate, or reduce behaviors associated with sexually transmitted disease	Infection Control Teaching: Safe Sex	Behavior Management: Sexual Behavior Modification Health Screening Health System Guidance — Impulse Control Training Risk Identification Self-Responsibility Facilitation

PART II - S

Continued

NOC-NIC LINKAGES FOR SEXUAL DYSFUNCTION

Outcome	Major Interventions	Suggested Interventions	
Sexual Functioning Definition: Integration of physical, socioemotional, and intellectual aspects of sexual expression and performance	Sexual Counseling	Body Image Enhancement Family Planning: Contraception Family Planning: Infertility Hormone Replacement Therapy Medication Management Premenstrual Syndrome (PMS) Management	Prenatal Care Self-Esteem Enhancement Self-Responsibility Facilitation Teaching: Safe Sex Teaching: Sexuality Values Clarification

NURSING DIAGNOSIS: Sexuality Patterns, Ineffective

Definition: Expressions of concern regarding own sexuality

NICS ASSOCIATED WITH DIAGNOSIS RELATED FACTORS

Behavior Modification: Social Skills Parent Education: Adolescent	Parent Education: Childrearing Family	Parenting Promotion	Teaching: Individual

NOC-NIC LINKAGES FOR SEXUALITY PATTERNS, INEFFECTIVE

Outcome	Major Interventions	Suggested Interventions	
Abuse Recovery: Sexual Definition: Extent of healing of physical and psychological injuries due to sexual abuse or exploitation	Abuse Protection Support Counseling Sexual Counseling	Active Listening Anger Control Assistance Anxiety Reduction Behavior Management: Sexual Guilt Work Facilitation Self-Awareness Enhancement	Self-Esteem Enhancement Spiritual Support Support Group Support System Enhancement Teaching: Sexuality Therapy Group
Physical Maturation: Female Definition: Normal physical changes in the female that occur with the transition from childhood to adulthood	Teaching: Safe Sex Teaching: Sexuality	Anxiety Reduction Behavior Management: Sexual Body Image Enhancement Parent Education: Adolescent	Premenstrual Syndrome (PMS) Management Self-Awareness Enhancement Self-Esteem Enhancement
Physical Maturation: Male Definition: Normal physical changes in the male that occur with the transition from childhood to adulthood	Teaching: Safe Sex Teaching: Sexuality	Anxiety Reduction Behavior Management: Sexual Body Image Enhancement	Parent Education: Adolescent Self-Awareness Enhancement Self-Esteem Enhancement

NOC-NIC LINKAGES FOR SEXUALITY PATTERNS, INEFFECTIVE		
Outcome	**Major Interventions**	**Suggested Interventions**
Sexual Identity Definition: Acknowledgment and acceptance of own sexual identity	Sexual Counseling	Anxiety Reduction Behavior Management: Sexual Body Image Enhancement Coping Enhancement Counseling Developmental Enhancement: Adolescent	Hormone Replacement Therapy Role Enhancement Self-Awareness Enhancement Self-Esteem Enhancement Support System Enhancement Teaching: Sexuality Values Clarification

NURSING DIAGNOSIS: Skin Integrity, Impaired

Definition: Altered epidermis and/or dermis

NICS ASSOCIATED WITH DIAGNOSIS RELATED FACTORS			
Chemotherapy Management Circulatory Precautions Environmental Management: Safety Fluid Management Fluid Monitoring	Heat Exposure Treatment Hypothermia Treatment Malignant Hyperthermia Precautions	Medication Management Nutrition Management Nutrition Therapy Nutritional Monitoring Peripheral Sensation Management	Pressure Management Pressure Ulcer Prevention Radiation Therapy Management Risk Identification

NOC-NIC LINKAGES FOR SKIN INTEGRITY, IMPAIRED		
Outcome	**Major Interventions**	**Suggested Interventions**
Allergic Response: Localized Definition: Severity of localized hypersensitive immune response to a specific environmental (exogenous) antigen	Pruritus Management Skin Care: Topical Treatments	Allergy Management Infection Protection Medication Administration	Medication Administration: Skin Skin Surveillance
Burn Healing Definition: Extent of healing of a burn site	Wound Care: Burns	Analgesic Administration Circulatory Precautions Exercise Therapy: Joint Mobility Infection Protection Medication Administration Medication Administration: Skin	Pain Management Skin Care: Donor Site Skin Care: Graft Site Skin Care: Topical Treatments Skin Surveillance

Continued

NOC-NIC LINKAGES FOR SKIN INTEGRITY, IMPAIRED

Outcome	Major Interventions	Suggested Interventions	
Tissue Integrity: Skin & Mucous Membranes			
Definition: Structural intactness and normal physiological function of skin and mucous membranes	Pressure Management Skin Surveillance	Amputation Care Cast Care: Maintenance Circulatory Care: Arterial Insufficiency Circulatory Care: Mechanical Assist Device Circulatory Care: Venous Insufficiency Circulatory Precautions Foot Care	Infection Protection Medication Administration: Skin Medication Management Ostomy Care Positioning Pressure Ulcer Care Radiation Therapy Management Skin Care: Topical Treatments Traction/Immobilization Care
Wound Healing: Primary Intention			
Definition: Extent of regeneration of cells and tissue following intentional closure	Incision Site Care Wound Care	Amputation Care Bleeding Reduction: Wound Cesarean Section Care Circulatory Precautions Infection Control: Intraoperative Infection Protection	Medication Administration Medication Administration: Skin Skin Care: Donor Site Skin Care: Graft Site Suturing Wound Care: Closed Drainage
Wound Healing: Secondary Intention			
Definition: Extent of regeneration of cells and tissue in an open wound	Pressure Ulcer Care Wound Care	Circulatory Care: Arterial Insufficiency Circulatory Care: Venous Insufficiency Circulatory Precautions Infection Control Infection Protection	Medication Administration: Skin Medication Management Skin Care: Topical Treatments Skin Surveillance Transcutaneous Electrical Nerve Stimulation (TENS) Wound Irrigation

NURSING DIAGNOSIS: Sleep Deprivation

Definition: Prolonged periods of time without sleep (sustained natural, periodic suspension of relative consciousness)

NICS ASSOCIATED WITH DIAGNOSIS RELATED FACTORS

Anxiety Reduction	Exercise Promotion	Pain Management	Relaxation Therapy
Dementia Management	Medication	Parenting Promotion	Urinary Incontinence
Environmental	Management		Care: Enuresis
Management			

NOC-NIC LINKAGES FOR SLEEP DEPRIVATION

Outcome	Major Interventions	Suggested Interventions	
Acute Confusion Level			
Definition: Severity of disturbance in consciousness and cognition that develops over a short period of time	Delirium Management Sleep Enhancement	Anxiety Reduction Calming Technique Energy Management Environmental Management: Comfort Hallucination Management	Medication Management Mood Management Music Therapy Reality Orientation Surveillance: Safety
Sleep			
Definition: Natural periodic suspension of consciousness during which the body is restored	Sleep Enhancement	Anxiety Reduction Environmental Management Environmental Management: Comfort Exercise Promotion Guided Imagery Massage Medication Management Meditation Facilitation	Music Therapy Nausea Management Pain Management Phototherapy: Mood/ Sleep Regulation Progressive Muscle Relaxation Relaxation Therapy Urinary Incontinence Care: Enuresis Vomiting Management
Symptom Severity			
Definition: Severity of perceived adverse changes in physical, emotional, and social functioning	Reality Orientation Sleep Enhancement	Anxiety Reduction Calming Technique Coping Enhancement Energy Management Guided Imagery Hallucination Management Massage	Medication Administration Medication Management Mood Management Pain Management Positioning Progressive Muscle Relaxation Relaxation Therapy

Critical reasoning note: The defining characteristics of the diagnosis are the symptoms that occur with prolonged lack of sleep; therefore outcomes that can be used to measure improvement of these symptoms are provided as well as an outcome to measure sleep.

PART II - S

NURSING DIAGNOSIS: Sleep Pattern, Disturbed

Definition: Time-limited disruption of sleep amount and quality due to external factors

NICS ASSOCIATED WITH DIAGNOSIS RELATED FACTORS			
Caregiver Support	Environmental Management	Environmental Management: Comfort	Respite Care

NOC-NIC LINKAGES FOR SLEEP PATTERN, DISTURBED		
Outcome	**Major Interventions**	**Suggested Interventions**
Sleep Definition: Natural periodic suspension of consciousness during which the body is restored	Environmental Management: Comfort Sleep Enhancement	Anxiety Reduction Autogenic Training Bathing Calming Technique Dementia Management Energy Management Environmental Management Exercise Promotion Hormone Replacement Therapy Kangaroo Care Massage Medication Administration Medication Management Medication Prescribing Meditation Facilitation Music Therapy Pain Management Phototherapy: Mood/ Sleep Regulation Positioning Progressive Muscle Relaxation Relaxation Therapy Security Enhancement Touch Urinary Incontinence Care: Enuresis

NURSING DIAGNOSIS: Sleep, Readiness for Enhanced

Definition: A pattern of natural, periodic suspension of consciousness that provides adequate rest, sustains a desired lifestyle, and can be strengthened

NOC-NIC LINKAGES FOR SLEEP, READINESS FOR ENHANCED		
Outcome	**Major Interventions**	**Suggested Interventions**
Sleep Definition: Natural periodic suspension of consciousness during which the body is restored	Sleep Enhancement	Anxiety Reduction Autogenic Training Calming Technique Environmental Management: Comfort Hormone Replacement Therapy Massage Medication Management Music Therapy Nausea Management Pain Management Phototherapy: Mood/ Sleep Regulation Premenstrual Syndrome (PMS) Management Progressive Muscle Relaxation Relaxation Therapy Security Enhancement

PART II - S

NURSING DIAGNOSIS: Social Interaction, Impaired

Definition: Insufficient or excessive quantity or ineffective quality of social exchange

NICS ASSOCIATED WITH DIAGNOSIS RELATED FACTORS			
Delusion Management	Dementia Management	Self-Awareness Enhancement	Visitation Facilitation

NOC-NIC LINKAGES FOR SOCIAL INTERACTION, IMPAIRED		
Outcome	**Major Interventions**	**Suggested Interventions**
Child Development: Adolescence Definition: Milestones of physical, cognitive, and psycho-social progression from 12 years through 17 years of age	Developmental Enhancement: Adolescent Socialization Enhancement	Behavior Management: Sexual Behavior Modification: Social Skills Family Integrity Promotion Family Process Maintenance Family Support	Recreation Therapy Self-Awareness Enhancement Self-Esteem Enhancement Support System Enhancement Therapeutic Play
Child Development: Middle Childhood Definition: Milestones of physical, cognitive, and psycho-social progression from 6 years through 11 years of age	Developmental Enhancement: Child	Behavior Management: Overactivity/Inattention Behavior Modification: Social Skills Family Integrity Promotion Family Support	Self-Awareness Enhancement Self-Esteem Enhancement Socialization Enhancement Therapeutic Play
Family Social Climate Definition: Supportive milieu as characterized by family member relationships and goals	Family Integrity Promotion Family Process Maintenance	Abuse Protection Support: Child Abuse Protection Support: Domestic Partner Abuse Protection Support: Elder Behavior Management: Overactivity/Inattention	Family Support Family Therapy Socialization Enhancement
Leisure Participation Definition: Use of relaxing, interest-ing, and enjoyable activities to promote well-being	Recreation Therapy Socialization Enhancement	Activity Therapy Animal-Assisted Therapy Anxiety Reduction	Behavior Modification: Social Skills Self-Esteem Enhancement
Play Participation Definition: Use of activities by a child from 1 year through 11 years of age to promote enjoy-ment, entertainment, and development	Socialization Enhancement Therapeutic Play	Activity Therapy Animal-Assisted Therapy	Behavior Modification: Social Skills Recreation Therapy

PART II - S

Continued

NOC-NIC LINKAGES FOR SOCIAL INTERACTION, IMPAIRED

Outcome	Major Interventions	Suggested Interventions	
Social Interaction Skills Definition: Personal behaviors that promote effective relationships	Behavior Modification: Social Skills	Active Listening Anger Control Assistance Anxiety Reduction Assertiveness Training Behavior Management: Sexual Communication Enhancement: Hearing Deficit Communication Enhancement: Speech Deficit	Dementia Management Developmental Enhancement: Adolescent Developmental Enhancement: Child Humor Recreation Therapy Reminiscence Therapy Visitation Facilitation
Social Involvement Definition: Social interactions with persons, groups, or organizations	Socialization Enhancement	Active Listening Activity Therapy Animal-Assisted Therapy Assertiveness Training Behavior Modification: Social Skills Communication Enhancement: Hearing Deficit Communication Enhancement: Speech Deficit	Developmental Enhancement: Adolescent Developmental Enhancement: Child Recreation Therapy Relocation Stress Reduction Reminiscence Therapy Therapeutic Play Support Group Support System Enhancement

NURSING DIAGNOSIS: Social Isolation

Definition: Aloneness experienced by the individual and perceived as imposed by others and as a negative or threatening state

NICS ASSOCIATED WITH DIAGNOSIS RELATED FACTORS

Behavior Modification: Social Skills Body Image Enhancement	Dementia Management Socialization Enhancement	Support System Enhancement Values Clarification

NOC-NIC LINKAGES FOR SOCIAL ISOLATION

Outcome	Major Interventions	Suggested Interventions	
Family Social Climate Definition: Supportive milieu as characterized by family member relationships and goals	Family Integrity Promotion	Attachment Promotion Behavior Modification: Social Skills Counseling Family Process Maintenance	Family Support Family Therapy Grief Work Facilitation: Perinatal Death Support System Enhancement

NOC-NIC LINKAGES FOR SOCIAL ISOLATION

Outcome	Major Interventions	Suggested Interventions	
Leisure Participation			
Definition: Use of relaxing, interesting, and enjoyable activities to promote well-being	Recreation Therapy	Activity Therapy Animal-Assisted Therapy	Exercise Promotion Socialization Enhancement
Loneliness Severity			
Definition: Severity of emotional, social, or existential isolation response	Behavior Modification: Social Skills Recreation Therapy Socialization Enhancement	Active Listening Activity Therapy Animal-Assisted Therapy Anxiety Reduction Assertiveness Training Communication Enhancement: Hearing Deficit Communication Enhancement: Speech Deficit Developmental Enhancement: Adolescent	Developmental Enhancement: Child Family Therapy Grief Work Facilitation Hope Inspiration Mood Management Self-Awareness Enhancement Self-Esteem Enhancement Support Group Support System Enhancement
Mood Equilibrium			
Definition: Appropriate adjustment of prevailing emotional tone in response to circumstances	Mood Management	Active Listening Anger Control Assistance Animal-Assisted Therapy Counseling Energy Management Grief Work Facilitation Guilt Work Facilitation Hope Inspiration Impulse Control Training	Medication Management Music Therapy Self-Esteem Enhancement Socialization Enhancement Spiritual Support Support System Enhancement Therapeutic Play Therapy Group
Play Participation			
Definition: Use of activities by a child from 1 year through 11 years of age to promote enjoyment, entertainment, and development	Developmental Enhancement: Child Socialization Enhancement	Activity Therapy Environmental Management Parent Education: Childrearing Family	Parenting Promotion Recreation Therapy Therapeutic Play
Social Interaction Skills			
Definition: Personal behaviors that promote effective relationships	Behavior Modification: Social Skills Socialization Enhancement	Anger Control Assistance Developmental Enhancement: Adolescent Developmental Enhancement: Child	Family Integrity Promotion Self-Awareness Enhancement Self-Esteem Enhancement

PART II - S

Continued

NOC-NIC LINKAGES FOR SOCIAL ISOLATION

Outcome	Major Interventions	Suggested Interventions	
Social Involvement Definition: Social interactions with persons, groups, or organizations	Socialization Enhancement	Activity Therapy Communication Enhancement: Hearing Deficit Communication Enhancement: Speech Deficit Counseling	Milieu Therapy Recreation Therapy Support Group Support System Enhancement Therapeutic Play Visitation Facilitation
Social Support Definition: Reliable assistance from others	Family Involvement Promotion Support System Enhancement	Caregiver Support Family Support Referral Respite Care	Socialization Enhancement Spiritual Support Support Group

NURSING DIAGNOSIS: Sorrow: Chronic

Definition: Cyclical, recurring, and potentially progressive pattern of pervasive sadness experienced (by a parent, caregiver, individual with chronic illness or disability) in response to continual loss, throughout the trajectory of an illness or disability

NICS ASSOCIATED WITH DIAGNOSIS RELATED FACTORS

Coping Enhancement
Environmental Management: Violence Prevention
Grief Work Facilitation
Resiliency Promotion

NOC-NIC LINKAGES FOR SORROW: CHRONIC

Outcome	Major Interventions	Suggested Interventions	
Acceptance: Health Status Definition: Reconciliation to significant change in health circumstances	Coping Enhancement Hope Inspiration	Anger Control Assistance Decision-Making Support Emotional Support Grief Work Facilitation Guilt Work Facilitation Mood Management	Resiliency Promotion Self-Esteem Enhancement Spiritual Support Support Group Truth Telling Values Clarification
Depression Level Definition: Severity of melancholic mood and loss of interest in life events	Hope Inspiration Mood Management	Activity Therapy Anger Control Assistance Animal-Assisted Therapy Emotional Support Forgiveness Facilitation Grief Work Facilitation Guilt Work Facilitation	Medication Management Sleep Enhancement Spiritual Support Substance Use Prevention Support Group Support System Enhancement

NOC-NIC LINKAGES FOR SORROW: CHRONIC

Outcome	Major Interventions	Suggested Interventions	
Depression Self-Control			
Definition: Personal actions to minimize melancholy and maintain interest in life events	Mood Management	Activity Therapy Behavior Modification Cognitive Restructuring Energy Management Grief Work Facilitation Guilt Work Facilitation Medication Management Risk Identification	Self-Modification Assistance Sleep Enhancement Substance Use Prevention Teaching: Prescribed Activity/Exercise Teaching: Prescribed Medication Teaching: Procedure/ Treatment Weight Management
Grief Resolution			
Definition: Adjustment to actual or impending loss	Grief Work Facilitation Grief Work Facilitation: Perinatal Death	Active Listening Anger Control Assistance Animal-Assisted Therapy Bibliotherapy Coping Enhancement Dying Care Emotional Support	Forgiveness Facilitation Guilt Work Facilitation Hope Inspiration Nutritional Monitoring Reminiscence Therapy Spiritual Support Support Group
Hope			
Definition: Optimism that is personally satisfying and life-supporting	Hope Inspiration Spiritual Support	Coping Enhancement Emotional Support Forgiveness Facilitation Mood Management	Self-Awareness Enhancement Self-Esteem Enhancement Support Group Support System Enhancement
Mood Equilibrium			
Definition: Appropriate adjustment of prevailing emotional tone in response to circumstances	Mood Management	Anger Control Assistance Emotional Support Hope Inspiration Humor Impulse Control Training Medication Management Meditation Facilitation Music Therapy	Sleep Enhancement Socialization Enhancement Spiritual Support Support Group Support System Enhancement Teaching: Prescribed Medication Teaching: Procedure/ Treatment
Psychosocial Adjustment: Life Change			
Definition: Adaptive psychosocial response of an individual to a significant life change	Coping Enhancement	Active Listening Anger Control Assistance Counseling Decision-Making Support Emotional Support Grief Work Facilitation Hope Inspiration	Mood Management Relocation Stress Reduction Self-Esteem Enhancement Socialization Enhancement Spiritual Support Support Group

PART II - S

NURSING DIAGNOSIS: Spiritual Distress

Definition: Impaired ability to experience and integrate meaning and purpose in life through connectedness with self, others, art, music, literature, nature, and/or a power greater than oneself

NICS ASSOCIATED WITH DIAGNOSIS RELATED FACTORS

Anxiety Reduction	Pain Management	Resiliency Promotion
Dying Care	Relocation Stress Reduction	Socialization Enhancement

NOC-NIC LINKAGES FOR SPIRITUAL DISTRESS

Outcome	Major Interventions	Suggested Interventions	
Dignified Life Closure Definition: Personal actions to maintain control during approaching end of life	Coping Enhancement Decision-Making Support	Active Listening Anger Control Assistance Anxiety Reduction Dying Care Emotional Support Family Involvement Promotion Forgiveness Facilitation Grief Work Facilitation Guilt Work Facilitation	Hope Inspiration Music Therapy Reminiscence Therapy Spiritual Growth Facilitation Spiritual Support Support System Enhancement Touch Truth Telling
Hope Definition: Optimism that is personally satisfying and life-supporting	Hope Inspiration Spiritual Support	Coping Enhancement Emotional Support Guilt Work Facilitation Spiritual Growth Facilitation	Support Group Support System Enhancement Values Clarification
Quality of Life Definition: Extent of positive perception of current life circumstances	Values Clarification	Coping Enhancement Hope Inspiration Mood Management Self-Awareness Enhancement	Self-Esteem Enhancement Self-Responsibility Facilitation Socialization Enhancement Spiritual Support
Social Involvement Definition: Social interactions with persons, groups, or organizations	Socialization Enhancement	Behavior Modification: Social Skills Family Involvement Promotion Recreation Therapy Religious Ritual Enhancement	Spiritual Support Support Group Support System Enhancement
Spiritual Health Definition: Connectedness with self, others, higher power, all life, nature, and the universe that transcends and empowers the self	Spiritual Growth Facilitation Spiritual Support	Active Listening Anger Control Assistance Forgiveness Facilitation Grief Work Facilitation Guilt Work Facilitation Hope Inspiration	Meditation Facilitation Religious Ritual Enhancement Self-Awareness Enhancement Self-Esteem Enhancement Socialization Enhancement Values Clarification

NURSING DIAGNOSIS: Spiritual Well-Being, Readiness for Enhanced

Definition: Ability to experience and integrate meaning and purpose in life through connectedness with self, others, art, music, literature, nature, and/or a power greater than oneself, that can be strengthened

NOC-NIC LINKAGES FOR SPIRITUAL WELL-BEING, READINESS FOR ENHANCED

Outcome	Major Interventions	Suggested Interventions	
Hope Definition: Optimism that is personally satisfying and life-supporting	Hope Inspiration Spiritual Growth Facilitation	Bibliotherapy Coping Enhancement Self-Awareness Enhancement	Self-Esteem Enhancement Spiritual Support Values Clarification
Personal Well-Being Definition: Extent of positive perception of one's health status	Spiritual Growth Facilitation Values Clarification	Bibliotherapy Coping Enhancement Forgiveness Facilitation Hope Inspiration Meditation Facilitation Music Therapy Religious Ritual Enhancement	Resiliency Promotion Role Enhancement Self-Awareness Enhancement Self-Esteem Enhancement Self-Modification Assistance Self-Responsibility Facilitation Spiritual Support
Spiritual Health Definition: Connectedness with self, others, higher power, all life, nature, and the universe that transcends and empowers the self	Spiritual Growth Facilitation Spiritual Support	Bibliotherapy Forgiveness Facilitation Hope Inspiration Meditation Facilitation Music Therapy Religious Addiction Prevention	Religious Ritual Enhancement Self-Awareness Enhancement Self-Esteem Enhancement Self-Modification Assistance Values Clarification

NURSING DIAGNOSIS: Stress Overload

Definition: Excessive amounts and types of demands that require action

NICS ASSOCIATED WITH DIAGNOSIS RELATED FACTORS

Coping Enhancement Environmental Management: Violence Prevention	Financial Resource Assistance Health Education Resiliency Promotion	Support System Enhancement Teaching: Individual

NOC-NIC LINKAGES FOR STRESS OVERLOAD

Outcome	Major Interventions	Suggested Interventions	
Agitation Level Definition: Severity of disruptive physiological and behavioral manifestations of stress or biochemical triggers	Anger Control Assistance Anxiety Reduction	Behavior Management Calming Technique Coping Enhancement Environmental Management: Violence Prevention Limit Setting	Medication Administration Mood Management Sleep Enhancement Vital Signs Monitoring Weight Management

Continued

PART II - S

NOC-NIC LINKAGES FOR STRESS OVERLOAD

Outcome	Major Interventions	Suggested Interventions	
Anxiety Level Definition: Severity of manifested apprehension, tension, or uneasiness arising from an unidentifiable source	Anxiety Reduction	Anger Control Assistance Behavior Management Calming Technique Coping Enhancement Decision-Making Support Mood Management Nausea Management	Presence Relaxation Therapy Security Enhancement Sleep Enhancement Spiritual Support Support System Enhancement
Coping Definition: Personal actions to manage stressors that tax an individual's resources	Anxiety Reduction Coping Enhancement	Anger Control Assistance Calming Technique Decision-Making Support Emotional Support Hope Inspiration	Mood Management Relaxation Therapy Resiliency Promotion Sleep Enhancement Support System Enhancement
Stress Level Definition: Severity of manifested physical or mental tension resulting from factors that alter an existing equilibrium	Anger Control Assistance Anxiety Reduction	Calming Technique Coping Enhancement Decision-Making Support Emotional Support Massage Mood Management	Nausea Management Relaxation Therapy Security Enhancement Sleep Enhancement Support System Enhancement

NURSING DIAGNOSIS: Surgical Recovery, Delayed

Definition: Extension of the number of postoperative days required to initiate and perform activities that maintain life, health, and well-being

NICS ASSOCIATED WITH DIAGNOSIS RELATED FACTORS

Anticipatory Guidance Incision Site Care	Infection Control: Intraoperative Pain Management	Preoperative Coordination Weight Management

NOC-NIC LINKAGES FOR SURGICAL RECOVERY, DELAYED

Outcome	Major Interventions	Suggested Interventions	
Ambulation Definition: Ability to walk from place to place independently with or without assistive device	Exercise Therapy: Ambulation	Energy Management Exercise Promotion: Stretching	Exercise Therapy: Joint Mobility Teaching: Prescribed Activity/Exercise

NOC-NIC LINKAGES FOR SURGICAL RECOVERY, DELAYED		
Outcome	Major Interventions	Suggested Interventions
Endurance Definition: Capacity to sustain activity	Energy Management Exercise Promotion	Environmental Management Environmental Management: Comfort Exercise Promotion: Strength Training Exercise Therapy: Ambulation	Exercise Therapy: Muscle Control Nutrition Management Nutritional Monitoring Self-Care Assistance Sleep Enhancement
Infection Severity Definition: Severity of infection and associated symptoms	Incision Site Care Infection Control	Amputation Care Discharge Planning Energy Management Fever Treatment Fluid Management Infection Protection Nutrition Therapy Nutritional Monitoring Pain Management	Pruritus Management Skin Care: Donor Site Skin Care: Graft Site Skin Surveillance Specimen Management Temperature Regulation Vital Signs Monitoring Wound Care Wound Care: Closed Drainage Wound Irrigation
Nausea & Vomiting Severity Definition: Severity of nausea, retching, and vomiting symptoms	Nausea Management Surveillance Vomiting Management	Diet Staging Electrolyte Monitoring Enteral Tube Feeding Environmental Management Fluid/Electrolyte Management Fluid Management	Fluid Monitoring Medication Administration Nutrition Management Nutritional Monitoring Total Parenteral Nutrition (TPN) Administration
Pain Level Definition: Severity of observed or reported pain	Pain Management	Analgesic Administration Analgesic Administration: Intraspinal Distraction Energy Management Environmental Management: Comfort Massage Medication Administration Medication Management	Music Therapy Positioning Sleep Enhancement Splinting Surveillance Transcutaneous Electrical Nerve Stimulation (TENS) Vital Signs Monitoring

Continued

PART II - S

NOC-NIC LINKAGES FOR SURGICAL RECOVERY, DELAYED

Outcome	Major Interventions	Suggested Interventions	
Post-Procedure Recovery Definition: Extent to which an individual returns to baseline function following a procedure(s) requiring anesthesia or sedation	Energy Management Pain Management	Analgesic Administration Bed Rest Care Cough Enhancement Fluid Management Incision Site Care Infection Protection Nausea Management Nutritional Monitoring Oral Health Maintenance Positioning	Respiratory Monitoring Self-Care Assistance Self-Efficacy Enhancement Sleep Enhancement Temperature Regulation Urinary Elimination Management Vital Signs Monitoring Wound Care: Closed Drainage
Wound Healing: Primary Intention Definition: Extent of regeneration of cells and tissue following intentional closure	Incision Site Care Wound Care: Closed Drainage	Bathing Cesarean Section Care Circulatory Precautions Fever Treatment Fluid Management Hyperglycemia Management Infection Control Infection Control: Intraoperative Infection Protection	Medication Administration Nutrition Management Nutrition Therapy Perineal Care Skin Surveillance Splinting Temperature Regulation Wound Care Wound Irrigation

Critical reasoning note: NOC does not have one outcome that covers surgical recovery, especially recovery following the first 24 hours; therefore a number of pertinent NOC outcomes to assess surgical recovery are provided. The outcome Post-Procedure Recovery, while not for major surgical procedures, covers a number of outcome indicators during the first 24 hours. Surgical recovery can be influenced by preoperative preparation. The outcome Pre-Procedure Readiness includes indicators that are important to consider for both diagnostic procedures and surgical interventions.

NURSING DIAGNOSIS: Swallowing, Impaired

Definition: Abnormal functioning of the swallowing mechanism associated with deficits in oral, pharyngeal, or esophageal structure or function

NICS ASSOCIATED WITH DIAGNOSIS RELATED FACTORS

Airway Management Behavior Management: Self-Harm Developmental Care	Enteral Tube Feeding Respiratory Monitoring	Transcutaneous Electrical Nerve Stimulation (TENS)

NOC-NIC LINKAGES FOR SWALLOWING, IMPAIRED

Outcome	Major Interventions	Suggested Interventions	
Aspiration Prevention Definition: Personal actions to prevent the passage of fluid and solid particles into the lung	Aspiration Precautions	Positioning Risk Identification Surveillance	Swallowing Therapy Teaching: Individual

Outcome	Major Interventions	Suggested Interventions	
NOC-NIC LINKAGES FOR SWALLOWING, IMPAIRED			
Swallowing Status Definition: Safe passage of fluids and/or solids from the mouth to the stomach	Swallowing Therapy	Aspiration Precautions Positioning	Referral Surveillance
Swallowing Status: Esophageal Phase Definition: Safe passage of fluids and/or solids from the pharynx to the stomach	Positioning Swallowing Therapy	Aspiration Precautions Oral Health Maintenance Pain Management	Surveillance Vomiting Management
Swallowing Status: Oral Phase Definition: Preparation, containment, and posterior movement of fluids and/or solids in the mouth	Swallowing Therapy	Aspiration Precautions Bottle Feeding Breastfeeding Assistance Feeding Oral Health Maintenance	Oral Health Restoration Positioning Self-Care Assistance: Feeding Surveillance
Swallowing Status: Pharyngeal Phase Definition: Safe passage of fluids and/or solids from the mouth to the esophagus	Aspiration Precautions Swallowing Therapy	Airway Suctioning Positioning	Surveillance

NURSING DIAGNOSIS: Thermoregulation, Ineffective

Definition: Temperature fluctuation between hypothermia and hyperthermia

NICS ASSOCIATED WITH DIAGNOSIS RELATED FACTORS			
Environmental Management			

Outcome	Major Interventions	Suggested Interventions	
NOC-NIC LINKAGES FOR THERMOREGULATION, INEFFECTIVE			
Thermoregulation Definition: Balance among heat production, heat gain, and heat loss	Temperature Regulation Temperature Regulation: Intraoperative	Environmental Management Fever Treatment Fluid Management Fluid Monitoring Heat Exposure Treatment	Hypothermia Treatment Malignant Hyperthermia Precautions Medication Administration Pain Management Vital Signs Monitoring

Continued

NOC-NIC LINKAGES FOR THERMOREGULATION, INEFFECTIVE

Outcome	Major Interventions	Suggested Interventions	
Thermoregulation: Newborn Definition: Balance among heat production, heat gain, and heat loss during the first 28 days of life	Newborn Monitoring Temperature Regulation	Acid-Base Management Acid-Base Monitoring Environmental Management Fever Treatment Fluid Management Fluid Monitoring	Heat Exposure Treatment Medication Administration Newborn Care Respiratory Monitoring Vital Signs Monitoring

Critical reasoning note: A number of the related factors, such as illness or treatment, are conditions that the nurse may be able to treat, but cannot necessarily prevent.

NURSING DIAGNOSIS: Tissue Integrity, Impaired

Definition: Damage to mucous membrane, corneal, integumentary, or subcutaneous tissues

NICS ASSOCIATED WITH DIAGNOSIS RELATED FACTORS

Circulatory Precautions Environmental Management Environmental Management: Safety	Exercise Therapy: Ambulation Fluid Management Fluid Monitoring	Nutrition Management Nutrition Therapy Nutritional Monitoring	Pressure Management Radiation Therapy Management Teaching: Individual

NOC-NIC LINKAGES FOR TISSUE INTEGRITY, IMPAIRED

Outcome	Major Interventions	Suggested Interventions	
Allergic Response: Localized Definition: Severity of localized hypersensitive immune response to a specific environmental (exogenous) antigen	Infection Protection Skin Care: Topical Treatments	Allergy Management Medication Administration Medication Administration: Ear Medication Administration: Enteral Medication Administration: Eye Medication Administration: Nasal	Medication Administration: Rectal Medication Administration: Skin Medication Administration: Vaginal Medication Management Pruritus Management Skin Surveillance
Ostomy Self-Care Definition: Personal actions to maintain ostomy for elimination	Ostomy Care Skin Surveillance	Infection Control Infection Protection Pressure Management Skin Care: Topical Treatments	Teaching: Individual Teaching: Procedure/ Treatment Teaching: Psychomotor Skill

NOC-NIC LINKAGES FOR TISSUE INTEGRITY, IMPAIRED		
Outcome	**Major Interventions**	**Suggested Interventions**
Tissue Integrity: Skin & Mucous Membranes Definition: Structural intactness and normal physiological function of skin and mucous membranes	Pressure Management Wound Care	Amputation Care Cast Care: Maintenance Circulatory Precautions Eye Care Foot Care Infection Protection Lower Extremity Monitoring Medication Administration: Ear Medication Administration: Enteral Medication Administration: Eye Medication Administration: Oral Medication Administration: Rectal Medication Administration: Skin Medication Administration: Vaginal Medication Management Oral Health Maintenance Oral Health Restoration Ostomy Care Perineal Care Positioning Pressure Ulcer Care Pressure Ulcer Prevention Radiation Therapy Management Rectal Prolapse Management Skin Surveillance Teaching: Foot Care Traction/Immobilization Care Urinary Incontinence Care
Wound Healing: Primary Intention Definition: Extent of regeneration of cells and tissue following intentional closure	Incision Site Care Wound Care	Amputation Care Cesarean Section Care Circulatory Precautions Infection Control: Intraoperative Infection Protection Medication Administration Skin Care: Donor Site Skin Care: Graft Site Suturing Wound Care: Closed Drainage
Wound Healing: Secondary Intention Definition: Extent of regeneration of cells and tissue in an open wound	Pressure Ulcer Care Wound Care	Circulatory Care: Arterial Insufficiency Circulatory Care: Venous Insufficiency Circulatory Precautions Infection Control Infection Protection Medication Administration: Oral Medication Administration: Skin Medication Management Total Parenteral Nutrition (TPN) Administration Transcutaneous Electrical Nerve Stimulation (TENS) Wound Irrigation

PART II - T

NURSING DIAGNOSIS: Tissue Perfusion: Peripheral, Ineffective

Definition: Decrease in blood circulation to the periphery that may compromise health

NICS ASSOCIATED WITH DIAGNOSIS RELATED FACTORS

Exercise Promotion Health Education	Smoking Cessation Assistance Teaching: Disease Process	Teaching: Individual Teaching: Procedure/ Treatment

NOC-NIC LINKAGES FOR TISSUE PERFUSION: PERIPHERAL, INEFFECTIVE

Outcome	Major Interventions	Suggested Interventions	
Circulation Status Definition: Unobstructed, unidirectional blood flow at an appropriate pressure through large vessels of the systemic and pulmonary circuits	Circulatory Care: Arterial Insufficiency Circulatory Care: Venous Insufficiency	Acid-Base Management Acid-Base Monitoring Circulatory Care: Mechanical Assist Device Circulatory Precautions Emergency Care Fluid /Electrolyte Management Fluid Management Fluid Monitoring Fluid Resuscitation Hemodynamic Regulation Hypovolemia Management Invasive Hemodynamic Monitoring	Laboratory Data Interpretation Lower Extremity Monitoring Neurological Monitoring Oxygen Therapy Peripheral Sensation Management Peripherally Inserted Central (PIC) Catheter Care Phlebotomy: Arterial Blood Sample Resuscitation Resuscitation: Neonate Shock Management Thrombolytic Therapy Management Vital Signs Monitoring
Fluid Overload Severity Definition: Severity of excess fluids in the intracellular and extracellular compartments of the body	Fluid/Electrolyte Management Fluid Management Hypervolemia Management	Acid-Base Management Acid-Base Monitoring Cardiac Care Circulatory Care: Venous Insufficiency Fluid Monitoring Hemodialysis Therapy Leech Therapy Lower Extremity Monitoring Medication Administration	Medication Management Oxygen Therapy Peritoneal Dialysis Therapy Positioning Pressure Management Pressure Ulcer Prevention Skin Surveillance
Sensory Function: Cutaneous Definition: Extent to which stimulation of the skin is correctly sensed	Peripheral Sensation Management	Circulatory Care: Arterial Insufficiency Circulatory Care: Venous Insufficiency Cutaneous Stimulation Foot Care Neurological Monitoring	Pain Management Positioning Pressure Ulcer Prevention Skin Surveillance Temperature Regulation

NOC-NIC LINKAGES FOR TISSUE PERFUSION: PERIPHERAL, INEFFECTIVE		
Outcome	**Major Interventions**	**Suggested Interventions**
Tissue Integrity: Skin & Mucous Membranes Definition: Structural intactness and normal physiological function of skin and mucous membranes	Circulatory Precautions Skin Surveillance	Amputation Care Bed Rest Care Cast Care: Maintenance Circulatory Care: Arterial Insufficiency Circulatory Care: Venous Insufficiency Cutaneous Stimulation Fluid Management Fluid Monitoring	Foot Care Medication Administration: Skin Medication Management Nutrition Management Positioning Pressure Management Pressure Ulcer Prevention Total Parenteral Nutrition (TPN) Administration
Tissue Perfusion: Peripheral Definition: Adequacy of blood flow through the small vessels of the extremities to maintain tissue function	Circulatory Care: Arterial Insufficiency Circulatory Care: Venous Insufficiency	Bedside Laboratory Testing Circulatory Care: Mechanical Assist Device Circulatory Precautions Embolus Care: Peripheral Embolus Precautions Emergency Care Exercise Promotion Fluid/Electrolyte Management Fluid Management Hypovolemia Management Intravenous (IV) Insertion Intravenous (IV) Therapy Laboratory Data Interpretation Lower Extremity Monitoring Medication Administration	Medication Management Phlebotomy: Arterial Blood Sample Phlebotomy: Venous Blood Sample Pneumatic Tourniquet Precautions Positioning Positioning: Wheelchair Pressure Ulcer Prevention Resuscitation Resuscitation: Neonate Shock Management Shock Management: Cardiac Shock Management: Vasogenic Shock Management: Volume Skin Surveillance Thrombolytic Therapy Management

PART II - T

NURSING DIAGNOSIS: Transfer Ability, Impaired

Definition: Limitation of independent movement between two nearby surfaces

NICS ASSOCIATED WITH DIAGNOSIS RELATED FACTORS

Communication Enhancement: Visual Deficit
Dementia Management
Environmental Management: Safety
Exercise Promotion
Exercise Promotion: Strength Training
Exercise Therapy: Balance
Exercise Therapy: Joint Mobility
Pain Management
Teaching: Prescribed Activity/Exercise
Weight Reduction Assistance

NOC-NIC LINKAGES FOR TRANSFER ABILITY, IMPAIRED

Outcome	Major Interventions	Suggested Interventions	
Balance Definition: Ability to maintain body equilibrium	Exercise Promotion: Strength Training Exercise Therapy: Balance	Body Mechanics Promotion Energy Management Environmental Management: Safety Exercise Promotion Exercise Therapy: Joint Mobility	Exercise Therapy: Muscle Control Fall Prevention Positioning Surveillance: Safety Teaching: Prescribed Activity/Exercise
Body Positioning: Self-Initiated Definition: Ability to change own body position independently with or without assistive device	Exercise Promotion: Strength Training Exercise Therapy: Muscle Control	Body Mechanics Promotion Energy Management Exercise Promotion Exercise Promotion: Stretching Exercise Therapy: Ambulation Exercise Therapy: Balance Exercise Therapy: Joint Mobility	Fall Prevention Pain Management Positioning Self-Care Assistance: Toileting Self-Care Assistance: Transfer Teaching: Prescribed Activity/Exercise Unilateral Neglect Management
Coordinated Movement Definition: Ability of muscles to work together voluntarily for purposeful movement	Exercise Promotion: Strength Training Exercise Therapy: Muscle Control	Body Mechanics Promotion Energy Management Exercise Promotion Exercise Promotion: Stretching Exercise Therapy: Balance Exercise Therapy: Joint Mobility	Medication Management Nutrition Management Pain Management Self-Care Assistance: Transfer Sleep Enhancement Weight Management

NOC-NIC LINKAGES FOR TRANSFER ABILITY, IMPAIRED		
Outcome	**Major Interventions**	**Suggested Interventions**
Transfer Performance Definition: Ability to change body location independently with or without assistive device	Exercise Promotion: Strength Training Self-Care Assistance: Transfer	Body Mechanics Promotion Energy Management Environmental Management: Safety Exercise Promotion Exercise Promotion: Stretching Exercise Therapy: Balance Exercise Therapy: Joint Mobility Exercise Therapy: Muscle Control Fall Prevention Pain Management Positioning Positioning: Wheelchair Self-Care Assistance Self-Care Assistance: Toileting Surveillance: Safety Teaching: Prescribed Activity/Exercise Teaching: Psychomotor Skill Weight Management

NURSING DIAGNOSIS: Unilateral Neglect

Definition: Impairment in sensory and motor response, mental representation and spatial attention of the body, and the corresponding environment characterized by inattention to one side and over-attention to the opposite side. Left side neglect is more severe and persistent than right side neglect.

NICS ASSOCIATED WITH DIAGNOSIS RELATED FACTORS		
Cerebral Edema Management Cerebral Perfusion Promotion	Communication Enhancement: Visual Deficit	Neurological Monitoring

NOC-NIC LINKAGES FOR UNILATERAL NEGLECT		
Outcome	**Major Interventions**	**Suggested Interventions**
Body Positioning: Self-Initiated Definition: Ability to change own body position independently with or without assistive device	Self-Care Assistance Unilateral Neglect Management	Exercise Promotion: Stretching Exercise Therapy: Ambulation Exercise Therapy: Balance Exercise Therapy: Muscle Control Fall Prevention Peripheral Sensation Management Positioning Teaching: Individual
Coordinated Movement Definition: Ability of muscles to work together voluntarily for purposeful movement	Exercise Therapy: Muscle Control	Exercise Promotion: Stretching Exercise Therapy: Ambulation Exercise Therapy: Balance Fall Prevention Unilateral Neglect Management

Continued

NOC-NIC LINKAGES FOR UNILATERAL NEGLECT		
Outcome	**Major Interventions**	**Suggested Interventions**
Heedfulness of Affected Side Definition: Personal actions to acknowledge, protect, and cognitively integrate affected body part(s) into self	Unilateral Neglect Management	Body Mechanics Promotion Environmental Management Environmental Management: Safety Exercise Therapy: Muscle Control
Self-Care: Activities of Daily Living (ADL) Definition: Ability to perform the most basic physical tasks and personal care activities independently with or without assistive device	Self-Care Assistance	Self-Care Assistance: Bathing/Hygiene Self-Care Assistance: Dressing/Grooming Self-Care Assistance: Feeding Self-Care Assistance: Toileting

NURSING DIAGNOSIS: Urinary Elimination, Impaired

Definition: Dysfunction in urine elimination

NICS ASSOCIATED WITH DIAGNOSIS RELATED FACTORS
Bladder Irrigation Infection Control

NOC-NIC LINKAGES FOR URINARY ELIMINATION, IMPAIRED		
Outcome	**Major Interventions**	**Suggested Interventions**
Urinary Elimination Definition: Collection and discharge of urine	Urinary Elimination Management	Fluid Management Fluid Monitoring Infection Protection Medication Administration Medication Management Pain Management Pelvic Muscle Exercise Pessary Management Prompted Voiding Self-Care Assistance: Toileting Specimen Management Tube Care: Urinary Urinary Bladder Training Urinary Catheterization Urinary Catheterization: Intermittent Urinary Incontinence Care Urinary Retention Care

Critical reasoning note: The interventions included for the general outcome of Impaired Urinary Elimination include those identified for specific urinary problems.

NURSING DIAGNOSIS: Urinary Elimination, Readiness for Enhanced

Definition: A pattern of urinary functions that is sufficient for meeting eliminatory needs and can be strengthened

NOC-NIC LINKAGES FOR URINARY ELIMINATION, READINESS FOR ENHANCED		
Outcome	**Major Interventions**	**Suggested Interventions**
Urinary Elimination Definition: Collection and discharge of urine	Urinary Elimination Management	Fluid Management Fluid Monitoring Infection Protection Medication Management	Pelvic Muscle Exercise Pessary Management Self-Care Assistance: Toileting Weight Management

NURSING DIAGNOSIS: Urinary Incontinence: Functional

Definition: Inability of usually continent person to reach toilet in time to avoid unintentional loss of urine

NICS ASSOCIATED WITH DIAGNOSIS RELATED FACTORS			
Delusion Management Dementia Management	Communication Enhancement: Visual Deficit	Mood Management	Relocation Stress Reduction

NOC-NIC LINKAGES FOR URINARY INCONTINENCE: FUNCTIONAL		
Outcome	**Major Interventions**	**Suggested Interventions**
Self-Care: Toileting Definition: Ability to toilet self independently with or without assistive device	Environmental Management Self-Care Assistance: Toileting	Communication Enhancement: Visual Deficit Environmental Management: Safety Exercise Therapy: Ambulation	Perineal Care Prompted Voiding Surveillance: Safety Urinary Incontinence Care
Urinary Continence Definition: Control of elimination of urine from the bladder	Prompted Voiding Urinary Habit Training	Environmental Management Fluid Management Pelvic Muscle Exercise Perineal Care	Self-Care Assistance: Toileting Urinary Incontinence Care

PART II - U

NURSING DIAGNOSIS: Urinary Incontinence: Overflow

Definition: Involuntary loss of urine associated with overdistension of the bladder

NICS ASSOCIATED WITH DIAGNOSIS RELATED FACTORS

Medication Management	Referral

NOC-NIC LINKAGES FOR URINARY INCONTINENCE: OVERFLOW

Outcome	Major Interventions	Suggested Interventions	
Medication Response Definition: Therapeutic and adverse effects of prescribed medication	Teaching: Prescribed Medication	Medication Administration Medication Management	Medication Reconciliation Surveillance
Urinary Continence Definition: Control of elimination of urine from the bladder	Urinary Catheterization: Intermittent Urinary Retention Care	Fluid Management Medication Management	Pessary Management Urinary Elimination Management Urinary Incontinence Care

NURSING DIAGNOSIS: Urinary Incontinence: Reflex

Definition: Involuntary loss of urine at somewhat predictable intervals when a specific bladder volume is reached

NICS ASSOCIATED WITH DIAGNOSIS RELATED FACTORS

Infection Control	Neurological Monitoring	Radiation Therapy Management	Vital Signs Monitoring

NOC-NIC LINKAGES FOR URINARY INCONTINENCE: REFLEX

Outcome	Major Interventions	Suggested Interventions	
Tissue Integrity: Skin & Mucous Membranes Definition: Structural intactness and normal physiological function of skin and mucous membranes	Urinary Incontinence Care	Bathing Perineal Care	Self-Care Assistance: Bathing/Hygiene
Urinary Continence Definition: Control of elimination of urine from the bladder	Urinary Catheterization: Intermittent	Fluid Management Fluid Monitoring Teaching: Procedure/ Treatment Tube Care: Urinary	Urinary Catheterization Urinary Incontinence Care Urinary Retention Care

NURSING DIAGNOSIS: Urinary Incontinence: Stress

Definition: Sudden leakage of urine with activities that increase intra-abdominal pressure

NICS ASSOCIATED WITH DIAGNOSIS RELATED FACTORS

Pelvic Muscle Exercise   Prenatal Care

NOC-NIC LINKAGES FOR URINARY INCONTINENCE: STRESS

Outcome	Major Interventions	Suggested Interventions	
Urinary Continence Definition: Control of elimination of urine from the bladder	Pelvic Muscle Exercise	Environmental Management: Safety Fluid Management Medication Management Perineal Care Pessary Management Postpartal Care	Self-Care Assistance: Toileting Teaching: Individual Teaching: Prescribed Medication Urinary Incontinence Care Weight Management

NURSING DIAGNOSIS: Urinary Incontinence: Urge

Definition: Involuntary passage of urine occurring soon after a strong sense of urgency to void

NICS ASSOCIATED WITH DIAGNOSIS RELATED FACTORS

Infection Control

NOC-NIC LINKAGES FOR URINARY INCONTINENCE: URGE

Outcome	Major Interventions	Suggested Interventions	
Self-Care: Toileting Definition: Ability to toilet self independently with or without assistive device	Self-Care Assistance: Toileting	Environmental Management: Safety Fluid Management Fluid Monitoring	Perineal Care Prompted Voiding Urinary Incontinence Care
Urinary Continence Definition: Control of elimination of urine from the bladder	Medication Management Urinary Bladder Training	Environmental Management Fluid Management Pelvic Muscle Exercise Perineal Care	Self-Care Assistance: Toileting Teaching: Prescribed Medication Urinary Habit Training Urinary Incontinence Care

NURSING DIAGNOSIS: Urinary Retention

Definition: Incomplete emptying of the bladder

NICS ASSOCIATED WITH DIAGNOSIS RELATED FACTORS

Urinary Catheterization

NOC-NIC LINKAGES FOR URINARY RETENTION

Outcome	Major Interventions	Suggested Interventions	
Urinary Elimination Definition: Collection and discharge of urine	Urinary Catheterization: Intermittent Urinary Retention Care	Fluid Management Fluid Monitoring Medication Administration Medication Management Self-Care Assistance: Toileting	Specimen Management Tube Care: Urinary Urinary Catheterization Urinary Elimination Management Urinary Incontinence Care

NURSING DIAGNOSIS: Ventilation, Impaired Spontaneous

Definition: Decreased energy reserves result in an individual's inability to maintain breathing adequate to support life

NICS ASSOCIATED WITH DIAGNOSIS RELATED FACTORS

Hyperglycemia Management   Hypoglycemia Management

NOC-NIC LINKAGES FOR VENTILATION, IMPAIRED SPONTANEOUS

Outcome	Major Interventions	Suggested Interventions	
Mechanical Ventilation Response: Adult Definition: Alveolar exchange and tissue perfusion are supported by mechanical ventilation	Mechanical Ventilation Management: Invasive Oxygen Therapy Respiratory Monitoring	Airway Management Airway Suctioning Anxiety Reduction Aspiration Precautions Bed Rest Care Calming Technique Chest Physiotherapy Coping Enhancement Emotional Support Energy Management Environmental Management: Comfort Environmental Management: Safety Fluid Management	Infection Control Infection Protection Mechanical Ventilatory Weaning Medication Management Oral Health Maintenance Patient Rights Protection Phlebotomy: Arterial Blood Sample Positioning Pressure Management Skin Surveillance Surveillance: Safety Technology Management Vital Signs Monitoring

NOC-NIC LINKAGES FOR VENTILATION, IMPAIRED SPONTANEOUS		
Outcome	**Major Interventions**	**Suggested Interventions**
Respiratory Status: Gas Exchange		
Definition: Alveolar exchange of carbon dioxide and oxygen to maintain arterial blood gas concentrations	Oxygen Therapy Respiratory Monitoring	Acid-Base Management Acid-Base Management: Respiratory Acidosis Acid-Base Management: Respiratory Alkalosis Acid-Base Monitoring Airway Insertion and Stabilization Airway Management Airway Suctioning Anxiety Reduction Aspiration Precautions Chest Physiotherapy Cough Enhancement / Energy Management Fluid/Electrolyte Management Fluid Management Fluid Monitoring Infection Control Infection Protection Intravenous (IV) Insertion Intravenous (IV) Therapy Laboratory Data Interpretation Phlebotomy: Arterial Blood Sample Resuscitation Ventilation Assistance
Respiratory Status: Ventilation		
Definition: Movement of air in and out of the lungs	Airway Management Artificial Airway Management Respiratory Monitoring Ventilation Assistance	Acid-Base Monitoring Airway Insertion and Stabilization Airway Suctioning Anxiety Reduction Aspiration Precautions Chest Physiotherapy Coping Enhancement Emergency Care Emotional Support Endotracheal Extubation / Energy Management Fluid Management Oxygen Therapy Phlebotomy: Arterial Blood Sample Positioning Resuscitation: Neonate Security Enhancement Surveillance Tube Care: Chest Vital Signs Monitoring
Vital Signs		
Definition: Extent to which temperature, pulse, respiration, and blood pressure are within normal range	Respiratory Monitoring Vital Signs Monitoring	Acid-Base Management Airway Management Anxiety Reduction Emergency Care Environmental Management Fluid/Electrolyte Management Fluid Management Infection Control Infection Protection / Intravenous (IV) Insertion Intravenous (IV) Therapy Medication Administration Medication Management Music Therapy Oxygen Therapy Pain Management Relaxation Therapy Ventilation Assistance

PART II - V

NURSING DIAGNOSIS: Ventilatory Weaning Response, Dysfunctional

Definition: Inability to adjust to lowered levels of mechanical ventilator support that interrupts and pro-longs the weaning process

NICS ASSOCIATED WITH DIAGNOSIS RELATED FACTORS			
Airway Suctioning	Environmental	Nutritional Monitoring	Self-Esteem
Anxiety Reduction	Management	Pain Management	Enhancement
Energy Management	Family Presence	Self-Efficacy	Sleep Enhancement
	Facilitation	Enhancement	Teaching: Individual
	Hope Inspiration		

NOC-NIC LINKAGES FOR VENTILATORY WEANING RESPONSE, DYSFUNCTIONAL		
Outcome	**Major Interventions**	**Suggested Interventions**
Anxiety Level		
Definition: Severity of manifested apprehension, tension, or uneasiness arising from an unidentifiable source	Anxiety Reduction Preparatory Sensory Information	Biofeedback Calming Technique Coping Enhancement Distraction Emotional Support Environmental Management: Comfort	Guided Imagery Medication Administration Music Therapy Presence Relaxation Therapy Security Enhancement
Mechanical Ventilation Weaning Response: Adult		
Definition: Respiratory and psychological adjustment to progressive removal of mechanical ventilation	Mechanical Ventilatory Weaning Respiratory Monitoring Vital Signs Monitoring	Acid-Base Management Airway Management Airway Suctioning Anxiety Reduction Artificial Airway Management Aspiration Precautions Calming Technique Distraction Emotional Support Endotracheal Extubation Energy Management	Environmental Management: Comfort Environmental Management: Safety Mechanical Ventilation Management: Invasive Medication Management Music Therapy Phlebotomy: Arterial Blood Sample Preparatory Sensation Information Presence Sleep Enhancement Surveillance

NOC-NIC LINKAGES FOR VENTILATORY WEANING RESPONSE, DYSFUNCTIONAL

Outcome	Major Interventions	Suggested Interventions	
Respiratory Status: Gas Exchange Definition: Alveolar exchange of carbon dioxide and oxygen to maintain arterial blood gas concentrations	Respiratory Monitoring Ventilation Assistance	Acid-Base Management: Respiratory Acidosis Acid-Base Management: Respiratory Alkalosis Acid-Base Monitoring Airway Management Airway Suctioning Anxiety Reduction Artificial Airway Management	Aspiration Precautions Chest Physiotherapy Cough Enhancement Energy Management Laboratory Data Interpretation Mechanical Ventilatory Weaning Oxygen Therapy Positioning Phlebotomy: Arterial Blood Sample
Respiratory Status: Ventilation Definition: Movement of air in and out of the lungs	Mechanical Ventilatory Weaning Respiratory Monitoring	Acid-Base Monitoring Airway Management Airway Suctioning Anxiety Reduction Artificial Airway Management Aspiration Precautions Calming Technique Cough Enhancement	Emotional Support Energy Management Environmental Management: Safety Oxygen Therapy Positioning Presence Relaxation Therapy Ventilation Assistance
Vital Signs Definition: Extent to which temperature, pulse, respiration, and blood pressure are within normal range	Respiratory Monitoring Vital Signs Monitoring	Airway Management Anxiety Reduction Environmental Management Environmental Management: Comfort Mechanical Ventilatory Weaning Medication Administration	Medication Management Music Therapy Oxygen Therapy Pain Management Relaxation Therapy Ventilation Assistance

NURSING DIAGNOSIS: Walking, Impaired

Definition: Limitation of independent movement within the environment on foot

NICS ASSOCIATED WITH DIAGNOSIS RELATED FACTORS

Communication Enhancement: Visual Deficit Dementia Management Energy Management	Environmental Management Exercise Promotion Exercise Promotion: Strength Training	Exercise Therapy: Balance Fall Prevention Mood Management	Pain Management Teaching: Prescribed Activity/Exercise Weight Reduction Assistance

Continued

NOC-NIC LINKAGES FOR WALKING, IMPAIRED

Outcome	Major Interventions	Suggested Interventions	
Ambulation Definition: Ability to walk from place to place independently with or without assistive device	Exercise Therapy: Ambulation	Body Mechanics Promotion Energy Management Environmental Management Environmental Management: Safety Exercise Promotion Exercise Promotion: Strength Training Exercise Promotion: Stretching Exercise Therapy: Balance	Exercise Therapy: Joint Mobility Exercise Therapy: Muscle Control Fall Prevention Lower Extremity Monitoring Medication Management Positioning Teaching: Prescribed Activity/Exercise
Balance Definition: Ability to maintain body equilibrium	Exercise Therapy: Ambulation Exercise Therapy: Balance	Energy Management Environmental Management: Safety Exercise Promotion: Strength Training Exercise Therapy: Joint Mobility	Exercise Therapy: Muscle Control Fall Prevention Teaching: Prescribed Activity/Exercise
Coordinated Movement Definition: Ability of muscles to work together voluntarily for purposeful movement	Exercise Therapy: Ambulation Exercise Therapy: Muscle Control	Body Mechanics Promotion Exercise Promotion Exercise Promotion: Strength Training	Exercise Promotion: Stretching Exercise Therapy: Balance
Endurance Definition: Capacity to sustain activity	Energy Management	Environmental Management Exercise Promotion Exercise Therapy: Ambulation Exercise Therapy: Balance Exercise Therapy: Joint Mobility	Exercise Therapy: Muscle Control Mutual Goal Setting Nutrition Management Sleep Enhancement Teaching: Prescribed Activity/Exercise
Joint Movement: Ankle, Hip, Knee Definition: Active range of motion of the _____ (specify joint) with self-initiated movement	Exercise Therapy: Joint Mobility	Energy Management Exercise Promotion Exercise Promotion: Strength Training	Exercise Promotion: Stretching Exercise Therapy: Ambulation Fall Prevention

NOC-NIC LINKAGES FOR WALKING, IMPAIRED

Outcome	Major Interventions	Suggested Interventions	
Mobility			
Definition: Ability to move purposefully in own environment independently with or without assistive device	Exercise Therapy: Ambulation	Analgesic Administration Body Mechanics Promotion Energy Management Environmental Management: Safety Exercise Promotion Exercise Promotion: Stretching	Exercise Promotion: Strength Training Exercise Therapy: Balance Exercise Therapy: Joint Mobility Exercise Therapy: Muscle Control Positioning Teaching: Prescribed Activity/Exercise

NURSING DIAGNOSIS: Wandering

Definition: Meandering, aimless, or repetitive locomotion that exposes the individual to harm; frequently incongruent with boundaries, limits, or obstacles

NICS ASSOCIATED WITH DIAGNOSIS RELATED FACTORS

Anxiety Reduction Behavior Modification Chemical Restraint Communication Enhancement: Visual Deficit	Constipation/Impaction Management Dementia Management Diarrhea Management Environmental Management	Mood Management Pain Management Prompted Voiding Reality Orientation	Relocation Stress Reduction Self-Care Assistance: Toileting Urinary Elimination Management

NOC-NIC LINKAGES FOR WANDERING

Outcome	Major Interventions	Suggested Interventions	
Elopement Occurrence			
Definition: Number of times in the past 24 hours/1 week/ 1 month (select one) that an individual with a cognitive impairment escapes a secure area	Elopement Precautions	Environmental Management: Safety	Surveillance: Safety
Elopement Propensity Risk			
Definition: The propensity of an individual with cognitive impairment to escape a secure area	Elopement Precautions	Anxiety Reduction Area Restriction Environmental Management: Safety	Patient Rights Protection Relocation Stress Reduction Surveillance: Safety

Continued

PART II - W

NOC-NIC LINKAGES FOR WANDERING

Outcome	Major Interventions	Suggested Interventions	
Fall Prevention Behavior Definition: Personal or family caregiver actions to minimize risk factors that might precipitate falls in the personal environment	Environmental Management: Safety Fall Prevention	Area Restriction Dementia Management Elopement Precautions	Self-Care Assistance Surveillance: Safety
Safe Home Environment Definition: Physical arrangements to minimize environmental factors that might cause physical harm or injury in the home	Elopement Precautions Environmental Management: Safety	Fall Prevention Family Involvement Promotion	Self-Care Assistance Surveillance: Safety
Safe Wandering Definition: Safe, socially acceptable moving about without apparent purpose in an individual with cognitive impairment	Dementia Management Elopement Precautions	Anxiety Reduction Area Restriction Calming Technique Distraction	Environmental Management: Safety Fall Prevention Reality Orientation Surveillance: Safety

Introduction to Linkages for Risk for Nursing Diagnoses

Major changes have been made in how the *risk nursing* diagnoses are constructed and presented. The diagnoses continue to be listed in alphabetical order, with the major concept stated first followed by the term *Risk for*. For example, *Risk for Imbalanced Fluid Volume* is presented as *Fluid Volume, Risk for Imbalanced*. The NANDA-I diagnoses that address risk do not include the same elements as the diagnoses that depict actual or health promotion patient states. These diagnoses include a definition and risk factors; defining characteristics are not part of a *risk nursing* diagnosis. As before, the definition of the diagnosis is provided along with the diagnostic name.

Previous editions provided outcomes that would be evaluated to determine if the problem that the patient was at risk for had occurred. For example, the suggested outcomes for *Activity Intolerance, Risk for,* included *Activity Tolerance, Endurance,* and *Energy Conservation,* the same outcomes as those for the diagnosis *Activity Intolerance.* The interventions linked to the outcome were those required to achieve the outcome and thus presupposed that some activity intolerance had occurred. As a result, both the outcomes and the interventions were often repetitious of those associated with actual or health promotion diagnoses in the preceding section.

CONSTRUCTION OF LINKAGES

To prevent repetition, the outcomes and the interventions that measure and treat the underlying risk factors associated with the NANDA-I diagnoses are presented in this edition. The risk factors associated with each diagnosis vary from a few to a lengthy list. For example, there are 7 risk factors with *Risk for Shock* and 66 with *Risk for Impaired*

Parenting; therefore the number of outcomes and interventions to address risk factors can vary from a few to many. There are instances in which the same outcome and/or intervention(s) might be related to more than one risk factor, as with hypoxemia and hypoxia with *Risk for Shock.* Risk factors can also vary by type; they can be environmental, physiological, psychological, genetic, or chemical factors. Risk factors are sometimes organized in groups that might be addressed by one or two outcomes and related interventions. For example, *Risk for Impaired Parenting* has risk factors grouped as Infant/Child, Knowledge, Physiological, Psychological, and Social. The outcome *Knowledge: Parenting* and the interventions *Parent Education: Adolescent, Parent Education: Childbearing Family,* and *Parent Education: Infant* can be related to more than one risk factor in the Knowledge group.

To avoid repetition of outcomes and interventions for each risk diagnosis and to prevent unwieldy lists of outcomes and interventions when there are a high number of risk factors, the NOC outcomes and NIC interventions are not linked to each risk factor. The outcome that would most likely be used to assess and measure if the risk state has occurred is listed without associated interventions. For example, *Parent-Infant Attachment* is the NOC outcome used to measure if impaired attachment actually occurs or is prevented for the diagnosis *Risk for Impaired Attachment.* Interventions commonly used to achieve the outcome can often be found within the previous section of actual or health promotion diagnoses. Based on the risk factors, a list of NOC outcomes and NIC interventions is provided. There are some outcomes and interventions that are appropriate for most *risk nursing* diagnoses; for example, the outcomes *Risk Detection* and *Risk Control* and the interventions *Risk Identification* and

Surveillance. These are not repeated with each diagnosis, but will be noted when they are an important outcome or intervention for a particular diagnosis.

Once the nurse has determined the risk factors pertinent to the patient/client, she or he can select the NOC outcomes and NIC interventions needed to address the risk factors for each risk nursing diagnosis. Two examples of how these NOC and NIC lists can be used with the list of risk factors follow. One of the risk factors listed for *Risk for Shock* is hypovolemia, a fluid volume deficit. Hypovolemia can be caused by prolonged inadequate fluid intake or by excessive fluid loss such as from vomiting, diarrhea, or hemorrhage. If the cause of the hypovolemia is hemorrhage, the outcome *Blood Loss Severity* might be selected and the intervention *Bleeding Reduction* or *Hemorrhage Control* selected depending upon the severity of the blood loss. With the diagnosis *Risk for Impaired Parenting,* the judgment might be that the risk factor is depression and *Mood Equilibrium* or *Depression Level* could be selected as an outcome and *Mood Management* and *Medication Management* as possible interventions. If the pertinent risk factor is lack of a social support network, *Social Support* might be selected as an outcome and *Support System Enhancement* as an intervention. Presenting the risk diagnoses in this fashion allows for the clinician to make clinical judgments at each step of the process and individualize the care for each patient/client. It also focuses on managing the risk factors to prevent the occurrence of the problem for which the patient/client is at risk.

PRESENTATION OF THE LINKAGES

Changes made in the construction of the linkages allow the linkages to be presented in a more succinct and hopefully useful manner. As with the actual and health promotion diagnoses, the risk nursing diagnosis and definition are presented. These are followed by the outcome(s) that can be used to assess and measure the occurrence of the patient state that is to be prevented or avoided. For example, with *Risk for Shock, Tissue Perfusion: Cellular* is suggested as an outcome consistent with the definition provided for shock, and *Parenting Performance* and *Parenting: Psychosocial Safety* are suggested as measures for the diagnosis *Risk for Impaired Parenting.* There is an occasional diagnosis with more than one or two outcomes to measure the occurrence of the risk state. *Risk for Delayed Development* can be assessed and measured by determining if the child reaches developmental milestones; therefore *Child Development* outcomes from 1 month to adolescence are all pertinent outcomes depending on the age of the child.

A list of NOC outcomes for the identified risk factors for each risk nursing diagnosis is presented next. The suggested outcomes are listed alphabetically, requiring the nurse to select the ones appropriate for the patient/client risk factor(s). The NIC interventions associated with the identified risk factors are listed next. Again, these are presented alphabetically, and need to be selected based on the risk factor and/or the outcome, as modeled previously. Because this is a major change in the presentation of this material, the authors would appreciate feedback from users as they implement and evaluate these linkages.

CASE STUDY 3

NANDA-I Risk for Nursing Diagnosis

Claudia S. is an 88-year-old woman who lives alone in an independent living unit in a retirement community. She has four daughters and nine grandchildren who visit on a regular basis. She no longer drives but has frequent contact with members of her church community. She spends her time reading, watching news and sports on television, and sewing lap robes that are donated to a local hospital. Claudia developed osteoarthritis after many years of active life on the family farm but is otherwise in good health with normal blood pressure and blood glucose level. She had bilateral knee replacements 15 years ago and now has degeneration of her right hip. She has elected not to have hip replacement surgery. She walks with the assistance of a cane and has a lift chair to help her stand up from a sitting position, but she declines to use the available walker. She has taken Tylenol 500 mg BID for several

CASE STUDY 3—cont'd

years to help control the pain. Lately her daughter has noticed that Claudia forgets to take her medication and has an increasing number of short-term memory lapses. The retirement community provides cleaning services twice a month and the family arranged for a noon meal to be delivered Monday through Friday. When Claudia disclosed she was not getting into the shower because she was afraid of falling, the family contacted the local visiting nurse association for assistance. After completing her assessment, the visiting nurse arranged for a home health aide to assist Claudia with bathing twice a week. The nurse identified the following priority nursing diagnosis with related outcomes and interventions:

NANDA-I Diagnosis:

Risk for Falls
Definition: Increased susceptibility to falling that may cause physical harm

Risk Factors
Age 65 or over
Lives alone
Use of assistive devices
Diminished mental status
Arthritis
Decreased lower extremity strength
Difficulty with gait
Impaired physical mobility

NOC Outcomes

Fall Prevention Behavior
Indicators
Uses assistive devices correctly
Uses safe transfer procedure
Eliminates clutter, spills, and glare from floors
Adjusts toilet height as needed
Adjusts chair height as needed
Uses grab bars as needed
Uses rubber mats in shower

NIC Interventions

Fall Prevention
Activities
Monitor gait, balance, and fatigue level with ambulation
Share with patient observations about gait and movement
Instruct patient about use of cane and walker
Encourage patient to use cane and walker
Maintain assistive devices in good working order
Place articles within easy reach of the patient
Provide elevated toilet seat for easy transfer
Provide chairs of proper height, with backrests and armrests for easy transfer
Educate family members about risk factors that contribute to falls and how these risks can be decreased
Suggest home adaptations to increase safety

Continued

PART II

CASE STUDY 3—cont'd

To assess and measure the actual occurrence of the risk nursing diagnosis, Risk for Falls, the nurse might select either *Falls Occurrence* or *Physical Injury Severity*.

Other NOCs Associated with the Risk Factors for Risk for Falls for Claudia
Acute Confusion Level
Ambulation
Cognition
Mobility
Transfer Performance

Other NICs Associated with the Prevention of Falls for Claudia
Body Mechanics Promotion
Environmental Management: Safety
Exercise Therapy: Ambulation
Reality Orientation

NOC and NIC Linked to Risk for Nursing Diagnoses

NURSING DIAGNOSIS: Activity Intolerance, Risk for

Definition: At risk for experiencing insufficient physiological or psychological energy to endure or complete required or desired daily activities

NOCS TO ASSESS AND MEASURE ACTUAL OCCURRENCE OF THE DIAGNOSIS

Activity Tolerance

Psychomotor Energy

NOCS ASSOCIATED WITH RISK FACTORS FOR ACTIVITY INTOLERANCE

Asthma Self-Management
Body Mechanics Performance
Cardiac Disease
   Self-Management
Cardiac Pump Effectiveness
Cardiopulmonary Status
Circulation Status
Coordinated Movement
Endurance
Energy Conservation

Fatigue Level
Health Promoting Behavior
Knowledge: Body Mechanics
Knowledge: Energy Conservation
Knowledge: Prescribed Activity
Multiple Sclerosis
   Self-Management
Nutritional Status: Energy
Physical Fitness

Respiratory Status
Respiratory Status: Gas
   Exchange
Respiratory Status: Ventilation
Risk Control
Risk Control: Cardiovascular
   Health
Risk Detection
Smoking Cessation Behavior

NICS ASSOCIATED WITH PREVENTION OF ACTIVITY INTOLERANCE

Asthma Management
Cardiac Precautions
Cardiac Care: Rehabilitative
Energy Management
Exercise Promotion
Exercise Promotion: Strength
   Training
Exercise Promotion: Stretching

Exercise Therapy: Ambulation
Exercise Therapy: Balance
Exercise Therapy: Joint Mobility
Exercise Therapy: Muscle Control
Nutrition Management
Pacemaker Management:
   Permanent
Respiratory Monitoring

Risk Identification
Self-Care Assistance: IADL
Smoking Cessation Assistance
Surveillance
Teaching: Prescribed
   Activity/Exercise
Vital Signs Monitoring

NURSING DIAGNOSIS: Aspiration, Risk for

Definition: At risk for entry of gastrointestinal secretions, oropharyngeal secretions, solids, or fluids, into tracheobronchial passages

NOCS TO ASSESS AND MEASURE ACTUAL OCCURRENCE OF THE DIAGNOSIS

Respiratory Status	Respiratory Status: Gas	Respiratory Status: Ventilation
Respiratory Status: Airway Patency	Exchange	

NOCS ASSOCIATED WITH RISK FACTORS FOR ASPIRATION

Aspiration Prevention	Nausea & Vomiting Control	Self Care: Non-Parenteral
Cognition	Nausea & Vomiting Severity	Medication
Cognitive Orientation	Neurological Status:	Swallowing Status
Gastrointestinal Function	Consciousness	Swallowing Status:
Immobility Consequences:	Post-Procedure Recovery	Esophageal Phase
Physiological	Risk Control	Swallowing Status:
Mechanical Ventilation	Risk Detection	Oral Phase
Response: Adult	Seizure Control	Swallowing Status:
Mechanical Ventilation Weaning	Self-Care: Eating	Pharyngeal Phase
Response: Adult		

NICS ASSOCIATED WITH PREVENTION OF ASPIRATION

Airway Management	Mechanical Ventilation	Risk Identification
Airway Suctioning	Management: Invasive	Sedation Management
Artificial Airway Management	Mechanical Ventilatory Weaning	Seizure Management
Aspiration Precautions	Medication Administration:	Self-Care Assistance:
Chest Physiotherapy	Enteral	Feeding
Cough Enhancement	Medication Administration: Oral	Surveillance
Dementia Management	Neurologic Monitoring	Swallowing Therapy
Enteral Tube Feeding	Positioning	Tube Care: Gastrointestinal
Feeding	Postanesthesia Care	Vomiting Management
Gastrointestinal Intubation	Respiratory Monitoring	
	Resuscitation: Neonate	

NURSING DIAGNOSIS: Attachment, Risk for Impaired

Definition: Disruption of the interactive process between parent/significant other, child/infant that fosters the development of a protective and nurturing reciprocal relationship

NOCS TO ASSESS AND MEASURE ACTUAL OCCURRENCE OF THE DIAGNOSIS

Parent-Infant Attachment

NOCS ASSOCIATED WITH RISK FACTORS FOR IMPAIRED ATTACHMENT

Anxiety Level	Child Development:	Preterm Infant Organization
Anxiety Self-Control	12 Months	Risk Control
Child Development: 1 Month	Knowledge: Parenting	Risk Detection
Child Development: 2 Months	Knowledge: Preterm	Stress Level
Child Development: 4 Months	Infant Care	Substance Addiction
Child Development:	Parenting Performance	Consequences
6 Months		

NICS ASSOCIATED WITH PREVENTION OF IMPAIRED ATTACHMENT

Anticipatory Guidance	Environmental Management:	Risk Identification
Anxiety Reduction	Attachment Process	Risk Identification: Childbearing
Attachment Promotion	Family Integrity Promotion:	Family
Childbirth Preparation	Childbearing Family	Substance Use Prevention
Coping Enhancement	Infant Care	Substance Use Treatment
Developmental Care	Parent Education:	Surveillance
Developmental Enhancement:	Childrearing Family	Teaching: Infant Stimulation
Child	Parent Education: Infant	0-4 Months
	Parenting Promotion	

PART II - A

NURSING DIAGNOSIS: Autonomic Dysreflexia, Risk for

Definition: At risk for life-threatening uninhibited response of the sympathetic nervous system, post spinal shock, in an individual with spinal cord injury or lesion at T6 or above (has been demonstrated in patients with injuries at T7 and T8)

NOCS TO ASSESS AND MEASURE ACTUAL OCCURRENCE OF THE DIAGNOSIS

Cardiopulmonary Status

Neurological Status: Autonomic

NOCS ASSOCIATED WITH RISK FACTORS FOR AUTONOMIC DYSREFLEXIA

Bone Healing
Bowel Elimination
Burn Recovery
Circulation Status
Gastrointestinal Function
Infection Severity
Medication Response
Pain Level

Risk Control
Risk Control: Hyperthermia
Risk Control: Hypothermia
Risk Control: Infectious
  Process
Risk Detection
Sensory Function: Cutaneous
Substance Withdrawal Severity

Symptom Severity: Premenstrual
  Syndrome (PMS)
Thermoregulation
Tissue Integrity: Skin & Mucous
  Membranes
Urinary Elimination
Wound Healing: Secondary
  Intention

NICS ASSOCIATED WITH PREVENTION OF AUTONOMIC DYSREFLEXIA

Bowel Management
Bowel Training
Circulatory Precautions
Constipation/Impaction
  Management
Dysreflexia Management
Embolus Care: Peripheral
Environmental Management:
  Safety
Exercise Therapy: Joint Mobility
Flatulence Reduction
High-Risk Pregnancy Care
Infection Control
Infection Protection
Intrapartal Care: High-Risk
  Delivery

Medication Management
Neurologic Monitoring
Pain Management
Positioning
Premenstrual Syndrome
  (PMS) Management
Pressure Management
Pressure Ulcer Care
Pressure Ulcer Prevention
Risk Identification
Sexual Counseling
Skin Surveillance
Substance Use Treatment:
  Drug Withdrawal

Surveillance
Surveillance: Late Pregnancy
Temperature Regulation
Thrombolytic Therapy
  Management
Urinary Catheterization
Urinary Catheterization:
  Intermittent
Urinary Elimination
  Management
Vital Signs Monitoring
Wound Care
Wound Care: Burns

NURSING DIAGNOSIS: Bleeding, Risk for

Definition: At risk for a decrease in blood volume that may compromise health

NOCS TO ASSESS AND MEASURE ACTUAL OCCURRENCE OF THE DIAGNOSIS

Blood Loss Severity   Circulation Status

NOCS ASSOCIATED WITH RISK FACTORS FOR BLEEDING

Blood Coagulation	Knowledge: Cancer	Maternal Status: Postpartum
Compliance Behavior:	Management	Medication Response
Prescribed Medication	Knowledge: Fall Prevention	Personal Safety Behavior
Fall Prevention Behavior	Knowledge: Medication	Physical Injury Severity
Falls Occurrence	Knowledge: Personal Safety	Risk Control
Gastrointestinal Function	Knowledge: Treatment Regimen	Risk Detection
Hemodialysis Access	Maternal Status: Antepartum	Treatment Behavior:
	Maternal Status: Intrapartum	Illness or Injury

NICS ASSOCIATED WITH PREVENTION OF BLEEDING

Bleeding Precautions	Chemotherapy Management	Risk Identification
Bleeding Reduction	Circumcision Care	Shock Prevention
Bleeding Reduction:	Dialysis Access Maintenance	Sports Injury Prevention:
Antepartum Uterus	Environmental Management:	Youth
Bleeding Reduction:	Safety	Surveillance
Gastrointestinal	Fall Prevention	Teaching: Prescribed Medication
Bleeding Reduction: Nasal	Incision Site Care	Teaching: Procedure/Treatment
Bleeding Reduction:	Medication Management	Thrombolytic Therapy
Postpartum Uterus	Postpartal Care	Management
Bleeding Reduction: Wound	Prenatal Care	Vehicle Safety Promotion

PART II - B

NURSING DIAGNOSIS: Blood Glucose Level, Risk for Unstable

Definition: Risk for variation of blood glucose/sugar levels from the normal range

NOCS TO ASSESS AND MEASURE ACTUAL OCCURRENCE OF THE DIAGNOSIS

Blood Glucose Level

NOCS ASSOCIATED WITH RISK FACTORS FOR UNSTABLE BLOOD GLUCOSE

Acceptance: Health Status
Activity Tolerance
Adherence Behavior:
   Healthy Diet
Compliance Behavior:
   Prescribed Diet
Compliance Behavior:
   Prescribed Medication
Depression Level
Diabetes Self-Management
Endurance
Knowledge: Diabetes
   Management

Knowledge: Diet
Knowledge: Medication
Knowledge: Prescribed Activity
Knowledge: Treatment Regimen
Mood Equilibrium
Nutritional Status
Nutritional Status: Biochemical
   Measures
Nutritional Status:
   Food & Fluid Intake

Nutritional Status:
   Nutrient Intake
Physical Fitness
Prenatal Health Behavior
Risk Control
Risk Detection
Stress Level
Weight Maintenance
   Behavior

NICS ASSOCIATED WITH PREVENTION OF UNSTABLE BLOOD GLUCOSE

Anxiety Reduction
Behavior Modification
Exercise Promotion
High-Risk Pregnancy Care
Hyperglycemia Management
Hypoglycemia Management
Medication Management
Mood Management

Nutritional Counseling
Nutritional Monitoring
Prenatal Care
Risk Identification
Self-Efficacy Enhancement
Self-Responsibility Facilitation
Surveillance

Teaching: Disease Process
Teaching: Prescribed Activity/
   Exercise
Teaching: Prescribed Diet
Teaching: Prescribed Medication
Teaching: Procedure/Treatment
Weight Management

NURSING DIAGNOSIS: Body Temperature, Risk for Imbalanced

Definition: At risk for failure to maintain body temperature within normal range

NOCS TO ASSESS AND MEASURE ACTUAL OCCURRENCE OF THE DIAGNOSIS

Thermoregulation	Thermoregulation: Newborn

NOCS ASSOCIATED WITH RISK FACTORS FOR IMBALANCED BODY TEMPERATURE

Activity Tolerance	Neurological Status: Autonomic	Risk Control: Hypothermia
Burn Healing	Newborn Adaptation	Risk Control: Infectious
Hydration	Physical Aging	Process
Immune Status	Physical Fitness	Risk Control: Sun Exposure
Infection Severity	Post-Procedure Recovery	Risk Detection
Infection Severity: Newborn	Risk Control	Weight Maintenance
Medication Response	Risk Control: Hyperthermia	Behavior

NICS ASSOCIATED WITH PREVENTION OF IMBALANCED BODY TEMPERATURE

Cerebral Edema Management	Kangaroo Care	Surveillance
Energy Management	Malignant Hyperthermia	Temperature Regulation
Environmental Management:	Precautions	Temperature Regulation:
Comfort	Medication Management	Intraoperative
Fluid Management	Newborn Care	Vital Signs Monitoring
Fluid Monitoring	Newborn Monitoring	Weight Management
Fluid Resuscitation	Postanesthesia Care	Wound Care: Burns
Infection Control	Risk Identification	
Infection Protection	Sedation Management	

PART II - B

NURSING DIAGNOSIS: Caregiver Role Strain, Risk for

Definition: Caregiver is vulnerable for felt difficulty in performing the family caregiver role

NOCS TO ASSESS AND MEASURE ACTUAL OCCURRENCE OF THE DIAGNOSIS

Caregiver Performance:
  Direct Care
Caregiver Performance:
  Indirect Care

Caregiver Role Endurance
Parenting Performance

NOCS ASSOCIATED WITH RISK FACTORS FOR CAREGIVER ROLE STRAIN

Abuse Cessation
Abuse Protection
Abusive Behavior Self-Restraint
Caregiver Emotional Health
Caregiver Home Care
  Readiness
Caregiver Lifestyle Disruption
Caregiver-Patient Relationship
Caregiver Physical Health
Caregiver Stressors
Cognition
Coping
Development: Young
  Adulthood
Development: Middle
  Adulthood
Drug Abuse Cessation
  Behavior

Family Coping
Family Functioning
Family Social Climate
Family Resiliency
Knowledge: Disease
  Process
Knowledge: Diet
Knowledge: Illness Care
Knowledge: Infant Care
Knowledge: Medication
Knowledge: Pain
  Management
Knowledge: Parenting
Knowledge: Prescribed
  Activity
Knowledge: Treatment
  Procedure

Knowledge: Treatment
  Regimen
Leisure Participation
Mood Equilibrium
Personal Resiliency
Risk Control
Risk Control: Drug Use
Risk Detection
Preterm Infant
  Organization
Role Performance
Social Support
Stress Level
Substance Addiction
  Consequences

NICS ASSOCIATED WITH PREVENTION OF CAREGIVER ROLE STRAIN

Abuse Protection Support
Anger Control Assistance
Anticipatory Guidance
Behavior Management
Caregiver Support
Cognitive Stimulation
Coping Enhancement
Developmental Care
Energy Management
Family Integrity Promotion
Family Integrity Promotion:
  Childbearing Family
Family Involvement
  Promotion
Family Mobilization
Family Support
Family Therapy
Financial Resource Assistance
Health System Guidance

Home Maintenance Assistance
Infant Care
Mood Management
Parent Education: Adolescent
Parent Education: Childrearing
  Family
Parent Education: Infant
Parenting Promotion
Reality Orientation
Recreation Therapy
Resiliency Promotion
Respite Care
Risk Identification
Role Enhancement
Socialization Enhancement
Substance Use Prevention
Substance Use Treatment
Substance Use Treatment:
  Drug Withdrawal

Support Group
Support System Enhancement
Surveillance
Teaching: Disease Process
Teaching: Infant Nutrition
  0-3 Months
Teaching: Infant Safety
  0-3 Months
Teaching: Infant Stimulation
  0-4 Months
Teaching: Prescribed
  Activity/Exercise
Teaching: Prescribed Diet
Teaching: Prescribed Medication
Teaching: Procedure/Treatment
Teaching: Psychomotor Skill

Critical reasoning note: Some of the risk factors pertain to the care recipient (e.g., Cognition/Cognitive Stimulation) and some to the care provider (e.g., Knowledge: Disease Process/Teaching Disease Process).

NURSING DIAGNOSIS: Confusion, Risk for Acute

Definition: At risk for reversible disturbances of consciousness, attention, cognition, and perception that develop over a short period of time

NOCS TO ASSESS AND MEASURE ACTUAL OCCURRENCE OF THE DIAGNOSIS

Acute Confusion Level

Cognitive Orientation

NOCS ASSOCIATED WITH RISK FACTORS FOR ACUTE CONFUSION

Alcohol Abuse Cessation
  Behavior
Cognition
Concentration
Drug Abuse Cessation Behavior
Electrolyte & Acid/Base Balance
Hydration
Infection Severity
Information Processing

Kidney Function
Medication Response
Memory
Mobility
Pain Level
Physical Aging
Post-Procedure Recovery
Risk Control

Risk Control: Alcohol Use
Risk Control: Drug Use
Risk Control: Infectious Process
Risk Detection
Sensory Function
Sleep
Substance Withdrawal Severity
Urinary Elimination

NICS ASSOCIATED WITH PREVENTION OF ACUTE CONFUSION

Acid-Base Management
Exercise Promotion
Fluid/Electrolyte Management
Fluid Management
Fluid Monitoring
Infection Protection
Medication Management
Pain Management

Postanesthesia Care
Reality Orientation
Risk Identification
Sleep Enhancement
Substance Use Treatment
Substance Use Treatment:
  Alcohol Withdrawal

Substance Use Treatment:
  Drug Withdrawal
Substance Use Treatment:
  Overdose
Surveillance
Urinary Retention Care

PART II - C

NURSING DIAGNOSIS: Constipation, Risk for

Definition: At risk for a decrease in normal frequency of defecation accompanied by difficult or incomplete passage of stool and/or passage of excessively hard, dry stool

NOCS TO ASSESS AND MEASURE ACTUAL OCCURRENCE OF THE DIAGNOSIS

Bowel Elimination

NOCS ASSOCIATED WITH RISK FACTORS FOR CONSTIPATION

Acute Confusion Level
Adherence Behavior: Healthy Diet
Compliance Behavior: Prescribed
    Diet
Electrolyte & Acid/Base Balance
Gastrointestinal Function
Hydration
Immobility Consequences:
    Physiological
Knowledge: Diet

Knowledge: Medication
Maternal Status: Antepartum
Medication Response
Mobility
Mood Equilibrium
Nutritional Status: Food
    & Fluid Intake
Physical Fitness
Psychomotor Energy

Risk Control
Risk Detection
Stress Level
Self-Care: Non-Parenteral
    Medication
Self-Care: Oral Hygiene
Self-Care: Toileting
Symptom Control
Weight Loss Behavior

NICS ASSOCIATED WITH PREVENTION OF CONSTIPATION

Anxiety Reduction
Bowel Management
Bowel Training
Constipation/Impaction
    Management
Diet Staging
Electrolyte Management
Exercise Promotion
Exercise Therapy: Ambulation
Fluid Management

Fluid Monitoring
Medication Administration: Oral
Medication Management
Medication Prescribing
Mood Management
Nutrition Management
Nutritional Counseling
Nutritional Monitoring
Oral Health Promotion

Prenatal Care
Reality Orientation
Risk Identification
Self-Care Assistance: Toileting
Surveillance
Teaching: Prescribed Diet
Teaching: Prescribed Medication
Weight Reduction Assistance

NURSING DIAGNOSIS: Contamination, Risk for

Definition: Accentuated risk of exposure to environmental contaminants in doses sufficient to cause adverse health effects

NOCS TO ASSESS AND MEASURE ACTUAL OCCURRENCE OF THE DIAGNOSIS

Gastrointestinal Function
Immune Status
Kidney Function

Neurological Status
Respiratory Status

Tissue Integrity: Skin & Mucous
Membranes

NOCS ASSOCIATED WITH RISK FACTORS FOR CONTAMINATION

Community Disaster Response
Community Risk Control:
Communicable Disease
Community Risk Control:
Lead Exposure
Immune Status
Infection Severity
Knowledge: Child Physical Safety

Knowledge: Health Behavior
Knowledge: Personal Safety
Maternal Status:
Antepartum
Nutritional Status:
Nutrient Intake
Personal Safety Behavior

Risk Control
Risk Control: Tobacco Use
Risk Detection
Safe Home Environment
Smoking Cessation Behavior

NICS ASSOCIATED WITH PREVENTION OF CONTAMINATION

Bioterrorism Preparedness
Community Disaster Preparedness
Environmental Management:
Community
Environmental Management:
Safety
Environmental Management:
Worker Safety
Environmental Risk Protection
Health Education
Health Policy Monitoring

Infection Control
Nutritional Counseling
Prenatal Care
Program Development
Risk Identification
Smoking Cessation
Assistance
Surveillance
Surveillance: Community
Teaching: Infant Safety
0-3 Months

Teaching: Infant Safety 4-6 Months
Teaching: Infant Safety 7-9 Months
Teaching: Infant Safety
10-12 Months
Teaching: Toddler Safety
13-18 Months
Teaching: Toddler Safety
19-24 Months
Teaching: Toddler Safety
25-36 Months

PART II - C

NURSING DIAGNOSIS: Development, Risk for Delayed

Definition: At risk for delay of 25% or more in one or more of the areas of social or self-regulatory behavior, or in cognitive, language, gross or fine motor skills

NOCS TO ASSESS AND MEASURE ACTUAL OCCURRENCE OF THE DIAGNOSIS

Child Development: 1 Month	Child Development: 12 Months	Child Development: 5 Years
Child Development: 2 Months	Child Development: 2 Years	Child Development: Middle
Child Development: 4 Months	Child Development: 3 Years	Childhood
Child Development: 6 Months	Child Development: 4 Years	Child Development: Adolescence

NOCS ASSOCIATED WITH RISK FACTORS FOR DELAYED DEVELOPMENT

Abusive Behavior Self-Restraint	Maternal Status: Antepartum	Risk Control
Caregiver Emotional Health	Neglect Recovery	Risk Control: Unintended
Drug Abuse Cessation Behavior	Newborn Adaptation	Pregnancy
Fetal Status: Antepartum	Nutritional Status	Risk Detection
Hyperactivity Level	Nutritional Status: Nutrient	Smoking Cessation Behavior
Infection Severity	Intake	Substance Addiction
Knowledge: Infant Care	Prenatal Health Behavior	Consequences
Knowledge: Parenting	Preterm Infant Organization	

NICS ASSOCIATED WITH PREVENTION OF DELAYED DEVELOPMENT

Abuse Protection Support: Child	Infection Protection	Surveillance
Behavior Management:	Intrapartal Care	Teaching: Infant Nutrition
Overactivity/Inattention	Intrapartal Care: High-Risk	0-3 Months
Caregiver Support	Delivery	Teaching: Infant Nutrition
Developmental Care	Mood Management	4-6 Months
Electronic Fetal Monitoring:	Newborn Monitoring	Teaching: Infant Nutrition
Antepartum	Parent Education: Childrearing	7-9 Months
Electronic Fetal Monitoring:	Family	Teaching: Infant Nutrition
Intrapartum	Parenting Promotion	10-12 Months
Family Planning: Contraception	Preconception Counseling	Teaching: Toddler Nutrition
Family Planning: Unplanned	Prenatal Care	13-18 Months
Pregnancy	Risk Identification	Teaching: Toddler Nutrition
Genetic Counseling	Risk Identification: Genetic	19-24 Months
High-Risk Pregnancy Care	Substance Use Treatment	

NURSING DIAGNOSIS: Disuse Syndrome, Risk for

Definition: At risk for deterioration of body systems as the result of prescribed or unavoidable musculoskeletal inactivity

NOCS TO ASSESS AND MEASURE ACTUAL OCCURRENCE OF THE DIAGNOSIS

Immobility Consequences: Physiological
Immobility Consequences: Psycho-
    Cognitive

NOCS ASSOCIATED WITH RISK FACTORS FOR DISUSE SYNDROME

Bone Healing	Neurological Status:	Pain Level
Burn Recovery	Consciousness	Risk Control
Heedfulness of Affected Side	Neurological Status: Spinal/	Risk Detection
Joint Movement: Passive	Sensory Motor Function	

NICS ASSOCIATED WITH PREVENTION OF DISUSE SYNDROME

Analgesic Administration	Intracranial Pressure (ICP)	Splinting
Bed Rest Care	Monitoring	Surveillance
Cast Care: Maintenance	Pain Management	Traction/Immobilization
Cerebral Edema Management	Physical Restraint	Care
Cerebral Perfusion Promotion	Positioning	Unilateral Neglect
Exercise Therapy: Joint Mobility	Positioning: Intraoperative	Management
Exercise Therapy: Muscle	Risk Identification	Wound Care: Burns
Control		

PART II - E

NURSING DIAGNOSIS: Electrolyte, Risk for Imbalance

Definition: At risk for change in serum electrolyte levels that may compromise health

NOCS TO ASSESS AND MEASURE ACTUAL OCCURRENCE OF THE DIAGNOSIS

Electrolyte & Acid/Base Balance

NOCS ASSOCIATED WITH RISK FACTORS FOR IMBALANCED ELECTROLYTE

Bowel Elimination	Gastrointestinal Function	Risk Control
Burn Healing	Hydration	Risk Detection
Burn Recovery	Kidney Function	Systemic Toxin Clearance:
Compliance Behavior:	Medication Response	Dialysis
Prescribed Diet	Nausea and Vomiting Severity	Wound Healing: Secondary
Fluid Balance	Nutritional Status: Biochemical	Intention
Fluid Overload Severity	Measures	

NICS ASSOCIATED WITH PREVENTION OF IMBALANCED ELECTROLYTE

Diarrhea Management	Hemodialysis Therapy	Risk Identification
Eating Disorders Management	Medication Management	Surveillance
Fluid/Electrolyte Management	Medication Reconciliation	Vomiting Management
Fluid Management	Nausea Management	Wound Care: Burns
Fluid Monitoring	Peritoneal Dialysis Therapy	Wound Care: Closed Drainage
Fluid Resuscitation		

NURSING DIAGNOSIS: Falls, Risk for

Definition: Increased susceptibility to falling that may cause physical harm

NOCS TO ASSESS AND MEASURE ACTUAL OCCURRENCE OF THE DIAGNOSIS

Falls Occurrence   Physical Injury Severity

NOCS ASSOCIATED WITH RISK FACTORS FOR FALLS

Acute Confusion Level
Agitation Level
Ambulation
Ambulation: Wheelchair
Balance
Blood Glucose Level
Bowel Continence
Bowel Elimination
Circulation Status
Client Satisfaction: Safety
Cognition
Coordinated Movement
Fall Prevention Behavior
Fatigue Level

Hearing Compensation
    Behavior
Hydration
Knowledge: Child Physical
    Safety
Knowledge: Fall Prevention
Medication Response
Mobility
Neurological Status: Peripheral
Parenting: Infant/Toddler
    Physical Safety
Physical Aging
Physical Fitness
Risk Control

Risk Control: Alcohol Use
Risk Detection
Safe Home Environment
Seizure Control
Self Care: Toileting
Sensory Function: Hearing
Sensory Function: Vision
Sleep
Transfer Performance
Urinary Continence
Vision Compensation
    Behavior
Vital Signs

NICS ASSOCIATED WITH PREVENTION OF FALLS

Body Mechanics Promotion
Bowel Incontinence Care
Circulatory Care: Arterial
    Insufficiency
Circulatory Care: Venous
    Insufficiency
Circulatory Precautions
Cognitive Stimulation
Delirium Management
Dementia Management
Diarrhea Management
Environmental Management:
    Safety
Exercise Promotion: Strength
    Training
Exercise Promotion: Stretching
Exercise Therapy: Ambulation
Exercise Therapy: Balance
Exercise Therapy: Joint Mobility

Exercise Therapy: Muscle
    Control
Fall Prevention
Fluid Management
Hyperglycemia Management
Hypoglycemia Management
Medication Management
Pain Management
Peripheral Sensation
    Management
Positioning: Wheelchair
Risk Identification
Seizure Precautions
Self-Care Assistance
Self-Care Assistance:
    Toileting
Self-Care Assistance:
    Transfer
Sleep Enhancement
Substance Use Prevention

Substance Use Treatment
Surveillance
Surveillance: Safety
Teaching: Infant Safety
    0-3 Months
Teaching: Infant Safety
    4-6 Months
Teaching: Infant Safety
    7-9 Months
Teaching: Infant Safety
    10-12 Months
Teaching: Toddler Safety
    13-18 Months
Teaching: Toddler Safety
    19-24 Months
Teaching: Toddler Safety
    25-36 Months
Urinary Incontinence Care
Vital Signs Monitoring

NURSING DIAGNOSIS: Fluid Volume, Risk for Deficient

Definition: At risk for experiencing vascular, cellular, or intracellular dehydration

NOCS TO ASSESS AND MEASURE ACTUAL OCCURRENCE OF THE DIAGNOSIS

Fluid Balance   Hydration

NOCS ASSOCIATED WITH RISK FACTORS FOR DEFICIENT FLUID VOLUME

Blood Glucose Level
Blood Loss Severity
Bowel Elimination
Breastfeeding Establishment: Infant
Breastfeeding Maintenance
Burn Healing
Electrolyte & Acid/Base Balance
Gastrointestinal Function

Infection Severity
Knowledge: Diet
Knowledge: Medication
Medication Response
Nausea & Vomiting Severity
Nutritional Status: Food &
 Fluid Intake
Risk Control
Risk Control: Hyperthermia

Risk Detection
Thermoregulation
Thermoregulation:
 Newborn
Urinary Elimination
Weight: Body Mass
Weight Gain Behavior
Weight Loss Behavior

NICS ASSOCIATED WITH PREVENTION OF DEFICIENT FLUID VOLUME

Bleeding Precautions
Bleeding Reduction
Bleeding Reduction: Antepartum
 Uterus
Bleeding Reduction: Gastrointestinal
Bleeding Reduction: Nasal
Bleeding Reduction: Postpartum Uterus
Bleeding Reduction: Wound
Blood Products Administration
Bottle Feeding
Breastfeeding Assistance
Diarrhea Management
Electrolyte Management:
 Hypernatremia
Electrolyte Monitoring
Fever Treatment
Fluid/Electrolyte Management

Fluid Management
Fluid Monitoring
Fluid Resuscitation
Heat Exposure Treatment
Hypovolemia Management
Infection Protection
Intravenous (IV) Insertion
Intravenous (IV) Therapy
Malignant Hyperthermia
 Precautions
Medication Management
Phlebotomy: Arterial Blood
 Sample
Phlebotomy: Cannulated Vessel
Phlebotomy: Venous Blood Sample
Risk Identification

Shock Management
Shock Management:
 Volume
Shock Prevention
Surveillance
Temperature Regulation
Tube Care: Chest
Tube Care: Gastrointestinal
Vital Signs Monitoring
Vomiting Management
Weight Gain Assistance
Weight Reduction
 Assistance
Wound Care: Burns
Wound Care: Closed
 Drainage

Critical reasoning note: Fluid volume deficit occurs when water and electrolytes are lost in the same proportion as they exist in normal body fluids, resulting in no change in the levels of serum electrolytes. Dehydration refers to a loss of water alone, resulting in increased sodium levels (Smeltzer, S. C., & Bare, B. G. [2004]. *Medical-surgical nursing* [Vol. I, p. 256]. Philadelphia: Lippincott, Williams & Wilkins.) Defining characteristics address primarily fluid volume deficit, but the definition and some of the characteristics include dehydration and loss of fluids through the gastrointestinal tract; therefore electrolytes are addressed in the outcomes and interventions.

NURSING DIAGNOSIS: Fluid Volume, Risk for Imbalanced

Definition: At risk for a decrease, increase, or rapid shift from one to the other of intravascular, interstitial, and/or intracellular fluid. This refers to body fluid loss, gain, or both

NOCS TO ASSESS AND MEASURE ACTUAL OCCURRENCE OF THE DIAGNOSIS

Fluid Balance	Fluid Overload Severity	Hydration

NOCS ASSOCIATED WITH RISK FACTORS FOR IMBALANCED FLUID VOLUME

Burn Healing	Knowledge: Congestive Heart	Risk Detection
Burn Recovery	Failure Management	Wound Healing: Primary Intention
Cardiac Pump Effectiveness	Physical Injury Severity	Wound Healing: Secondary
Gastrointestinal Function	Post-Procedure Recovery	Intention
Infection Severity	Risk Control	

NICS ASSOCIATED WITH PREVENTION OF IMBALANCED FLUID VOLUME

Fever Treatment	Infection Control	Surveillance
Fluid/Electrolyte Management	Infection Protection	Tube Care: Gastrointestinal
Fluid Management	Invasive Hemodynamic Monitoring	Wound Care
Fluid Monitoring	Risk Identification	Wound Care: Burns
Gastrointestinal Intubation	Shock Management: Vasogenic	
Hemodynamic Regulation		

NURSING DIAGNOSIS: Gastrointestinal Motility, Risk for Dysfunctional

Definition: Risk for increased, decreased, ineffective, or lack of peristaltic activity within the gastrointestinal system

NOCS TO ASSESS AND MEASURE ACTUAL OCCURRENCE OF THE DIAGNOSIS

Gastrointestinal Function

NOCS ASSOCIATED WITH RISK FACTORS FOR DYSFUNCTIONAL GASTROINTESTINAL MOTILITY

Adherence Behavior:	Knowledge: Diet	Risk Control: Infectious
Healthy Diet	Medication Response	Process
Anxiety Level	Mobility	Risk Detection
Compliance Behavior:	Physical Aging	Stress Level
Prescribed Diet	Physical Fitness	Tissue Perfusion:
Diabetes Self-Management	Preterm Infant	Abdominal
Infection Severity	Organization	Organs
Knowledge: Diabetes	Risk Control	
Management		

NICS ASSOCIATED WITH PREVENTION OF DYSFUNCTIONAL GASTROINTESTINAL MOTILITY

Anxiety Reduction	Infection Protection	Surveillance
Developmental Care	Medication Management	Teaching: Disease Process
Diet Staging	Nutrition Management	Teaching: Prescribed Diet
Exercise Promotion	Nutrition Therapy	Teaching: Prescribed Medication
Exercise Therapy: Ambulation	Nutritional Counseling	Tube Care: Gastrointestinal
Gastrointestinal Intubation	Nutritional Monitoring	
Infection Control	Risk Identification	

NURSING DIAGNOSIS: Grieving, Complicated, Risk for

Definition: At risk for a disorder that occurs after the death of a significant other, in which the experience of distress accompanying bereavement fails to follow normative expectations and manifests in functional impairment

NOCS TO ASSESS AND MEASURE ACTUAL OCCURRENCE OF THE DIAGNOSIS

Grief Resolution

NOCS ASSOCIATED WITH RISK FACTORS FOR COMPLICATED GRIEVING

Anxiety Level	Depression Level	Risk Detection
Anxiety Self-Control	Depression Self-Control	Social Support
Comfort Status: Psychospiritual	Mood Equilibrium	Suffering Severity
Comfort Status: Sociocultural	Personal Resiliency	
Coping	Risk Control	

NICS ASSOCIATED WITH PREVENTION OF COMPLICATED GRIEVING

Active Listening	Grief Work Facilitation: Perinatal	Risk Identification
Anxiety Resolution	Death	Spiritual Growth Facilitation
Coping Enhancement	Guilt Work Facilitation	Spiritual Support
Family Integrity Promotion	Hope Inspiration	Support Group
Forgiveness Facilitation	Mood Management	Support System Enhancement
Grief Work Facilitation	Presence	Surveillance
	Resiliency Promotion	

PART II - G

NURSING DIAGNOSIS: Growth, Risk for Disproportionate

Definition: At risk for growth above the 97th percentile or below the 3rd percentile for age, crossing two percentile channels

NOCS TO ASSESS AND MEASURE ACTUAL OCCURRENCE OF THE DIAGNOSIS

Growth

Physical Maturation: Female

Physical Maturation: Male

Weight: Body Mass

NOCS ASSOCIATED WITH RISK FACTORS FOR DISPROPORTIONATE GROWTH

Abuse Cessation
Abuse Protection
Adherence Behavior: Healthy Diet
Aggression Self-Control
Alcohol Abuse Cessation Behavior
Appetite
Breastfeeding Maintenance
Community Disaster Response
Community Risk Control: Lead Exposure
Compliance Behavior: Prescribed Diet

Drug Abuse Cessation Behavior
Infection Severity
Infection Severity: Newborn
Knowledge: Health Resources
Knowledge: Infant Care
Knowledge: Preconception Maternal Health
Knowledge: Pregnancy
Knowledge: Preterm Infant Care
Neglect Cessation

Nutritional Status: Food & Fluid Intake
Nutritional Status: Nutrient Intake
Prenatal Health Behavior
Preterm Infant Organization
Risk Control
Risk Detection
Substance Addiction Consequences
Weight Gain Behavior
Weight Loss Behavior

NICS ASSOCIATED WITH PREVENTION OF DISPROPORTIONATE GROWTH

Abuse Protection Support: Child
Anger Control Assistance
Attachment Promotion
Behavior Modification
Bottle Feeding
Breastfeeding Assistance
Community Disaster Preparedness
Developmental Care
Eating Disorders Management
Environmental Management: Violence Prevention
Financial Resource Assistance
Health Education
Health Screening
Infection Control

Lactation Counseling
Learning Facilitation
Nutrition Management
Nutrition Therapy
Nutritional Monitoring
Preconception Counseling
Prenatal Care
Parent Education: Infant
Risk Identification
Risk Identification: Genetic
Substance Use Prevention
Substance Use Treatment
Surveillance
Teaching: Infant Nutrition 0-3 Months

Teaching: Infant Nutrition 4-6 Months
Teaching: Infant Nutrition 7-9 Months
Teaching: Infant Nutrition 10-12 Months
Teaching: Prescribed Diet
Teaching: Toddler Nutrition 13-18 Months
Teaching: Toddler Nutrition 19-24 Months
Teaching: Toddler Nutrition 25-36 Months
Weight Gain Assistance
Weight Management
Weight Reduction Assistance

NURSING DIAGNOSIS: Human Dignity, Risk for Compromised

Definition: At risk for perceived loss of respect and honor

NOCS TO ASSESS AND MEASURE ACTUAL OCCURRENCE OF THE DIAGNOSIS

Client Satisfaction: Protection of Rights

Dignified Life Closure

NOCS ASSOCIATED WITH RISK FACTORS FOR COMPROMISED HUMAN DIGNITY

Bowel Continence	Client Satisfaction: Physical Care	Participation in Health Care Decisions
Client Satisfaction	Client Satisfaction: Psychological Care	Personal Autonomy
Client Satisfaction: Caring	Comfort Status: Physical	Risk Control
Client Satisfaction: Communication	Comfort Status: Psychospiritual	Risk Detection
Client Satisfaction: Cultural Needs Fulfillment	Comfort Status: Sociocultural	Urinary Continence

NICS ASSOCIATED WITH PREVENTION OF COMPROMISED HUMAN DIGNITY

Admission Care	Decision-Making Support	Patient Rights Protection
Anticipatory Guidance	Discharge Planning	Risk Identification
Bowel Incontinence Care	Health System Guidance	Surveillance
Culture Brokerage		

NURSING DIAGNOSIS: Infant Behavior, Risk for Disorganized

Definition: Risk for alteration in integrating and modulation of the physiological and behavioral systems of functioning (i.e. autonomic, motor, state-organization, self-regulatory, and attentional-interactional systems)

NOCS TO ASSESS AND MEASURE ACTUAL OCCURRENCE OF THE DIAGNOSIS

Child Development: 1 Month	Child Development: 4 Months	Child Development: 12 Months
Child Development: 2 Months	Child Development: 6 Months	

NOCS ASSOCIATED WITH RISK FACTORS FOR DISORGANIZED INFANT BEHAVIOR

Comfort Status: Environment	Knowledge: Preterm Infant Care	Preterm Infant Organization
Coordinated Movement	Neurological Status	Risk Control
Discomfort Level	Pain Level	Risk Detection
Knowledge: Infant Care		

NICS ASSOCIATED WITH PREVENTION OF DISORGANIZED INFANT BEHAVIOR

Circumcision Care	Newborn Monitoring	Teaching: Infant Safety 10-12 Months
Developmental Care	Pain Management	
Environmental Management: Attachment Process	Positioning	Teaching: Infant Stimulation 0-4 Months
	Risk Identification	
Environmental Management: Comfort	Surveillance	Teaching: Infant Stimulation 5-8 Months
	Teaching: Infant Safety 0-3 Months	
Infant Care	Teaching: Infant Safety 4-6 Months	Teaching: Infant Stimulation 9-12 Months
Kangaroo Care	Teaching: Infant Safety 7-9 Months	
Neurologic Monitoring		

PART II - I

NURSING DIAGNOSIS: Infection, Risk for

Definition: At increased risk for being invaded by pathogenic organisms

NOCS TO ASSESS AND MEASURE ACTUAL OCCURRENCE OF THE DIAGNOSIS

Infection Severity

Infection Severity: Newborn

NOCS ASSOCIATED WITH RISK FACTORS FOR INFECTION

Burn Healing
Community Risk Control:
　Communicable Disease
Gastrointestinal Function
Immune Status
Immunization Behavior
Maternal Status: Antepartum
Maternal Status: Intrapartum
Maternal Status: Postpartum
Medication Response

Nutritional Status: Nutrient
　Intake
Oral Hygiene
Physical Injury Severity
Respiratory Status: Airway
　Patency
Risk Control
Risk Control: Infectious
　Process

Risk Control: Sexually
　Transmitted Diseases (STD)
Risk Detection
Smoking Cessation Behavior
Tissue Integrity: Skin &
　Mucous Membranes
Wound Healing: Primary
　Intention
Wound Healing: Secondary
　Intention

NICS ASSOCIATED WITH PREVENTION OF INFECTION

Amputation Care
Cesarean Section Care
Circumcision Care
Communicable Disease
　Management
Cough Enhancement
Immunization/Vaccination
　Management
Incision Site Care
Infection Control
Infection Control: Intraoperative
Infection Protection
Intrapartal Care

Intrapartal Care: High-Risk
　Delivery
Medication Management
Nutrition Therapy
Nutritional Monitoring
Oral Health Promotion
Oral Health Restoration
Perineal Care
Postpartal Care
Pregnancy Termination Care
Pressure Ulcer Care
Pressure Ulcer Prevention
Pruritus Management
Risk Identification

Skin Care: Donor Site
Skin Care: Graft Site
Skin Surveillance
Smoking Cessation
　Assistance
Surveillance
Teaching: Safe Sex
Tube Care: Urinary
Wound Care
Wound Care: Burns
Wound Care: Closed
　Drainage
Wound Irrigation

NURSING DIAGNOSIS: Injury, Risk for

Definition: At risk of injury as a result of environmental conditions interacting with the individual's adaptive and defensive resources

NOCS TO ASSESS AND MEASURE ACTUAL OCCURRENCE OF THE DIAGNOSIS

Falls Occurrence

Physical Injury Severity

NOCS ASSOCIATED WITH RISK FACTORS FOR INJURY

Abuse Protection
Allergic Response: Systemic
Balance
Blood Coagulation
Client Satisfaction: Safety
Cognitive Orientation
Community Risk Control:
   Communicable Disease
Fall Prevention Behavior
Fatigue Level
Immune Status
Immunization Behavior
Information Processing

Knowledge: Child Physical
   Safety
Knowledge: Fall Prevention
Knowledge: Personal Safety
Mobility
Nutritional Status: Nutrient
   Intake
Parenting: Adolescent Physical
   Safety
Parenting: Early/Middle
   Childhood Physical Safety
Parenting: Infant/Toddler
   Physical Safety

Parenting: Psychosocial Safety
Personal Safety Behavior
Risk Control
Risk Detection
Safe Home Environment
Safe Wandering
Self-Care Status
Sensory Function
Sensory Function: Hearing
Sensory Function: Vision
Tissue Integrity: Skin & Mucous
   Membranes
Transfer Performance

NICS ASSOCIATED WITH PREVENTION OF INJURY

Abuse Protection Support
Abuse Protection Support:
   Child
Abuse Protection Support:
   Domestic Partner
Abuse Protection Support:
   Elder
Allergy Management
Bleeding Precautions
Communicable Disease
   Management
Delusion Management
Dementia Management
Energy Management
Environmental Management:
   Safety
Environmental Management:
   Violence Prevention
Exercise Promotion
Exercise Therapy: Ambulation
Fall Prevention

Immunization/Vaccination
   Management
Impulse Control Training
Infection Control
Laser Precautions
Latex Precautions
Malignant Hyperthermia
   Precautions
Medication Management
Nutrition Therapy
Nutritional Monitoring
Parent Education: Adolescent
Parent Education: Childbearing
   Family
Parent Education: Infant
Physical Restraint
Pressure Management
Pressure Ulcer Care
Pressure Ulcer Prevention
Reality Orientation
Risk Identification
Security Enhancement

Seizure Precautions
Sports-Injury Prevention:
   Youth
Surveillance
Surveillance: Safety
Teaching: Infant Safety
   0-3 Months
Teaching: Infant Safety
   4-6 Months
Teaching: Infant Safety
   7-9 Months
Teaching: Infant Safety
   10-12 Months
Teaching: Toddler Safety
   13-18 Months
Teaching: Toddler Safety
   19-24 Months
Teaching: Toddler Safety
   25-36 Months
Thrombolytic Therapy
   Management

PART II - I

NURSING DIAGNOSIS: Latex Allergy Response, Risk for

Definition: Risk for hypersensitivity to natural latex rubber products

NOCS TO ASSESS AND MEASURE ACTUAL OCCURRENCE OF THE DIAGNOSIS

Allergic Response: Localized
Tissue Integrity: Skin & Mucous
  Membranes

NOCS ASSOCIATED WITH RISK FACTORS FOR LATEX ALLERGY RESPONSE

Asthma Self-Management	Knowledge: Asthma Management	Risk Detection
Compliance Behavior:	Risk Control	
Prescribed Diet		

NICS ASSOCIATED WITH PREVENTION OF LATEX ALLERGY RESPONSE

Allergy Management	Environmental Risk Protection	Surveillance
Environmental Management	Latex Precautions	Teaching: Prescribed Diet
Environmental Management:	Risk Identification	
Worker Safety		

NURSING DIAGNOSIS: Liver Function, Risk for Impaired

Definition: At risk for a decrease in liver function that may compromise health

NOCS TO ASSESS AND MEASURE ACTUAL OCCURRENCE OF THE DIAGNOSIS

Blood Coagulation   Medication Response

NOCS ASSOCIATED WITH RISK FACTORS FOR IMPAIRED LIVER FUNCTION

Alcohol Abuse Cessation	Medication Response	Risk Control: Infectious
Behavior	Risk Control	Process
Drug Abuse Cessation Behavior	Risk Control: Alcohol Use	Risk Control: Sexually
Infection Severity	Risk Control: Drug Use	Transmitted Diseases (STD)
Knowledge: Medication		Risk Detection

NICS ASSOCIATED WITH PREVENTION OF IMPAIRED LIVER FUNCTION

Infection Control	Substance Use Treatment:	Teaching: Individual
Infection Protection	Alcohol Withdrawal	Teaching: Prescribed
Medication Management	Substance Use Treatment:	Medication
Risk Identification	Drug Withdrawal	
Substance Use Treatment	Surveillance	

Critical reasoning note: NOC currently does not have an outcome that is a measure of liver function although an outcome is in development. We have listed two of the common outcomes that might occur with liver failure. Others, such as Blood Loss Severity, Fluid Overload Severity, Nutritional Status, Neurological Status: Consciousness, and Tissue Integrity: Skin & Mucous Membranes, might be considered.

NURSING DIAGNOSIS: Loneliness, Risk for

Definition: At risk for experiencing discomfort associated with a desire or need for more contact with others

NOCS TO ASSESS AND MEASURE ACTUAL OCCURRENCE OF THE DIAGNOSIS

Loneliness Severity

NOCS ASSOCIATED WITH RISK FACTORS FOR LONELINESS

Adaptation to Physical Disability
Caregiver Stressors
Family Functioning
Family Integrity
Family Social Climate
Grief Resolution
Leisure Participation

Neglect Cessation
Parent-Infant Attachment
Parenting Performance
Play Participation
Psychosocial Adjustment:
    Life Change

Risk Control
Risk Detection
Social Interaction Skills
Social Involvement
Social Support

NICS ASSOCIATED WITH PREVENTION OF LONELINESS

Activity Therapy
Animal-Assisted Therapy
Attachment Promotion
Behavior Modification:
    Social Skills
Caregiver Support
Emotional Support
Family Integrity Promotion
Family Integrity Promotion:
    Childbearing Family

Family Process Maintenance
Family Support
Grief Work Facilitation
Parenting Promotion
Recreation Therapy
Relocation Stress Reduction
Risk Identification
Sibling Support

Socialization Enhancement
Support Group
Support System Enhancement
Surveillance
Visitation Facilitation

PART II - L

NURSING DIAGNOSIS: Maternal/Fetal Dyad, Risk for Disturbed

Definition: At risk for disruption of the symbiotic maternal/fetal dyad as a result of comorbid or pregnancy-related conditions

NOCS TO ASSESS AND MEASURE ACTUAL OCCURRENCE OF THE DIAGNOSIS

Fetal Status: Antepartum	Maternal Status: Antepartum

NOCS ASSOCIATED WITH RISK FACTORS FOR DISTURBED MATERNAL/FETAL DYAD

Abuse Protection	Knowledge: Cardiac Disease	Nausea & Vomiting
Alcohol Abuse Cessation	Management	Severity
Behavior	Knowledge: Diabetes	Prenatal Health
Asthma Self-Management	Management	Behavior
Blood Glucose Level	Knowledge: Diet	Risk Control
Cardiac Disease	Knowledge: Hypertension	Risk Detection
Self-Management	Management	Seizure Control
Cardiopulmonary Status	Knowledge: Medication	Smoking Cessation
Diabetes Self-Management	Knowledge: Preconception	Behavior
Drug Abuse Cessation Behavior	Maternal Health	Surveillance
Knowledge: Asthma Manage-	Knowledge: Pregnancy	Vital Signs
ment	Medication Response	

NICS ASSOCIATED WITH PREVENTION OF DISTURBED MATERNAL/FETAL DYAD

Abuse Protection Support:	Preconception Counseling	Substance Use Treatment:
Domestic Partner	Prenatal Care	Drug Withdrawal
Asthma Management	Respiratory Monitoring	Surveillance
Bleeding Reduction:	Risk Identification	Surveillance: Late Pregnancy
Antepartum Uterus	Seizure Management	Teaching: Disease Process
Cardiac Care	Seizure Precautions	Teaching: Prescribed Diet
Cardiac Precautions	Smoking Cessation	Teaching: Prescribed
Electronic Fetal Monitoring:	Assistance	Medication
Antepartum	Substance Use Treatment	Ultrasonography: Limited
High-Risk Pregnancy Care	Substance Use Treatment:	Obstetric
Medication Management	Alcohol Withdrawal	Vital Signs Monitoring
Nausea Management		Vomiting Management

NURSING DIAGNOSIS: Nutrition: Imbalanced, Risk for More than Body Requirements

Definition: At risk for an intake of nutrients that exceeds metabolic needs

NOCS TO ASSESS AND MEASURE ACTUAL OCCURRENCE OF THE DIAGNOSIS

Nutritional Status: Food & Fluid Intake	Nutritional Status: Nutrient Intake	Weight: Body Mass

NOCS ASSOCIATED WITH RISK FACTORS FOR IMBALANCED NUTRITION, MORE THAN BODY REQUIREMENTS

Adherence Behavior: Healthy Diet	Knowledge: Infant Care	Risk Detection
Compliance Behavior: Prescribed Diet	Knowledge: Weight Management	Stress Level
Knowledge: Diet	Risk Control	Weight Maintenance Behavior

NICS ASSOCIATED WITH PREVENTION OF IMBALANCED NUTRITION, MORE THAN BODY REQUIREMENTS

Anxiety Reduction	Risk Identification	Teaching: Toddler Nutrition 13-18 Months
Behavior Modification	Self-Modification Assistance	Teaching: Toddler Nutrition 19-24 Months
Nutrition Management	Surveillance	Teaching: Toddler Nutrition 25-36 Months
Nutritional Counseling	Teaching: Infant Nutrition 0-3 Months	Weight Management
Nutritional Monitoring	Teaching: Infant Nutrition 4-6 Months	Weight Reduction Assistance
	Teaching: Infant Nutrition 7-9 Months	
	Teaching: Infant Nutrition 10-12 Months	
	Teaching: Prescribed Diet	

NURSING DIAGNOSIS: Parenting, Risk for Impaired

Definition: Risk for inability of the primary caretaker to create, maintain, or regain an environment that promotes the optimum growth and development of the child

NOCS TO ASSESS AND MEASURE ACTUAL OCCURRENCE OF THE DIAGNOSIS

Parenting Performance   Parenting: Psychosocial Safety

NOCS ASSOCIATED WITH RISK FACTORS FOR IMPAIRED PARENTING

Abusive Behavior Self-Restraint
Aggression Self-Control
Caregiver Emotional Health
Caregiver Physical Health
Caregiver Stressors
Child Development: 1 Month
Child Development: 2 Months
Child Development: 4 Months
Child Development: 6 Months
Child Development: 12 Months
Child Development: 2 Years
Child Development: 3 Years
Child Development: 4 Years
Child Development: 5 Years
Child Development: Middle
  Childhood

Child Development: Adolescence
Cognition
Coping
Decision-Making
Depression Level
Depression Self-Control
Distorted Thought Self-Control
Family Coping
Family Normalization
Family Social Climate
Fatigue Level
Health Beliefs: Perceived
  Resources
Hyperactivity Level
Information Processing
Knowledge: Health Resources

Knowledge: Infant Care
Knowledge: Parenting
Knowledge: Preterm Infant
  Care
Mood Equilibrium
Parent-Infant Attachment
Personal Resiliency
Risk Control
Risk Control: Alcohol Use
Risk Control: Drug Use
Risk Detection
Self-Esteem
Sleep
Social Interaction Skills
Social Support
Stress Level

NICS ASSOCIATED WITH PREVENTION OF IMPAIRED PARENTING

Abuse Protection Support: Child
Anger Control Assistance
Anticipatory Guidance
Anxiety Reduction
Attachment Promotion
Behavior Management:
  Overactivity/Inattention
Behavior Modification: Social Skills
Caregiver Support
Childbirth Preparation
Coping Enhancement
Decision-Making Support
Developmental Enhancement:
  Adolescent
Developmental Enhancement: Child
Energy Management

Environmental Management:
  Attachment Process
Family Integrity Promotion
Family Integrity Promotion:
  Childbearing Family
Family Involvement Promotion
Family Process Maintenance
Financial Resource Assistance
Health Education
Health Literacy Enhancement
Home Maintenance Assistance
Learning Facilitation
Learning Readiness
  Enhancement
Mood Management
Normalization Promotion

Parent Education: Adolescent
Parent Education: Childrearing
  Family
Parent Education: Infant
Parenting Promotion
Prenatal Care
Resiliency Promotion
Respite Care
Risk Identification
Self-Esteem Enhancement
Sleep Enhancement
Substance Use Prevention
Substance Use Treatment
Support Group
Support System Enhancement
Surveillance

Critical reasoning note: Some of the risk factors pertain to the infant/child, such as developmental delay or premature birth, and some pertain to the primary caregiver such as deficient knowledge or depression.

NURSING DIAGNOSIS: Perioperative-Positioning Injury, Risk for

Definition: At risk for inadvertent anatomical and physical changes as a result of posture or equipment used during an invasive/surgical procedure

NOCS TO ASSESS AND MEASURE ACTUAL OCCURRENCE OF THE DIAGNOSIS
Physical Injury Severity

NOCS ASSOCIATED WITH RISK FACTORS FOR PERIOPERATIVE-POSITIONING INJURY

Acute Confusion Level
Aspiration Prevention
Circulation Status
Cognitive Orientation
Fluid Overload Severity
Immobility Consequences:
   Physiological

Post-Procedure Recovery
Risk Control
Risk Detection
Sensory Function
Thermoregulation

Tissue Integrity: Skin
   & Mucous Membranes
Tissue Perfusion: Cellular
Tissue Perfusion: Peripheral
Weight: Body Mass

NICS ASSOCIATED WITH PREVENTION OF PERIOPERATIVE-POSITIONING INJURY

Aspiration Precautions
Cerebral Perfusion Promotion
Circulatory Precautions
Delirium Management
Embolus Precautions
Fluid Management
Infection Control:
   Intraoperative

Nutrition Therapy
Peripheral Sensation
   Management
Positioning: Intraoperative
Pressure Management
Reality Orientation

Risk Identification
Skin Surveillance
Surgical Precautions
Surveillance
Temperature Regulation:
   Intraoperative

NURSING DIAGNOSIS: Peripheral Neurovascular Dysfunction, Risk for

Definition: At risk for disruption in circulation, sensation, or motion of an extremity

NOCS TO ASSESS AND MEASURE ACTUAL OCCURRENCE OF THE DIAGNOSIS
Neurological Status: Peripheral   Sensory Function: Cutaneous   Tissue Perfusion: Peripheral

NOCS ASSOCIATED WITH RISK FACTORS FOR DYSFUNCTION PERIPHERAL NEUROVASCULAR

Bone Healing
Burn Healing
Burn Recovery

Circulation Status
Immobility Consequences:
   Physiological

Physical Injury Severity
Risk Control
Risk Detection

NICS ASSOCIATED WITH PREVENTION OF DYSFUNCTION PERIPHERAL NEUROVASCULAR

Bed Rest Care
Cast Care: Maintenance
Cast Care: Wet
Circulatory Care: Arterial
   Insufficiency
Circulatory Care:
   Venous Insufficiency
Circulatory Precautions
Cutaneous Stimulation
Embolus Care: Peripheral

Embolus Precautions
Lower Extremity Monitoring
Neurologic Monitoring
Peripheral Sensation
   Management
Physical Restraint
Pneumatic Tourniquet
   Precautions
Positioning
Positioning: Neurologic

Positioning: Wheelchair
Pressure Management
Pressure Ulcer Prevention
Risk Identification
Splinting
Surveillance
Traction/Immobilization Care
Wound Care: Burns

PART II - P

NURSING DIAGNOSIS: Poisoning, Risk for

Definition: Accentuated risk of accidental exposure to, or ingestion of, drugs or dangerous products in doses sufficient to cause poisoning

NOCS TO ASSESS AND MEASURE ACTUAL OCCURRENCE OF THE DIAGNOSIS

Symptom Severity

NOCS ASSOCIATED WITH RISK FACTORS FOR POISONING

Acute Confusion Level	Parenting: Early/Middle Childhood Physical Safety	Risk Control: Drug Use
Cognition		Risk Detection
Community Risk Control: Lead Exposure	Parenting: Infant/Toddler Physical Safety	Safe Home Environment
Knowledge: Child Physical Safety	Personal Safety Behavior	Self-Care: Non-Parenteral Medication
	Physical Safety	Self-Care: Parental Medication
Knowledge: Medication	Risk Control	Sensory Function: Vision
Knowledge: Personal Safety	Risk Control: Alcohol Use	Vision Compensation Behavior
Mood Equilibrium		
Parenting: Adolescent Physical Safety		

NICS ASSOCIATED WITH PREVENTION OF POISONING

Communication Enhancement: Visual Deficit	Mood Management	Teaching: Infant Safety 7-9 Months
Delirium Management	Parent Education: Adolescent	Teaching: Infant Safety 10-12 Months
Dementia Management	Parent Education: Childrearing Family	Teaching: Prescribed Medication
Environmental Management: Safety	Parent Education: Infant	Teaching: Toddler Safety 13-18 Months
Environmental Management: Worker Safety	Risk Identification	Teaching: Toddler Safety 19-24 Months
	Substance Use Prevention	
Health Education	Substance Use Treatment	Teaching: Toddler Safety 25-36 Months
Medication Management	Surveillance	
Medication Reconciliation	Surveillance: Safety	

NURSING DIAGNOSIS: Post-Trauma Syndrome, Risk for

Definition: At risk for sustained maladaptive response to a traumatic, overwhelming event

NOCS TO ASSESS AND MEASURE ACTUAL OCCURRENCE OF THE DIAGNOSIS

Abuse Recovery
Comfort Status: Psychospiritual

NOCS ASSOCIATED WITH RISK FACTORS FOR POST-TRAUMA SYNDROME

Anxiety Level	Personal Resiliency	Self-Esteem
Coping	Risk Control	Social Support
Health Beliefs: Perceived Threat	Risk Detection	Stress Level

NICS ASSOCIATED WITH PREVENTION OF POST-TRAUMA SYNDROME

Anxiety Reduction	Guilt Work Facilitation	Self-Esteem Enhancement
Coping Enhancement	Hope Inspiration	Spiritual Support
Counseling	Resiliency Promotion	Support Group
Family Mobilization	Risk Identification	Support System Enhancement
	Security Enhancement	Surveillance

NURSING DIAGNOSIS: Powerlessness, Risk for

Definition: At risk for perceived lack of control over a situation and/or one's ability to significantly affect on outcome

NOCS TO ASSESS AND MEASURE ACTUAL OCCURRENCE OF THE DIAGNOSIS

Health Beliefs: Perceived Control Participation in Health Care Decisions	Personal Autonomy	Self-Direction of Care

NOCS ASSOCIATED WITH RISK FACTORS FOR POWERLESSNESS

Adaptation to Physical Disability	Immobility Consequences: Psycho-Cognitive	Knowledge: Treatment Regimen
Body Image	Knowledge: Diet	Personal Resiliency
Coping	Knowledge: Disease Process	Physical Injury Severity
Dignified Life Closure	Knowledge: Health Resources	Risk Control
Health Beliefs: Perceived Ability to Perform	Knowledge: Medication	Risk Detection
Health Beliefs: Perceived Resources	Knowledge: Treatment Procedure	Self-Esteem

NICS ASSOCIATED WITH PREVENTION OF POWERLESSNESS

Anticipatory Guidance	Health System Guidance	Self-Esteem Enhancement
Assertiveness Training	Learning Facilitation	Surveillance
Body Image Enhancement	Mood Management	Teaching: Disease Process
Coping Enhancement	Resiliency Promotion	Teaching: Prescribed Diet
Dying Care	Risk Identification	Teaching: Prescribed Medication
Financial Resource Assistance	Self-Efficacy Enhancement	Teaching: Procedure/Treatment

NURSING DIAGNOSIS: Religiosity, Risk for Impaired

Definition: At risk for an impaired ability to exercise reliance on religious beliefs and/or participate in rituals of a particular faith tradition

NOCS TO ASSESS AND MEASURE ACTUAL OCCURRENCE OF THE DIAGNOSIS

Comfort Status: Psychospiritual	Spiritual Health

NOCS ASSOCIATED WITH RISK FACTORS FOR IMPAIRED RELIGIOSITY

Acceptance: Health Status	Fear Level	Risk Control
Anxiety Level	Loneliness Severity	Risk Detection
Client Satisfaction: Cultural Needs Fulfillment	Pain: Disruptive Effects	Social Involvement
Coping	Pain Level	Social Support
Depression Level	Psychosocial Adjustment: Life Change	Suffering Severity

NICS ASSOCIATED WITH PREVENTION OF IMPAIRED RELIGIOSITY

Anxiety Reduction	Religious Ritual Enhancement	Socialization Enhancement
Coping Enhancement	Relocation Stress Reduction	Spiritual Growth Facilitation
Culture Brokerage	Risk Identification	Support System Enhancement
Family Mobilization	Security Enhancement	Surveillance
Pain Management		

PART II - R

NURSING DIAGNOSIS: Relocation Stress Syndrome, Risk for

Definition: At risk for physiological and/or psychosocial disturbance following transfer from one environment to another

NOCS TO ASSESS AND MEASURE ACTUAL OCCURRENCE OF THE DIAGNOSIS

Personal Health Status

Psychosocial Adjustment:
  Life Change

NOCS ASSOCIATED WITH RISK FACTORS FOR RELOCATION STRESS SYNDROME

Cognition
Coping
Discharge Readiness:
  Supported Living
Family Participation in
  Professional Care

Grief Resolution
Personal Autonomy
Personal Health Status

Risk Control
Risk Detection
Social Support

NICS ASSOCIATED WITH PREVENTION OF RELOCATION STRESS SYNDROME

Anticipatory Guidance
Coping Enhancement
Counseling
Dementia Management
Discharge Planning
Emotional Support

Family Involvement Promotion
Grief Work Facilitation
Patient Rights Protection
Relocation Stress Reduction
Risk Identification
Self-Efficacy Enhancement

Spiritual Support
Support System Enhancement
Surveillance
Transport: Interfacility
Visitation Facilitation

NURSING DIAGNOSIS: Renal Perfusion, Risk for Ineffective

Definition: At risk for a decrease in blood circulation to the kidney that may compromise health

NOCS TO ASSESS AND MEASURE ACTUAL OCCURRENCE OF THE DIAGNOSIS

Kidney Function

Tissue Perfusion:
    Abdominal Organs

NOCS ASSOCIATED WITH RISK FACTORS FOR INEFFECTIVE RENAL PERFUSION

Blood Loss Severity
Burn Healing
Burn Recovery
Cardiopulmonary Status
Circulation Status
Diabetes Self-Management
Electrolyte & Acid/Base Balance
Fluid Balance
Fluid Overload Severity

Hydration
Immune Hypersensitivity
    Response
Infection Severity
Knowledge: Congestive Heart
    Failure Management
Knowledge: Diabetes
    Management
Knowledge: Hypertension
    Management
Knowledge: Infection
    Management

Medication Response
Nutritional Status: Biochemical
    Measures
Physical Injury Severity
Risk Control
Risk Detection
Safe Home Environment
Smoking Cessation Behavior
Vital Signs

NICS ASSOCIATED WITH PREVENTION OF INEFFECTIVE RENAL PERFUSION

Acid-Base Management:
    Metabolic Acidosis
Bleeding Reduction
Bleeding Reduction:
    Gastrointestinal
Blood Products Administration
Chemotherapy Management
Circulatory Care: Arterial
    Insufficiency
Embolus Care: Peripheral
Embolus Precautions
Environmental Management:
    Safety

Fluid Management
Hemodynamic Regulation
Hemorrhage Control
Hypovolemia Management
Infection Control
Medication Management
Oxygen Therapy
Risk Identification
Shock Management
Shock Prevention
Smoking Cessation
    Assistance

Surveillance
Teaching: Disease Process
Teaching: Prescribed Diet
Teaching: Prescribed
    Medication
Teaching: Procedure/Treatment
Thrombolytic Therapy
    Management
Urinary Elimination
    Management
Vital Signs Monitoring
Wound Care: Burns

PART II - R

NURSING DIAGNOSIS: Resilience, Risk for Compromised

Definition: At risk for decreased ability to sustain a pattern of positive responses to an adverse situation or crisis

NOCS TO ASSESS AND MEASURE ACTUAL OCCURRENCE OF THE DIAGNOSIS

Personal Resiliency

NOCS ASSOCIATED WITH RISK FACTORS FOR COMPROMISED RESILIENCE

Acceptance: Health Status
Adaptation to Physical Disability
Anxiety Level
Client Satisfaction:
   Case Management
Client Satisfaction:
   Continuity of Care
Client Satisfaction:
   Symptom Control

Dignified Life Closure
Grief Resolution
Hope
Pain Level
Psychosocial Adjustment:
   Life Change
Risk Control

Risk Control: Unplanned
   Pregnancy
Risk Detection
Stress Level
Suffering Severity
Symptom Control
Symptom Severity

NICS ASSOCIATED WITH PREVENTION OF COMPROMISED RESILIENCE

Anxiety Reduction
Anticipatory Guidance
Behavior Modification
Calming Technique
Case Management
Crisis Intervention
Culture Brokerage
Dying Care
Family Planning: Unplanned
   Pregnancy

Grief Work Facilitation
Grief Work Facilitation:
   Perinatal Death
Guilt Work Facilitation
Health System Guidance
Hope Inspiration
Multidisciplinary Care
   Conference

Relaxation Therapy
Relocation Stress Reduction
Risk Identification
Self-Efficacy Enhancement
Self-Responsibility Facilitation
Surveillance
Sustenance Support

NURSING DIAGNOSIS: Self-Esteem: Situational Low, Risk for

Definition: At risk for developing negative perception of self-worth in response to a current situation (specify)

NOCS TO ASSESS AND MEASURE ACTUAL OCCURRENCE OF THE DIAGNOSIS

Self-Esteem

NOCS ASSOCIATED WITH RISK FACTORS FOR SITUATIONAL LOW SELF-ESTEEM

Abuse Cessation
Abuse Protection
Abuse Recovery
Abuse Recovery: Emotional
Abuse Recovery: Financial
Abuse Recovery: Physical
Abuse Recovery: Sexual
Adaptation to Physical
  Disability
Body Image

Child Development:
  Middle Childhood
Child Development: Adolescence
Coping
Development: Late Adulthood
Development: Middle Adulthood
Development: Young Adulthood
Grief Resolution
Health Beliefs: Perceived Control
Neglect Cessation

Neglect Recovery
Personal Autonomy
Personal Health Status
Personal Resiliency
Psychosocial Adjustment:
  Life Change
Risk Control
Risk Detection
Role Performance
Sexual Identity

NICS ASSOCIATED WITH PREVENTION OF SITUATIONAL LOW SELF-ESTEEM

Abuse Protection Support
Assertiveness Training
Behavior Modification
Body Image Enhancement
Bowel Incontinence Care:
  Encopresis
Coping Enhancement
Developmental Enhancement:
  Adolescent
Developmental Enhancement:
  Child

Grief Work Facilitation
Grief Work Facilitation:
  Perinatal Death
Guilt Work Facilitation
Relocation Stress Reduction
Resiliency Promotion
Risk Identification
Role Enhancement
Self-Awareness Enhancement

Self-Esteem Enhancement
Self-Responsibility Facilitation
Surveillance
Sustenance Support
Teaching: Sexuality
Urinary Incontinence Care:
  Enuresis
Values Clarification

PART II - S

NURSING DIAGNOSIS: Self-Mutilation, Risk for

Definition: At risk for deliberate self-injurious behavior causing tissue damage with the intent of causing nonfatal injury to attain relief of tension

NOCS TO ASSESS AND MEASURE ACTUAL OCCURRENCE OF THE DIAGNOSIS

Self-Mutilation Restraint

NOCS ASSOCIATED WITH RISK FACTORS FOR SELF-MUTILATION

Abuse Protection
Abuse Recovery
Abuse Recovery: Emotional
Abuse Recovery: Physical
Abuse Recovery: Sexual
Aggression Self-Control
Agitation Level
Alcohol Abuse Cessation
    Behavior
Anxiety Level
Body Image
Child Adaptation to
    Hospitalization

Child Development:
    Adolescence
Child Development:
    Middle Childhood
Coping
Depression Level
Distorted Thought Self-Control
Drug Abuse Cessation Behavior
Family Functioning
Family Integrity
Health Beliefs: Perceived
    Control
Identity
Impulse Self-Control

Mood Equilibrium
Nutritional Status: Nutrient
    Intake
Personal Autonomy
Risk Control
Risk Detection
Self-Esteem
Sexual Identity
Social Interaction Skills
Social Involvement
Stress Level
Substance Addiction
    Consequences

NICS ASSOCIATED WITH PREVENTION OF SELF-MUTILATION

Abuse Protection Support
Abuse Protection Support:
    Child
Active Listening
Anger Control Assistance
Anxiety Reduction
Area Restriction
Behavior Management
Behavior Management:
    Self-Harm
Behavior Modification
Body Image Enhancement
Calming Technique
Cognitive Restructuring
Coping Enhancement
Counseling
Delusion Management

Developmental Enhancement:
    Adolescent
Developmental Enhancement:
    Child
Emotional Support
Environmental Management:
    Safety
Environmental Management:
    Violence Prevention
Grief Work Facilitation
Guilt Work Facilitation
Family Integrity Promotion
Family Integrity Promotion:
    Childbearing Family
Family Therapy
Impulse Control Training

Limit Setting
Mood Management
Nutritional Counseling
Patient Contracting
Risk Identification
Self-Awareness Enhancement
Self-Esteem Enhancement
Self-Modification Assistance
Sexual Counseling
Socialization Enhancement
Substance Use Treatment
Surveillance
Therapy Group

NURSING DIAGNOSIS: Shock, Risk for

Definition: At risk for an inadequate blood flow to the body's tissues, which may lead to life-threatening cellular dysfunction

NOCS TO ASSESS AND MEASURE ACTUAL OCCURRENCE OF THE DIAGNOSIS
Tissue Perfusion: Cellular

NOCS ASSOCIATED WITH RISK FACTORS FOR SHOCK

Blood Loss Severity	Infection Severity: Newborn	Risk Control: Infectious
Blood Transfusion Reaction	Respiratory Status: Gas	Process
Circulation Status	Exchange	Risk Detection
Hemodialysis Access	Risk Control	Vital Signs
Infection Severity		

NICS ASSOCIATED WITH PREVENTION OF SHOCK

Bleeding Precautions	Blood Products	Infection Protection
Bleeding Reduction	Administration	Oxygen Therapy
Bleeding Reduction:	Circulatory Care:	Respiratory Monitoring
Antepartum Uterus	Arterial Insufficiency	Risk Identification
Bleeding Reduction:	Circulatory Care:	Shock Prevention
Gastrointestinal	Venous Insufficiency	Surveillance
Bleeding Reduction: Nasal	Embolus Care: Pulmonary	Vital Signs Monitoring
Bleeding Reduction:	Hemorrhage Control	
Postpartum Uterus	Hypovolemia Management	
Bleeding Reduction: Wound	Infection Control	

PART II - S

NURSING DIAGNOSIS: Skin Integrity, Risk for Impaired

Definition: At risk for skin being adversely altered

NOCS TO ASSESS AND MEASURE ACTUAL OCCURRENCE OF THE DIAGNOSIS

Tissue Integrity: Skin & Mucous
  Membranes

NOCS ASSOCIATED WITH RISK FACTORS FOR IMPAIRED SKIN INTEGRITY

Allergic Response: Localized
Body Positioning: Self-Initiated
Breastfeeding Establishment:
  Maternal
Circulation Status
Fluid Overload Severity
Hydration
Immobility Consequences:
  Physiological
Immune Status
Infection Severity
Infection Severity: Newborn

Immune Hypersensitivity
  Response
Medication Response
Neurological Status:
  Peripheral
Nutritional Status
Nutritional Status:
  Nutrient Intake
Ostomy Self-Care
Risk Control
Risk Control: Hyperthermia
Risk Control: Hypothermia

Risk Control: Infectious
  Process
Risk Control: Sun Exposure
Risk Detection
Self-Mutilation Restraint
Sensory Function:
  Cutaneous
Tissue Perfusion: Cellular
Tissue Perfusion:
  Peripheral
Urinary Continence
Weight: Body Mass

NICS ASSOCIATED WITH PREVENTION OF IMPAIRED SKIN INTEGRITY

Bathing
Bed Rest Care
Bowel Incontinence Care
Cast Care: Maintenance
Cast Care: Wet
Circulatory Care: Arterial
  Insufficiency
Circulatory Care: Venous
  Insufficiency
Circulatory Precautions
Eating Disorders Management
Fluid/Electrolyte Management
Fluid Management
Foot Care
Incision Site Care
Infection Control

Infection Protection
Lactation Counseling
Latex Precautions
Lower Extremity Monitoring
Medication Administration:
  Skin
Medication Management
Nutrition Management
Nutrition Therapy
Ostomy Care
Perineal Care
Pneumatic Tourniquet
  Precautions
Positioning
Positioning: Intraoperative
Pressure Management

Pressure Ulcer Prevention
Pruritus Management
Radiation Therapy
  Management
Risk Identification
Skin Care: Topical Treatments
Skin Surveillance
Surveillance
Teaching: Foot Care
Total Parenteral Nutrition
  (TPN) Administration
Traction/Immobilization Care
Tube Care: Gastrointestinal
Weight Gain Assistance
Weight Reduction Assistance

NURSING DIAGNOSIS: Spiritual Distress, Risk for

Definition: At risk for an impaired ability to experience and integrate meaning and purpose in life through connectedness with self, others, art, music, literature, nature, and/or a power greater than oneself

NOCS TO ASSESS AND MEASURE ACTUAL OCCURRENCE OF THE DIAGNOSIS
Spiritual Health

NOCS ASSOCIATED WITH RISK FACTORS FOR SPIRITUAL DISTRESS

Acceptance: Health Status
Adaptation to Physical Disability
Alcohol Abuse Cessation Behavior
Anxiety Level
Client Satisfaction:
   Cultural Needs Fulfillment
Comfort Status: Psychospiritual
Comfort Status: Sociocultural
Comfortable Death
Community Disaster Readiness

Coping
Depression Level
Dignified Life Closure
Drug Abuse Cessation Behavior
Grief Resolution
Hope
Loneliness Severity
Mood Equilibrium
Pain: Adverse Psychological
   Response

Pain: Disruptive Effects
Psychosocial Adjustment:
   Life Change
Risk Control
Risk Detection
Self-Esteem
Social Interaction Skills
Social Involvement
Stress Level
Suffering Severity

NICS ASSOCIATED WITH PREVENTION OF SPIRITUAL DISTRESS

Anxiety Reduction
Behavior Modification: Social Skills
Community Disaster Preparedness
Conflict Mediation
Coping Enhancement
Culture Brokerage
Dying Care
Environmental Management:
   Comfort
Forgiveness Facilitation

Grief Work Facilitation
Grief Work Facilitation:
   Perinatal Death
Hope Inspiration
Mood Management
Pain Management
Religious Ritual
   Enhancement
Relocation Stress Reduction
Reminiscence Therapy

Risk Identification
Self-Awareness
   Enhancement
Self-Esteem Enhancement
Socialization Enhancement
Spiritual Support
Substance Use Treatment
Support System
   Enhancement
Surveillance

PART II - S

NURSING DIAGNOSIS: Sudden Infant Death Syndrome, Risk for

Definition: Presence of risk factors for sudden death of an infant under 1 year of age

NOCS TO ASSESS AND MEASURE ACTUAL OCCURRENCE OF THE DIAGNOSIS

*See critical reasoning note below

NOCS ASSOCIATED WITH RISK FACTORS FOR SUDDEN INFANT DEATH SYNDROME

Knowledge: Infant Care	Prenatal Health Behavior	Risk Control: Tobacco Use
Knowledge: Preterm Infant Care	Preterm Infant Organization	Risk Detection
Maternal Status: Antepartum	Risk Control	Smoking Cessation Behavior
Parenting: Infant/Toddler	Risk Control: Hyperthermia	Thermoregulation: Newborn
Physical Safety		

NICS ASSOCIATED WITH PREVENTION OF SUDDEN INFANT DEATH SYNDROME

Developmental Care	Risk Identification:	Teaching: Infant Safety
Infant Care	Childbearing Family	4-6 Months
Parent Education: Infant	Smoking Cessation	Teaching: Infant Safety
Prenatal Care	Assistance	7-9 Months
Risk Identification	Surveillance	Teaching: Infant Safety
	Teaching: Infant Safety	10-12 Months
	0-3 Months	Temperature Regulation

Critical reasoning note: The outcome for this diagnosis would be that the infant does not experience sudden infant death. NOC does not have an outcome that directly fits the diagnosis; continued life could be measured using the Child Development outcomes from 1 month to 12 months.

NURSING DIAGNOSIS: Suffocation, Risk for

Definition: Accentuated risk of accidental suffocation (inadequate air available for inhalation)

NOCS TO ASSESS AND MEASURE ACTUAL OCCURRENCE OF THE DIAGNOSIS

Respiratory Status: Ventilation

NOCS ASSOCIATED WITH RISK FACTORS FOR SUFFOCATION

Aspiration Prevention	Neurological Status:	Risk Control
Asthma Self-Management	Consciousness	Risk Detection
Body Positioning: Self-Initiated	Parenting: Infant/Toddler	Safe Home Environment
Knowledge: Child Physical	Physical Safety	Sensory Function:
Safety	Personal Safety Behavior	Taste & Smell
Knowledge: Infant Care	Physical Injury Severity	Substance Addiction
Knowledge: Personal Safety	Post-Procedure Recovery	Consequences
Knowledge: Preterm	Respiratory Status:	Suicide Self-Restraint
Infant Care	Airway Patency	Swallowing Status

NICS ASSOCIATED WITH PREVENTION OF SUFFOCATION

Airway Management	Positioning	Teaching: Infant Safety 0-3 Months
Artificial Airway Management	Postanesthesia Care	Teaching: Infant Safety 4-6 Months
Aspiration Precautions	Respiratory Monitoring	Teaching: Infant Safety 7-9 Months
Asthma Management	Risk Identification	Teaching: Infant Safety 10-12 Months
Environmental Management:	Substance Use Treatment:	Teaching: Toddler Safety 13-18 Months
Safety	Overdose	Teaching: Toddler Safety 19-24 Months
Impulse Control Training	Suicide Prevention	Teaching: Toddler Safety 25-36 Months
Infant Care	Surveillance	
Parent Education: Infant	Swallowing Therapy	

PART II - S

NURSING DIAGNOSIS: Suicide, Risk for

Definition: At risk for self-inflicted, life-threatening injury

NOCS TO ASSESS AND MEASURE ACTUAL OCCURRENCE OF THE DIAGNOSIS

Suicide Self-Restraint

NOCS ASSOCIATED WITH RISK FACTORS FOR SUICIDE

Abuse Recovery
Abuse Recovery: Emotional
Abuse Recovery: Financial
Abuse Recovery: Physical
Abuse Recovery: Sexual
Acceptance: Health Status
Adaptation to Physical Disability
Alcohol Abuse Cessation
  Behavior
Child Development: Adolescence
Depression Level
Development: Late Adulthood
Development: Young Adulthood

Drug Abuse Cessation Behavior
Family Functioning
Family Integrity
Grief Resolution
Hope
Impulse Self-Control
Loneliness Severity
Mood Equilibrium
Pain: Adverse Psychological
  Response
Pain: Disruptive Effects
Personal Autonomy
Personal Resiliency

Personal Well-Being
Psychosocial Adjustment:
  Life Change
Role Performance
Risk Control
Risk Detection
Sexual Identity
Social Involvement
Social Support
Student Health Status
Substance Addiction
  Consequences
Suffering Severity

NICS ASSOCIATED WITH PREVENTION OF SUICIDE

Abuse Protection Support: Child
Behavior Management: Self-Harm
Counseling
Crisis Intervention
Delusion Management
Environmental Management:
  Safety
Family Integrity Promotion
Family Therapy
Financial Resource Assistance
Grief Work Facilitation

Guilt Work Facilitation
Hallucination Management
Hope Inspiration
Impulse Control Training
Limit Setting
Mood Management
Pain Management
Patient Contracting
Phototherapy: Mood/Sleep
  Regulation
Relocation Stress Reduction

Risk Identification
Role Enhancement
Socialization Enhancement
Substance Use Treatment
Suicide Prevention
Support Group
Support System
  Enhancement
Surveillance
Teaching: Sexuality
Therapy Group

PART II - S

NURSING DIAGNOSIS: Tissue Perfusion: Cardiac, Risk for Decreased

Definition: Risk for decrease in cardiac (coronary) circulation

NOCS TO ASSESS AND MEASURE ACTUAL OCCURRENCE OF THE DIAGNOSIS

Circulation Status
Tissue Perfusion: Cardiac

NOCS ASSOCIATED WITH RISK FACTORS FOR DECREASED CARDIAC TISSUE PERFUSION

Adherence Behavior:
  Healthy Diet
Cardiac Pump Effectiveness
Compliance Behavior:
  Prescribed Diet
Compliance Behavior:
  Prescribed Medication
Diabetes Self-Management
Drug Abuse Cessation
  Behavior
Hydration

Knowledge: Conception
  Prevention
Knowledge: Diabetes
  Management
Knowledge: Diet
Knowledge: Health Behavior
Knowledge: Hypertension
  Management
Knowledge: Medication
Knowledge: Weight
  Management

Medication Response
Physical Fitness
Respiratory Status:
  Gas Exchange
Risk Control
Risk Detection
Smoking Cessation
  Behavior
Weight Loss Behavior

NICS ASSOCIATED WITH PREVENTION OF DECREASED CARDIAC TISSUE PERFUSION

Cardiac Precautions
Exercise Promotion
Family Planning:
  Contraception
Fluid Management
Fluid Resuscitation
Health Education

Medication Management
Nutritional Counseling
Oxygen Therapy
Risk Identification
Smoking Cessation
  Assistance
Substance Use Treatment

Surveillance
Teaching: Prescribed Diet
Teaching: Prescribed
  Medication
Vital Signs Monitoring
Weight Reduction
  Assistance

NURSING DIAGNOSIS: Tissue Perfusion: Cerebral, Risk for Ineffective

Definition: Risk for a decrease in cerebral tissue circulation

NOCS TO ASSESS AND MEASURE ACTUAL OCCURRENCE OF THE DIAGNOSIS

Tissue Perfusion: Cerebral

NOCS ASSOCIATED WITH RISK FACTORS FOR INEFFECTIVE CEREBRAL TISSUE PERFUSION

Blood Coagulation
Cardiac Pump Effectiveness
Circulation Status
Knowledge: Cardiac Disease
  Management

Knowledge: Hypertension
  Management
Medication Response
Neurological Status
Physical Injury Severity

Risk Control
Risk Detection
Substance Addiction
  Consequences

NICS ASSOCIATED WITH PREVENTION OF INEFFECTIVE CEREBRAL TISSUE PERFUSION

Bleeding Precautions
Cardiac Care
Cardiac Care: Acute
Cardiac Precautions
Cerebral Edema Management
Circulatory Care: Arterial
  Insufficiency
Circulatory Care: Venous
  Insufficiency
Defibrillator Management:
  External
Defibrillator Management:
  Internal

Embolus Care: Peripheral
Embolus Care: Pulmonary
Embolus Precautions
Hemodynamic Regulation
Intracranial Pressure (ICP)
  Monitoring
Medication Management
Neurologic Monitoring
Pacemaker Management:
  Permanent
Pacemaker Management:
  Temporary

Risk Identification
Substance Use Treatment
Surveillance
Teaching: Disease Process
Teaching: Prescribed Diet
Teaching: Prescribed Medication
Teaching: Procedure/Treatment
Thrombolytic Therapy
  Management

PART II - T

NURSING DIAGNOSIS: Tissue Perfusion, Gastrointestinal, Risk for Ineffective

Definition: At risk for decrease in gastrointestinal circulation

NOCS TO ASSESS AND MEASURE ACTUAL OCCURRENCE OF THE DIAGNOSIS

Tissue Perfusion:
  Abdominal Organs

NOCS ASSOCIATED WITH RISK FACTORS FOR INEFFECTIVE GASTROINTESTINAL TISSUE PERFUSION

Alcohol Abuse Cessation
  Behavior
Blood Coagulation
Blood Loss Severity
Cardiac Pump Effectiveness
Circulation Status
Diabetes Self-Management

Drug Abuse Cessation Behavior
Fluid Overload Severity
Gastrointestinal Function
Kidney Function
Knowledge: Cardiac Disease
  Management
Knowledge: Diabetes
  Management

Medication Response
Risk Control
Risk Detection
Smoking Cessation
  Behavior
Substance Addiction
  Consequences

NICS ASSOCIATED WITH PREVENTION OF INEFFECTIVE GASTROINTESTINAL TISSUE PERFUSION

Bleeding Precautions
Bleeding Reduction
Bleeding Reduction:
  Gastrointestinal
Cardiac Care
Cardiac Care: Acute
Cardiac Precautions
Circulatory Care: Arterial
  Insufficiency
Circulatory Care: Venous
  Insufficiency

Fluid Management
Hemodynamic Regulation
Medication Management
Pacemaker Management:
  Permanent
Pacemaker Management:
  Temporary
Risk Identification
Smoking Cessation
  Assistance

Substance Use Treatment
Surveillance
Teaching: Disease Process
Teaching: Prescribed Diet
Teaching: Prescribed
  Medication
Teaching: Procedure/Treatment
Thrombolytic Therapy
  Management

NURSING DIAGNOSIS: Trauma, Risk for

Definition: Accentuated risk of accidental tissue injury (e.g., wound, burn, fracture)

NOCS TO ASSESS AND MEASURE ACTUAL OCCURRENCE OF THE DIAGNOSIS

Falls Occurrence
Physical Injury Severity

Tissue Integrity: Skin & Mucous
  Membranes

NOCS ASSOCIATED WITH RISK FACTORS FOR TRAUMA

Acute Confusion Level
Agitation Level
Alcohol Abuse Cessation
  Behavior
Balance
Cognition
Community Risk Control:
  Violence
Community Violence Level
Coordinated Movement
Elopement Propensity Risk
Fall Prevention Behavior

Knowledge: Child Physical
  Safety
Knowledge: Fall Prevention
Knowledge: Personal Safety
Neurological Status: Peripheral
Parenting: Adolescent Physical
  Safety
Parenting: Early/Middle
  Childhood Physical Safety
Parenting: Infant/Toddler
  Physical Safety
Personal Safety Behavior
Physical Fitness

Risk Control
Risk Control: Alcohol Use
Risk Control: Drug Use
Risk Control: Sun Exposure
Risk Detection
Safe Home Environment
Safe Wandering
Sensory Function: Vision
Substance Withdrawal
  Severity
Vision Compensation
  Behavior

NICS ASSOCIATED WITH PREVENTION OF TRAUMA

Communication Enhancement:
  Visual Deficit
Delirium Management
Dementia Management
Elopement Precautions
Environmental Management:
  Safety
Environmental Management:
  Violence Prevention
Environmental Management:
  Worker Safety
Exercise Promotion
Exercise Promotion: Strength
  Training
Exercise Therapy: Balance
Exercise Therapy: Muscle
  Control
Fall Prevention
Health Education
Laser Precautions

Parent Education: Adolescent
Parent Education: Childrearing
  Family
Parent Education: Infant
Peripheral Sensation
  Management
Physical Restraint
Radiation Therapy
  Management
Reality Orientation
Risk Identification
Risk Identification:
  Childbearing Family
Sports-Injury Prevention:
  Youth
Substance Use Treatment
Substance Use Treatment:
  Alcohol Withdrawal
Substance Use Treatment:
  Drug Withdrawal

Surgical Precautions
Surveillance
Surveillance: Safety
Teaching: Infant Safety
  0-3 Months
Teaching: Infant Safety
  4-6 Months
Teaching: Infant Safety
  7-9 Months
Teaching: Infant Safety
  10-12 Months
Teaching: Toddler Safety
  13-18 Months
Teaching: Toddler Safety
  19-24 Months
Teaching: Toddler Safety
  25-36 Months
Vehicle Safety Promotion

NURSING DIAGNOSIS: Urinary Incontinence: Urge, Risk for

Definition: At risk for involuntary loss of urine associated with a sudden, strong sensation or urinary urgency

NOCS TO ASSESS AND MEASURE ACTUAL OCCURRENCE OF THE DIAGNOSIS

Urinary Continence

NOCS ASSOCIATED WITH RISK FACTORS FOR URINARY INCONTINENCE: URGE

Alcohol Abuse Cessation Behavior	Neurological Status: Spinal Sensory/Motor Function	Risk Control: Infectious Process
Infection Severity	Risk Control	Risk Detection
Knowledge: Medication	Risk Control: Alcohol Use	Self-Care: Toileting
Medication Response		

NICS ASSOCIATED WITH PREVENTION OF URINARY INCONTINENCE: URGE

Fluid Management	Risk Identification	Teaching: Prescribed Medication
Infection Control	Self-Care Assistance: Toileting	Urinary Elimination Management
Medication Management	Substance Use Treatment	Urinary Habit Training
Pelvic Muscle Exercise	Surveillance	
Pessary Management		
Prompted Voiding		

NURSING DIAGNOSIS: Vascular Trauma, Risk for

Definition: At risk for damage to a vein and its surrounding tissues related to the presence of a catheter and/or infused solutions

NOCS TO ASSESS AND MEASURE ACTUAL OCCURRENCE OF THE DIAGNOSIS

Hemodialysis Access

NOCS ASSOCIATED WITH RISK FACTORS FOR VASCULAR TRAUMA

Allergic Response: Localized	Risk Detection	Tissue Integrity: Skin & Mucous Membranes
Risk Control	Self-Care: Parenteral Medication	

NICS ASSOCIATED WITH PREVENTION OF VASCULAR TRAUMA

Allergy Management	Medication Administration: Intravenous (IV)	Risk Identification
Dialysis Access Maintenance	Peripherally Inserted Central (PIC) Catheter Care	Skin Surveillance
Intravenous (IV) Insertion	Phlebotomy: Cannulated Vessel	Surveillance
Intravenous (IV) Therapy		Venous Access Device (VAD) Maintenance
Invasive Hemodynamic Monitoring		

NURSING DIAGNOSIS: Violence: Other-Directed, Risk for

Definition: At risk for behaviors in which an individual demonstrates that he or she can be physically, emotionally, and/or sexually harmful to others

NOCS TO ASSESS AND MEASURE ACTUAL OCCURRENCE OF THE DIAGNOSIS

Abusive Behavior Self-Restraint   Aggression Self-Control

NOCS ASSOCIATED WITH RISK FACTORS FOR OTHER-DIRECTED VIOLENCE

Abuse Recovery: Emotional
Abuse Recovery: Physical
Abuse Recovery: Sexual
Acute Confusion Level
Agitation Level
Alcohol Abuse Cessation
    Behavior
Cognition
Depression Level

Distorted Thought Self-Control
Drug Abuse Cessation Behavior
Hyperactivity Level
Impulse Self-Control
Maternal Status: Antepartum
Maternal Status: Intrapartum
Neurological Status

Risk Control
Risk Control: Alcohol Use
Risk Control: Drug Use
Risk Detection
Seizure Control
Stress Level
Suicide Self-Restraint

NICS ASSOCIATED WITH PREVENTION OF OTHER-DIRECTED VIOLENCE

Abuse Protection Support
Abuse Protection Support:
    Child
Anger Control Assistance
Anxiety Reduction
Behavior Management
Behavior Management:
    Overactivity/Inattention
Behavior Management:
    Sexual
Behavior Modification
Delusion Management

Dementia Management
Dementia Management:
    Bathing
Environmental Management:
    Violence Prevention
Fire-Setting Precautions
Hallucination Management
Impulse Control Training
Intrapartal Care
Mood Management
Mutual Goal Setting

Neurologic Monitoring
Prenatal Care
Reality Orientation
Risk Identification
Seizure Management
Substance Use Prevention
Substance Use Treatment
Suicide Prevention
Surveillance
Therapeutic Play

PART II - V

NURSING DIAGNOSIS: Violence: Self-Directed, Risk for

Definition: At risk for behaviors in which an individual demonstrates that he or she can be physically, emotionally, and/or sexually harmful to self

NOCS TO ASSESS AND MEASURE ACTUAL OCCURRENCE OF THE DIAGNOSIS

Self-Mutilation Restraint   Suicide Self-Restraint

NOCS ASSOCIATED WITH RISK FACTORS FOR SELF-DIRECTED VIOLENCE

Agitation Level	Identity	Risk Detection
Anxiety Level	Impulse Self-Control	Sexual Functioning
Coping	Loneliness Severity	Social Interaction Skills
Depression Level	Mood Equilibrium	Social Involvement
Depression Self-Control	Personal Health Status	Social Support
Distorted Thought Self-Control	Personal Well-Being	Stress Level
Family Functioning	Risk Control	Substance Addiction
Family Integrity	Risk Control: Alcohol Use	Consequences
Hope	Risk Control: Drug Use	Will to Live

NICS ASSOCIATED WITH PREVENTION OF SELF-DIRECTED VIOLENCE

Anger Control Assistance	Family Integrity Promotion	Substance Use Treatment:
Anxiety Reduction	Family Therapy	Alcohol Withdrawal
Behavior Management:	Hallucination Management	Substance Use Treatment:
Self-Harm	Hope Inspiration	Drug Withdrawal
Behavior Modification:	Impulse Control Training	Substance Use Treatment:
Social Skills	Limit Setting	Overdose
Calming Technique	Mood Management	Suicide Prevention
Cognitive Restructuring	Patient Contracting	Support Group
Conflict Mediation	Phototherapy: Mood/Sleep	Support System Enhancement
Coping Enhancement	Regulation	Surveillance
Counseling	Recreation Therapy	Surveillance: Safety
Crisis Intervention	Risk Identification	Teaching: Safe Sex
Delusion Management	Self-Awareness Enhancement	Therapy Group
Dementia Management	Self-Modification Assistance	
Environmental Management:	Socialization Enhancement	
Safety	Substance Use Treatment	
Environmental Management:		
Violence Prevention		

Introduction to Linkages for Clinical Conditions

This section of the book includes NOC and NIC links with 10 common, often costly, clinical conditions. The purpose of the section is to illustrate how NOC outcomes and NIC interventions can be linked to clinical diagnoses when a classification other than NANDA-I is used. This may occur because NANDA-I currently does not have a diagnosis covering the condition or because another classification is selected as a basis for developing interventions and outcomes for generic care plans. In the latter case, the care plan may contain NANDA-I diagnoses as well as patient outcomes and nursing interventions. However, the outcomes and interventions selected may not use a standardized nursing terminology, but reflect local terms used in the organization. For that reason we have developed these conditions for the purpose of illustrating how NOC outcomes and NIC interventions can be used with other classifications of clinical conditions.

The clinical conditions presented in this section are Asthma, Chronic Obstructive Pulmonary Disease, Colon and Rectal Cancer, Depression, Diabetes Mellitus, Heart Failure, Hypertension, Pneumonia, Stroke, and Total Joint Replacement: Knee/Hip. Each condition is introduced with a brief statement that describes the condition followed by information about the prevalence, incidence, cost, and (as indicated) mortality associated with the condition. This information illustrates the importance of these clinical conditions in terms of numbers of patients requiring care and the personal and national costs associated with the conditions, because of either the chronic nature or the prevalence of the condition. A brief description of the risk factors and the condition follows; this can include the course of the condition/disease, the diagnosis, the symptoms, the treatment, and/or the implications for nursing. Information presented about the clinical condition is selective and

in no way provides a complete review of symptomatology, diagnostic tests, disease course, treatment, complications, and prognosis. The brief discussion of the clinical condition is provided to illustrate the impact these conditions have on health care system resources and the importance of prevention and treatment in providing quality, cost-effective care that will enhance the patient's health and quality of life.

The conditions are presented alphabetically using the clinical condition names identified in the preceding paragraph. Following overview of the clinical conditions and references, a generic care plan is presented. These plans vary in terms of depth, that is, the number of outcomes and interventions provided; the portion of the clinical condition covered, that is, diagnostic phase, acute phase, chronic or rehabilitative phase; and the applicability of the plan for all organizations and settings. In general, the care plans do not address care for a patient in an intensive care unit, immediately following an intrusive procedure or surgery, or during rehabilitation. They also do not address considerations for age, gender, socioeconomic status, or culture because these may differ from organization to organization. They do illustrate the various ways in which NOC outcomes and NIC interventions can be used in the development of generic and individual care plans for patients with these 10 diagnoses.

The NOC outcomes are presented in alphabetical order rather than in order of importance or the sequence in which they might be used. One clinical condition, colon cancer, has two plans of care provided-one for prevention in patients at risk and one for patients following a diagnosis of colon cancer. A number of the care plans include outcomes and interventions that are applicable following discharge from an acute care setting or following a diagnosis, such as asthma, that requires the patient to learn how to perform self-care.

Before the clinical conditions, a less generalized and more complete care plan for the patient with stroke is presented. The plan is for ischemic stroke only and it uses all three of the languages: NANDA-I, NOC, and NIC. It includes selected indicators and the measurement scales for the outcome. The plan *Coordinated Care Path Ischemic Stroke: Outcome Sheet* was developed by Kimberly M. Pattee, RN, BSN, for a 232-bed community hospital—Mercy

Hospital in Iowa City, Iowa. The plan is an excellent illustration of the use of NANDA-I diagnoses, NOC outcomes, and NIC interventions in a care plan for newly diagnosed stroke patients. The plan is a guideline that can be altered to meet individual patient needs. It will assist in the evaluation of evidence-based care for the individual patient and the patient population. We thank Mercy staff for developing this plan and allowing us to share it with others who are engaged in the process of quality improvement.

Sample Care Path for a Clinical Condition: Coordinated Care Path for Ischemic Stroke

Date: _____
[ ] See Additional Care Plan

Plan of Care Discussed with Patient/Significant Other: _____

Note: If goals are not at established TARGET level by discharge indicate reason using all applicable:

A = Died	D = Patient Compliance Issues
B = Chronic Condition	E = Transfer to Rehab/SNF/ECF
C = D/C with Home Services	F = Left AMA

G = Learning Barrier
H = Physical Limitation Transfer
I = Transfer to Other Acute Care Hospital
PN = See Care Plan Progress Notes for Further Explanation

Nursing Diagnosis	OUTCOMES					TARGET	Evaluation — Date and Initial			
							Admit/Start	D/C	INIT.	Reason
1. Risk for Impaired Skin Integrity Interventions: • Skin Surveillance • Pressure Management										
Tissue Integrity: Skin and Mucous Membranes Indicators: • Skin temperature is WNL • Skin elasticity is WNL • Skin on all areas is intact	Severely Compromised 1	Substantially Compromised 2	Moderately Compromised 3	Mildly Compromised 4	Not Compromised 5					
Sensory Functions: Indicators: • Ability to sense skin stimulation • Ability to sense position changes of head and body	Severe Deviation From Normal Range 1	Substantial Deviation From Normal Range 2	Moderate Deviation From Normal Range 3	Mild Deviation From Normal Range 4	No Deviation From Normal Range 5					
2. Potential for Confusion: Acute Interventions: • Anxiety Reduction • Cerebral Perfusion Promotion • Delirium Management • Fall Prevention • Neurological Monitoring • Reality Orientation										
Cognition: Indicators: • Is attentive to events in immediate area • Concentrates for appropriate amount of time on situation	Severely Compromised 1	Substantially Compromised 2	Moderately Compromised 3	Mildly Compromised 4	Not Compromised 5					
Cognitive Orientation Indicators: • Identifies self • Identifies primary significant other • Identifies current place, day, month, year, and season of year	Severely Compromised 1	Substantially Compromised 2	Moderately Compromised 3	Mildly Compromised 4	Not Compromised 5					

INIT.	SIGNATURE	DISCL.	INIT.	SIGNATURE	DISCL.	INIT.	SIGNATURE	DISCL.	INIT.

PART III

Continued

PART III

Sample Care Path for a Clinical Condition: Coordinated Care Path for Ischemic Stroke—cont'd

OUTCOMES

Note: If goals are not met at established TARGET level by discharge indicate reason using all applicable:

A = Died
B = Chronic Condition
C = D/C with Home Services
D = Patient Compliance Issues
E = Transfer to SNF or ECF
F = Left AMA
G = Learning Barrier
H = Physical Limitation Transfer
I = Transfer to Other Acute Care Hospital
PN = See Care Plan Progress Notes for Further Explanation

Nursing Diagnosis		1	2	3	4	5	TARGET	Evaluation Date and Initial (Admit/Start · D/C · Reason)

2. Potential for Confusion: Acute (cont'd)

Interventions:
- Anxiety Reduction
- Cerebral Perfusion Promotion
- Delirium Management
- Fall Prevention
- Neurological Monitoring
- Reality Orientation

Neurological Status: Consciousness

Indicators:
- Opens eyes to external stimuli
- Obeys commands/requests
- Motor responses to noxious stimuli

	Severely Compromised 1	Substantially Compromised 2	Moderately Compromised 3	Mildly Compromised 4	Not Compromised 5

Indicators:
- Seizure activity
- Abnormal flexion (decorticate)
- Abnormal extension (decerebrate)

	Severe 1	Substantial 2	Moderate 3	Mild 4	None 5

3. Ineffective Cerebral Tissue Perfusion: Actual or Potential

Interventions:
- Neurological Monitoring
- Memory Training
- Reality Orientation

Neurological Status: Cranial Sensory/Motor Function

Indicators:
- Facial movement is symmetrical
- Swallow reflex is intact
- Gag reflex is intact
- Shoulder movement is equal bilaterally
- Speech is at pre-stroke levels
- Vision is at pre-stroke levels

	Severely Compromised 1	Substantially Compromised 2	Moderately Compromised 3	Mildly Compromised 4	Not Compromised 5

Indicators:
- Dizziness
- Vertigo
- Involuntary head movement
- Hoarseness
- Loss of sensation
- Tingling

	Severe 1	Substantial 2	Moderate 3	Mild 4	None 5

INIT. / DISCL. / SIGNATURE

Sample Care Path for a Clinical Condition: Coordinated Care Path for Ischemic Stroke—cont'd

Note: If goals are not at established TARGET level by discharge indicate reason using all applicable:

A = Died	D = Patient Compliance Issues	G = Learning Barrier
B = Chronic Condition	E = Transfer to SNF or ECF	H = Physical Limitation Transfer
C = D/C with Home Services	F = Left AMA	I = Transfer to Other Acute Care Hospital
		PN = See Care Plan Progress Notes for Further Explanation

OUTCOMES

Nursing Diagnosis	1	2	3	4	5	TARGET	Evaluation Date and Initial — Admit/Start	D/C	Reason
3. Ineffective Cerebral Tissue Perfusion: Actual or Potential (cont'd)									
Interventions: • Neurological Monitoring • Memory Training • Reality Orientation									
Memory — Indicators: • Recalls immediate information accurately	Severely Compromised 1	Substantially Compromised 2	Moderately Compromised 3	Mildly Compromised 4	Not Compromised 5				
Concentration — Indicators: • Maintains attention • Responds appropriately to visual cues • Responds appropriately to language cues • Appropriately asks for assistance	Severely Compromised 1	Substantially Compromised 2	Moderately Compromised 3	Mildly Compromised 4	Not Compromised 5				
4. Fluid Volume Deficit: Actual or Potential									
Swallowing Status — Indicators: • Able to handle oral secretions • Timely swallow reflex • Maintains head and neck in correct position for swallow	Severely Compromised 1	Substantially Compromised 2	Moderately Compromised 3	Mildly Compromised 4	Not Compromised 5				
• Choking with swallowing • Gagging with swallowing • Coughing with swallowing • Discomfort with swallowing	Severe 1	Substantial 2	Moderate 3	Mild 4	None 5				
5. Altered Nutritional Status: Actual or Potential — Interventions: • Fluid Management • IV Therapy • Nutritional Monitoring • Nutritional Management • Self-care Assistance: Feeding									
Nutritional Status — Indicators: • Food intake is sufficient for body requirements	Not Adequate 1	Slightly Adequate 2	Moderately Adequate 3	Substantially Adequate 4	Totally Adequate 5				
Hydration — Indicators: • Skin turgor • Moist oral mucous membranes	Severely Compromised 1	Substantially Compromised 2	Moderately Compromised 3	Mildly Compromised 4	Not Compromised 5				
INIT. / SIGNATURE	SIGNATURE	DISCL	INIT.	SIGNATURE	INIT.		DISCL.	INIT.	

PART III

Continued

PART III

Sample Care Path for a Clinical Condition: Coordinated Care Path for Ischemic Stroke—cont'd

OUTCOMES

Note: If goals are not at established TARGET level by discharge indicate reason using all applicable:

A = Died
B = Chronic Condition
C = D/C with Home Services
D = Patient Compliance Issues
E = Transfer to SNF or ECF
F = Left AMA
G = Learning Barrier
H = Physical Limitation Transfer
I = Transfer to Other Acute Care Hospital
PN = See Care Plan Progress Notes for Further Explanation

Nursing Diagnosis	Indicators	1	2	3	4	5	TARGET	Evaluation Date and Initial — Admit/Start	D/C	Reason
4. Fluid Volume Deficit: Actual or Potential (cont'd)										
5. Altered Nutritional Status: Actual or Potential (cont'd) Interventions: • Fluid Management • IV Therapy • Nutritional Monitoring • Nutritional Management • Self-care Assistance: Feeding	Indicators: • Thirst • Dark urine • Decreased blood pressure • Rapid, thready pulse • Muscle cramps or twitching (not seizure activity)	Severe 1	Substantial 2	Moderate 3	Mild 4	None 5				
6. Impaired Urinary Elimination: Actual or Potential Interventions: • Urinary Elimination Management • Self-care Assistance, Toileting	Urinary Continence Indicators: • Recognizes urge to void • Responds to urge in timely manner • Gets to toilet between urge and passage of urine • Voids >150ml urine each time.	Never Demonstrated 1	Rarely Demonstrated 2	Sometimes Demonstrated 3	Often Demonstrated 4	Consistently Demonstrated 5				
	• Urine leakage between voidings • Urine leakage with increased abdominal pressure (sneezing, coughing, laughing, lifting) • Wets any clothing during day • Wets any clothing or bedding during night	Consistently Demonstrated 1	Often Demonstrated 2	Sometimes Demonstrated 3	Rarely Demonstrated 4	Never Demonstrated 5				
7. Impaired Bowel Elimination: Actual or Potential Interventions: • Bowel Management • Self-care Assistance • Toileting	Bowel Elimination Indicators: • Recognizes urge to defecate • Maintains control of passage of stool • Responds to urge in timely manner • Gets to toilet between urge and evacuation of stool	Never Demonstrated 1	Rarely Demonstrated 2	Sometimes Demonstrated 3	Often Demonstrated 4	Consistently Demonstrated 5				
INIT.	SIGNATURE	INIT.	DISCL	SIGNATURE	INIT.	DISCL	SIGNATURE	DISCL.	INIT.	

Sample Care Path for a Clinical Condition: Coordinated Care Path for Ischemic Stroke—cont'd

Note: If goals are not at established **TARGET** level by discharge **indicate reason using all applicable:**

A = Died	D = Patient Compliance Issues	G = Learning Barrier
B = Chronic Condition	E = Transfer to SNF or ECF	H = Physical Limitation Transfer
C = D/C with Home Services	F = Left AMA	I = Transfer to Other Acute Care Hospital
		PN = See Care Plan Progress Notes for Further Explanation

OUTCOMES

Nursing Diagnosis						Evaluation Date and Initial		
						Admit/Start	D/C	Reason
7. Impaired Bowel Elimination: Actual or Potential (cont'd) Interventions: • Bowel Management • Self-care Assistance • Toileting	Indicators: • Diarrhea • Constipation • Soils any clothing during day • Soils any clothing or bedding during night	Consistently Demonstrated 1	Often Demonstrated 2	Sometimes Demonstrated 3	Rarely Demonstrated 4	Never Demonstrated 5		
8. Impaired Communication: Verbal, Visual, Auditory Interventions: • Active Listening • Communication Enhancement: Speech Deficit • Communication Enhancement: Visual Deficit • Communication Enhancement: Hearing Deficit	**Verbal** Indicators: • Uses spoken language • Clarity of speech • Interpretation of spoken language	Severely Compromised 1	Substantially Compromised 2	Moderately Compromised 3	Mildly Compromised 4	Not Compromised 5		
	Visual • Floaters in eyes • Flashes of light • Halos around lights • Double vision • Blurred vision • Distorted vision	Severe 1	Substantial 2	Moderate 3	Mild 4	None 5		
	Auditory Indicators: • Tinnitus • New loss of or decrease in hearing	Severe 1	Substantial 2	Moderate 3	Mild 4	None 5		
9. Pain, Acute: Actual or Potential Interventions: • Pain Management	**Pain Level** Indicators: • Reported pain • Moaning and crying • Restlessness • Muscle tension • Headaches	Severe 1	Substantial 2	Moderate 3	Mild 4	None 5		
INIT.	SIGNATURE	DISCL.	INIT.	SIGNATURE	DISCL.	INIT.	SIGNATURE	DISCL.	INIT.

(Copyright Mercy Hospital, Iowa City, IA. Courtesy of Kimberly M. Pattee at Mercy Hospital, 500 East Market Street, Iowa City, IA 52245.)

PART III

Continued

Sample Care Path for a Clinical Condition: Coordinated Care Path for Ischemic Stroke—cont'd

Note: If goals are not at established TARGET level by discharge Indicate reason using all applicable:

A = Died
B = Chronic Condition
C = D/C with Home Services
D = Patient Compliance Issues
E = Transfer to SNF or ECF
F = Left AMA
G = Learning Barrier
H = Physical Limitation Transfer
I = Transfer to Other Acute Care Hospital
PN = See Care Plan Progress Notes for Further Explanation

Nursing Diagnosis	TARGET	OUTCOMES					Evaluation — Date and Initial		
							Admit/Start	D/C	Reason
10. Impaired Mobility: Potential or Actual Interventions: • Bedrest Care • Exercise Therapy: Ambulation, Joint Mobility, Muscle Control • Positioning		**Mobility** Indicators: • Balance • Coordination • Gait • Joint movement • Walking	Severely Compromised 1	Substantially Compromised 2	Moderately Compromised 3	Mildly Compromised 4	Not Compromised 5		
		• Moves from lying to sitting • Moves from sitting to lying • Moves from sitting to standing • Moves from standing to sitting • Bends at waist while standing • Moves from side to side while lying	Severely Compromised 1	Substantially Compromised 2	Moderately Compromised 3	Mildly Compromised 4	Not Compromised 5		
		Transfer Performance Indicators: • Transfers from bed to chair • Transfers from chair to bed • Transfers from bed to commode • Transfers from commode to bed	Severely Compromised 1	Substantially Compromised 2	Moderately Compromised 3	Mildly Compromised 4	Not Compromised 5		
		Ambulation Indicators: • Bears weight • Walks with effective gait • Walks up steps • Walks down steps • Walks around room	Consistently Demonstrated 1	Often Demonstrated 2	Sometimes Demonstrated 3	Rarely Demonstrated 4	Never Demonstrated 5		
		Neurological Status: Central Motor Control Indicators: • Able to maintain walking balance at pre-stroke level • Able to maintain sitting posture at pre-stroke level • Able to maintain standing posture at pre-stroke level	Severely Compromised 1	Substantially Compromised 2	Moderately Compromised 3	Mildly Compromised 4	Not Compromised 5		

INIT.	DISCL.	INIT.	SIGNATURE	DISCL.	INIT.	SIGNATURE	DISCL.	INIT.	SIGNATURE	INIT.

Sample Care Path for a Clinical Condition: Coordinated Care Path for Ischemic Stroke—cont'd

Note: If goals are not at established TARGET level by discharge Indicate reason using all applicable:

A = Died	D = Patient Compliance Issues
B = Chronic Condition	E = Transfer to SNF or ECF
C = D/C with Home Services	F = Left AMA

G = Learning Barrier
H = Physical Limitation Transfer
I = Transfer to Other Acute Care Hospital
PN = See Care Plan Progress Notes for Further Explanation

Nursing Diagnosis	OUTCOMES					TARGET	Evaluation Date and Initial		
							Admit/Start	D/C	Reason
13. Disturbed Body Image, Actual or Potential **14. Grieving, Actual or Anticipatory** **15. Low Self-Esteem, Actual or Potential** Interventions: • Body Image Enhancement • Self-Esteem Enhancement • Coping Enhancement • Emotional Support • Family Support • Grief Work Facilitation									
Adaptation to Physical Disability Indicators: • Verbalizes ability to adjust to disability • Adapts to functional limitations • Identifies plan to meet activities of daily living • Accepts need for physical assistance • Reports decrease in stress related to disability	Never Demonstrated 1	Rarely Demonstrated 2	Sometimes Demonstrated 3	Often Demonstrated 4	Consistently Demonstrated 5				
Body Image Indicators: • Satisfaction with body function • Adjustment to changes in physical appearance • Adjustment to changes in body function • Adjustment to changes in health status • Willingness to use strategies to enhance function	Never Positive 1	Rarely Positive 2	Sometimes Positive 3	Often Positive 4	Consistently Positive 5				
Family Coping Indicators: • Involves family members in decision making • Expresses feelings and emotions freely among members • Seeks family assistance when appropriate	Never Demonstrated 1	Rarely Demonstrated 2	Sometimes Demonstrated 3	Often Demonstrated 4	Consistently Demonstrated 5				
Grief Resolution Indicators: • Verbalizes reality of loss • Maintains grooming and hygiene • Reports absence of sleep disturbance • Progresses through stages of grief • Expresses positive expectations about the future	Never Demonstrated 1	Rarely Demonstrated 2	Sometimes Demonstrated 3	Often Demonstrated 4	Consistently Demonstrated 5				
INIT.	SIGNATURE	DISCL.	INIT.	SIGNATURE	DISCL.	INIT.	SIGNATURE	DISCL.	INIT.

PART III

Continued

PART III

Sample Care Path for a Clinical Condition: Coordinated Care Path for Ischemic Stroke—cont'd

Note: If goals are not at established TARGET level by discharge indicate reason using all applicable:

A = Died
B = Chronic Condition
C = D/C with Home Services
D = Patient Compliance Issues
E = Transfer to SNF or ECF
F = Left AMA
G = Learning Barrier
H = Physical Limitation Transfer
I = Transfer to Other Acute Care Hospital
PN = See Care Plan Progress Notes for Further Explanation

Nursing Diagnosis	OUTCOMES (TARGET)					Evaluation Date and Initial		
						Admit/Start	D/C	Reason

13. Disturbed Body Image, Actual or Potential
14. Grieving, Actual or Anticipatory
15. Low Self-Esteem, Actual or Potential

Interventions:
- Body Image Enhancement
- Self-Esteem Enhancement
- Coping Enhancement
- Emotional Support
- Family Support
- Grief Work Facilitation

Adaptation to Physical Disability

Indicators:
- Verbalizes ability to adjust to disability
- Adapts to functional limitations
- Identifies plan to meet activities of daily living
- Accepts need for physical assistance
- Reports decrease in stress related to disability

Never Demonstrated 1	Rarely Demonstrated 2	Sometimes Demonstrated 3	Often Demonstrated 4	Consistently Demonstrated 5

Body Image

Indicators:
- Satisfaction with body function
- Adjustment to changes in physical appearance
- Adjustment to changes in body function
- Adjustment to changes in health status
- Willingness to use strategies to enhance function

Never Positive 1	Rarely Positive 2	Sometimes Positive 3	Often Positive 4	Consistently Positive 5

Family Coping

Indicators:
- Involves family members in decision making
- Expresses feelings and emotions freely among members
- Seeks family assistance when appropriate

Never Demonstrated 1	Rarely Demonstrated 2	Sometimes Demonstrated 3	Often Demonstrated 4	Consistently Demonstrated 5

Grief Resolution

Indicators:
- Verbalizes reality of loss
- Maintains grooming and hygiene
- Reports absence of sleep disturbance
- Progresses through stages of grief
- Expresses positive expectations about the future

Never Demonstrated 1	Rarely Demonstrated 2	Sometimes Demonstrated 3	Often Demonstrated 4	Consistently Demonstrated 5

INIT.	SIGNATURE	DISCL.	INIT.	DISCL.	INIT.	SIGNATURE	DISCL.	INIT.

Sample Care Path for a Clinical Condition: Coordinated Care Path for Ischemic Stroke—cont'd

Note: If goals are not at established TARGET level by discharge Indicate reason using all applicable:

A = Died
B = Chronic Condition
C = D/C with Home Services
D = Patient Compliance Issues
E = Transfer to SNF or ECF
F = Left AMA
G = Learning Barrier
H = Physical Limitation Transfer
I = Transfer to Other Acute Care Hospital
PN = See Care Plan Progress Notes for Further Explanation

OUTCOMES

Nursing Diagnosis							Evaluation Date and Initial		
						TARGET	Admit/Start	D/C	Reason

13. Disturbed Body Image, Actual or Potential
14. Grieving, Actual or Anticipatory (cont'd)
15. Low Self-Esteem, Actual or Potential

Interventions:
- Body Image Enhancement
- Self-Esteem Enhancement
- Coping Enhancement
- Emotional Support
- Family Support
- Grief Work Facilitation

Psychosocial Adjustment: Life Change

Indicators:
- Sets realistic goals
- Reports feeling useful
- Verbalizes optimism about present and future
- Uses effective coping strategies
- Reports feeling socially engaged

| Never Demonstrated 1 | Rarely Demonstrated 2 | Sometimes Demonstrated 3 | Often Demonstrated 4 | Consistently Demonstrated 5 |

Self-Esteem

Indicators:
- Verbalizations of self-acceptance
- Acceptance of self limitations
- Maintenance of eye contact
- Open communication
- Maintenance of grooming and/or hygiene
- Feelings about self-worth

| Never Positive 1 | Rarely Positive 2 | Sometimes Positive 3 | Often Positive 4 | Consistently Positive 5 |

16. Ineffective Airway Clearance, Actual or Potential

Interventions:
- Airway management
- Aspiration precautions
- Positioning

Respiratory Status: Airway Patency

Indicators:
- Ease of breathing
- Respiratory rate
- Respiratory rhythm
- Moves sputum out of airway
- Moves blockage out of airway

| Severely Compromised 1 | Substantially Compromised 2 | Moderately Compromised 3 | Mildly Compromised 4 | Not Compromised 5 |

Indicators:
- Anxiety related to breathing
- Fear
- Choking
- Adventitious breath sounds

| Severe 1 | Substantial 2 | Moderate 3 | Mild 4 | None 5 |

INIT.	SIGNATURE	DISCL.	INIT.	SIGNATURE	DISCL.	INIT.	SIGNATURE	DISCL.	INIT.

(Copyright Mercy Hospital, Iowa City, IA. Courtesy of Kimberly M. Pattee at Mercy Hospital, 500 East Market Street, Iowa City, IA 52245.)

PART III

NOC and NIC Linked to Clinical Conditions
Asthma

Asthma is a common, chronic disorder of the airways that is complex and characterized by variable recurring symptoms (National Heart, Lung, and Blood Institute [NHLBI], 2007). Inflammation causes the membranes that line the airways to swell (mucosal edema), the smooth muscle that encircles the bronchioles to contract (bronchospasm), and mucus production to increase, forming bronchial plugs (Smeltzer, Bare, Hinkle, & Cheever, 2008). The inflammatory changes lead to airway narrowing resulting in symptoms of wheezing, breathlessness, chest tightness, dyspnea, and coughing that can range from mild to severe.

PREVALENCE, MORTALITY, AND COST

It is estimated that approximately 38.4 million Americans have been diagnosed with asthma during their lifetime. It is a leading cause of chronic illness among children. In 2008, 8.7 million school-aged children were reported to have asthma and 3.2 million had an asthma attack within the previous year (American Lung Association, 2010). The prevalence of asthma increased markedly between 1980 and 2000 but has risen less rapidly since 2000 (Martinez, 2008). It is estimated that the number of people with asthma will grow by more than 100 million by 2025 (American Academy of Allergy Asthma & Immunology, 2010). Asthma accounts for more than 4000 deaths each year and is a contributing factor in approximately 7000 other deaths each year. Death rates are higher among females and among African Americans (Asthma and Allergy Foundation of America, n.d.). In addition to asthma's negative effects on health, there is an economic toll associated with asthma. The estimated annual economic cost of asthma for 2010 is $20.7 billion with indirect costs such as lost productivity accounting for $5.1 billion. The largest direct medical expenditures are prescription drugs, amounting to $5 billion annually (American Lung Association, 2010).

RISK FACTORS

Chronic exposure to airway irritants and allergens is the predisposing factor both for developing asthma and for causing exacerbations. Identification and avoidance of substances and environmental factors that precipitate exacerbations are major steps in asthma control. Common precipitating factors include allergens, respiratory tract infections, hyperventilation with exercise, weather changes, and exposure to respiratory irritants such as tobacco smoke and chemicals.

COURSE OF THE DISEASE

Asthma can progress from mild intermittent attacks to severe persistent attacks with continual symptoms (Smeltzer, Bare, Hinkle, & Cheever, 2008). If the patient has mild intermittent asthma, symptoms occur less than two times a week and the patient is asymptomatic between attacks. If asthma occurs more frequently and has some impact on activity level, primarily when exacerbations occur, it may be diagnosed as mild persistent or moderate persistent asthma. Severe persistent asthma is characterized by continual symptoms, frequent exacerbations, and limitations in physical activity. An asthma exacerbation may begin with progressive symptoms over a few days or may occur abruptly. If the exacerbation is allowed to progress, tachycardia, diaphoresis, hypoxemia, and central cyanosis may occur.

Chronic inflammation can cause fibrotic changes in the airway that further decrease airway diameter and may lead to irreversible limitation of airflow eventually resulting in death if a severe asthmatic episode occurs. Status asthmaticus—severe persistent asthma that does not respond to conventional treatment—is another cause of death. Several risk factors are associated with death from asthma, including the following:

- History of sudden, severe exacerbations or prior intubations and admissions to intensive care units
- Two or more hospitalizations within the past year and/or three or more emergency department visits
- Excessive use of short-acting beta-adrenergic inhalers
- Recent withdrawal from use of systemic corticosteroids
- Comorbidities of cardiovascular disease, chronic obstructive pulmonary disease (COPD), or psychiatric disease
- Low socioeconomic status and urban residence (Smeltzer, Bare, Hinkle, & Cheever, 2008)

Federal guidelines for the diagnosis and management of asthma recommend four components essential for its effective management. These are (1) measures of assessment and monitoring to diagnose the severity of asthma and to achieve control, (2) education, (3) control of environmental factors and comorbid conditions, and (4) pharmacological therapy (NHLBI, 2007).

Major aspects of care include the removal of excessive secretions by employment of mucus-thinning agents and postural drainage techniques (which helps prevent respiratory tract infections) and the use of antimicrobial drugs as indicated. Pharmacological therapy includes long-acting medications to control persistent asthma and quick-relief medications to treat exacerbations. Control of persistent asthma is achieved with the use of antiinflammatory drugs, particularly corticosteroids, and long-acting bronchodilators. Exacerbations are treated with short-acting bronchodilators, such as beta-2 agonists and anticholinergics, and oxygen as needed. Because it is the patient's responsibility to manage the disease, patient education about the disease and its prevention and treatment is an essential aspect of care. The patient should be instructed in the proper use of a peak flow monitor to assess airflow during expiration as well as the actions to take if peak airflow decreases.

USE OF NOC AND NIC FOR PATIENTS WITH ASTHMA

Nursing has a major role in patient education, especially assisting the patient to identify and avoid risk factors and teaching the patient strategies to manage the disease. The patient should learn how to monitor and control the environment to avoid secondary smoke, allergens, and chemical irritants. If the patient smokes, he or she will need education to understand the negative effects of smoking and the beneficial effects of smoking cessation; it may also be necessary to help the patient find the optimal programs or methods for smoking cessation. Using medications correctly and monitoring medication responses are also part of patient education. If the disease becomes persistent, the patient will need to learn methods of clearing the respiratory tract to increase air exchange and prevent infection. The outcomes in the following generic care plan are suggested for helping the patient control his or her asthma and manage mild to moderate exacerbations. Exacerbations are best managed by an educated patient who can initiate early treatment (NHLBI, 2007). Should hypoxemia occur, short-term oxygen therapy may be required. If an exacerbation is severe or the patient develops status asthmaticus, the patient may require care in an intensive care unit and may need assisted ventilation. A plan for acute care will need to be followed in those cases.

REFERENCES

American Academy of Allergy Asthma and Immunology. (2010). *Asthma statistics.* <http://www.aaaai.org/media/statistics/asthma-statistics.asp> Accessed 25.03.10.

American Lung Association. (2010). *Trends in asthma morbidity and mortality.* Washington, DC: Author.

Asthma and Allergy Foundation of America. (n.d.). *Asthma facts and figures.* <http://www.aafa.org/display.cfm?id=8&sub=42> Accessed 29.03.10.

Martinez, F. D. (2008). Trends in asthma prevalence, admission rates, and asthma deaths. *Respiratory Care, 53*(5), 561–567.

National Heart, Lung, and Blood Institute (NHLBI). (2007). *Expert panel report 3: Guidelines for the diagnosis and management of asthma.* Bethesda, MD: Author.

Smeltzer, S. C., Bare, B. G., Hinkle, J. L., & Cheever, K. H. (2008). *Brunner and Suddarth's textbook of medical-surgical nursing* (11th ed., pp. 709–718). Philadelphia: Lippincott Williams & Wilkins.

PART III - A

NOC-NIC LINKAGES FOR ASTHMA		
Outcome	**Major Interventions**	**Suggested Interventions**

Asthma Self-Management
Definition:
Personal actions to prevent or reverse inflammatory condition resulting in bronchial constriction of the airways
	Asthma
	  Management
		Medication
		  Management
		Mutual Goal Setting
			Respiratory
			  Monitoring
			Risk Identification

Infection Severity
Definition:
Severity of infection and associated symptoms
	Infection Control
	Infection Protection
		Chest Physiotherapy
		Cough Enhancement
		Fever Treatment
			Fluid Management
			Medication Adminis-
			  tration: Inhalation
			Medication
			  Administration: Oral

Knowledge: Asthma Management
Definition:
Extent of understanding conveyed about asthma, its treatment, and the prevention of complications
	Teaching: Disease
	  Process
	Teaching:
	  Prescribed
	  Medication
	Teaching: Procedure/
	  Treatment
		Health Education
		Learning Facilitation
			Learning Readiness
			  Enhancement
			Teaching: Prescribed
			  Activity/Exercise

Medication Response
Definition:
Therapeutic and adverse effects of prescribed medication
	Surveillance
	Teaching:
	  Prescribed
	  Medication
		Medication Administra-
		  tion: Inhalation
		Medication Administra-
		  tion: Oral
			Medication
			  Reconciliation

Respiratory Status: Airway Patency
Definition:
Open, clear tracheobron-chial passages for air exchange
	Airway
	  Management
	Asthma
	  Management
		Airway Suctioning
		Anxiety Reduction
		Aspiration Precautions
			Cough Enhancement
			Respiratory
			  Monitoring

Respiratory Status: Ventilation
Definition:
Movement of air in and out of the lungs
	Airway
	  Management
	Asthma
	  Management
		Airway Suctioning
		Aspiration Precautions
		Chest Physiotherapy
			Cough Enhancement
			Positioning
			Respiratory
			  Monitoring

Risk Control
Definition:
Personal actions to prevent, eliminate, or reduce modifiable health threats
	Risk Identification	Environmental
		  Management
		Health Education
		Immunization/Vaccination
		  Management
			Infection Control
			Surveillance

Smoking Cessation Behavior
Definition:
Personal actions to eliminate tobacco use
	Smoking Cessation
	  Assistance
		Health Education
		Risk Identification
			Teaching: Disease
			  Process

Chronic Obstructive Pulmonary Disease (COPD)

Chronic obstructive pulmonary disease (COPD) includes chronic bronchitis and emphysema, conditions that obstruct airflow from the lungs; both of these conditions are irreversible. Chronic bronchitis is characterized by inflammation, excess mucous production, and smooth muscle constriction; the end result is a narrowed bronchial lumen and mucous plugs that obstruct airflow. In emphysema chronically overdistended alveoli lead to destruction of the alveolar walls and impaired gas exchange at the alveolar level. There are two main types of emphysema, but both can result in hypoxemia, hypercapnia, and the use of accessory muscles in breathing as the work of breathing becomes more difficult. Centrilobular emphysema can lead to right-sided heart failure with the resulting symptoms of heart failure, including peripheral edema.

PREVALENCE, MORTALITY, AND COST

COPD is a leading cause of death and disability. It is the fourth leading cause of death in the United States and is projected to be the third leading cause of death for both males and females by the year 2020 (COPD International, 2004). It is the only major disease with an increasing death rate. It is estimated that 16 million Americans have been diagnosed and another 14 million may be in the early stages of the disease and are undiagnosed (COPD International, 2004). In 2000 COPD was responsible for 119,000 deaths, 726,000 hospitalizations, and 1.5 million visits to emergency departments (COPD International, 2004; Schoenstadt, 2009). Because it is a chronic, progressive disease it often results in lost time from work and eventual disability. The total estimated cost for COPD in the United States in 2002 was $32.1 billion, consisting of $18 billion in direct costs and $14.1 billion in indirect costs (COPD International, 2004).

RISK FACTORS

Smoking is considered the most common cause of COPD, accounting for more than 80% of those diagnosed with COPD and 90% of COPD-related deaths (COPD International, 2008). Environmental factors such as chemicals, dust, and fumes as well as second-hand smoke can contribute to COPD. Other risk factors include allergies and asthma, periodontal disease, and frequent respiratory tract infections. These risk factors can be exacerbating factors if the disease is present. Genetic abnormalities have more recently been identified as risk factors (COPD International, 2004; Smeltzer, Bare, Hinkle, & Cheever, 2008).

COURSE OF THE DISEASE

The primary presenting symptoms are usually cough, excessive sputum production, and dyspnea on exertion. Wheezing and chest tightness are common, early symptoms of emphysema (Mayo Clinic Staff, 2009; Smeltzer, Bare, Hinkle, & Cheever, 2008). As the work of breathing increases, energy depletion and weight loss secondary to difficulty eating may occur. The patient may be unable to participate in even mild exercise, and eventually unable to work as the disease progresses. Based on diagnostic findings and symptoms, the disease is staged as mild, moderate, or severe. Complications can include respiratory tract infections, hypertension, heart problems, and depression (Mayo Clinic Staff, 2009).

Treatment includes risk reduction techniques; medication administration, especially bronchodilators and corticosteroids, and antibiotics if inflammation is present; oxygen therapy; pulmonary rehabilitation; and surgery (Smeltzer et al., 2008). Pulmonary rehabilitation includes educational, psychosocial, and behavioral components as well as physiological aspects. Surgery can include volume reduction surgery and lung transplantation if criteria are met. Nursing has a major role assisting the patient reduce risks, manage symptoms, prevent complications, and cope with the effects of the disease. Nurses are active participants in pulmonary rehabilitation programs, and in some cases the program may be carried out primarily at home once the patient is taught pulmonary exercises. Nurses play a major role in assisting the patient maintain physical conditioning with breathing and general exercises as tolerated, adequate nutrition, self-care activities, and coping strategies to deal with the anger and depression that can accompany disease progression. Family members will also need education and support to cope with the changes in the patient's functional and emotional status and with the caregiver's role as the patient's condition deteriorates.

USE OF NOC AND NIC FOR PATIENTS WITH COPD

Because COPD is progressive, outcomes and interventions will change as the disease progresses and symptoms change. In addition to the outcomes suggested in the generic care plan, the following outcomes might also be considered: *Aspiration Prevention; Comfort Status: Physical; Comfort Status: Psychospiritual; Comfort Status: Sociocultural; Compliance Behavior: Prescribed Diet; Compliance Behavior: Prescribed Medication; Family Normalization; Fatigue; Personal Well-Being; Quality of Life; Symptom Control; Symptom Severity; Suffering Severity; Treatment Behavior: Illness or Injury;* and *Weight Management.* Caregiver outcomes, although not included in the generic care plan, are important if the patient is receiving care at home. Additional NICs that might be considered are *Aspiration Precautions, Chest Physiotherapy, Cough Enhancement, Medication Administration,* and *Ventilation Assistance.* The care plan includes outcomes and interventions used in the early stages of the disease and does not address complications and end of life care.

REFERENCES

COPD International. (2004). *COPD statistical information.* <http://www.copd-international.com/library/statistics.htm> Accessed 29.03.10.

COPD International. (2008). *COPD.* <http://www.copd-international.com/COPD.htm COPD> Accessed 29.03.10.

Mayo Clinic Staff. (2009). *COPD.* <http://www.mayoclinic.com/health/copd/ds00916> Accessed 29.03.10.

Schoenstadt, A. (2009). *COPD statistics.* <http://Copd.emedtv.com/copd/copd-statistics.html> Accessed 29.03.10.

Smeltzer, S. C., Bare, B. G., Hinkle, J. L., & Cheever, K. H. (2008). *Brunner and Suddarth's textbook of medical-surgical nursing* (11th ed., pp. 686–701). Philadelphia: Lippincott Williams & Wilkins.

NOC-NIC LINKAGES FOR CHRONIC OBSTRUCTIVE PULMONARY DISEASE (COPD)		
Outcome	**Major Interventions**	**Suggested Interventions**
Activity Tolerance Definition: Physiological response to energy-consuming movements with daily activities	Activity Therapy Respiratory Monitoring	Exercise Promotion Exercise Therapy: Ambulation Oxygen Therapy Pain Management	Smoking Cessation Assistance Teaching: Prescribed Activity/Exercise
Adaptation to Physical Disability Definition: Adaptive response to a significant functional challenge due to a physical disability	Anticipatory Guidance Coping Enhancement	Counseling Emotional Support Grief Work Facilitation	Support Group Support System Enhancement
Comfort Status Definition: Overall physical, psychospiritual, sociocultural, and environmental ease and safety of an individual	Environmental Management: Comfort Pain Management	Airway Management Anxiety Reduction Energy Management Emotional Support	Positioning Relaxation Therapy Spiritual Support

NOC-NIC LINKAGES FOR CHRONIC OBSTRUCTIVE PULMONARY DISEASE (COPD)		
Outcome	**Major Interventions**	**Suggested Interventions**
Compliance Behavior Definition: Personal actions to promote wellness, recovery, and rehabilitation recommended by a health professional	Self-Efficacy Enhancement Self-Responsibility Facilitation	Behavior Modification Culture Brokerage Health System Guidance Nutritional Counseling Self-Modification Assistance Teaching: Disease Process	Teaching: Prescribed Activity/Exercise Teaching: Prescribed Medication Teaching: Procedure/ Treatment Teaching: Psychomotor Skill
Coping Definition: Personal actions to manage stressors that tax an individual's resources	Coping Enhancement	Anger Control Assistance Anticipatory Guidance Anxiety Reduction	Relaxation Therapy Self-Modification Assistance
Depression Level Definition: Severity of melancholic mood and loss of interest in life events	Mood Management	Counseling Emotional Support Grief Work Facilitation Hope Inspiration Medication Administration	Medication Management Music Therapy Spiritual Support Support System Enhancement
Energy Conservation Definition: Personal actions to manage energy for initiating and sustaining activity	Energy Management	Environmental Management Sleep Enhancement	Teaching: Prescribed Activity/Exercise
Immunization Behavior Definition: Personal actions to obtain immunization to prevent a communicable disease	Immunization/ Vaccination Management	Cough Enhancement Fluid Management Health Education	Medication Administration Risk Identification Teaching: Disease Process
Infection Severity Definition: Severity of infection and associated symptoms	Infection Control Infection Protection	Chest Physiotherapy	Fever Treatment
Knowledge: Disease Process Definition: Extent of understanding conveyed about a specific disease process and prevention of complications	Teaching: Disease Process	Learning Facilitation	Learning Readiness Enhancement
Knowledge: Energy Conservation Definition: Extent of understanding conveyed about energy conservation techniques	Teaching: Prescribed Activity/Exercise	Energy Management Learning Facilitation	Learning Readiness Enhancement Sleep Enhancement

PART III - C

Continued

NOC-NIC LINKAGES FOR CHRONIC OBSTRUCTIVE PULMONARY DISEASE (COPD)		
Outcome	**Major Interventions**	**Suggested Interventions**
Knowledge: Medication Definition: Extent of understanding conveyed about the safe use of medication	Teaching: Prescribed Medication	Learning Facilitation Learning Readiness Enhancement Teaching: Procedure/ Treatment
Knowledge: Treatment Procedure Definition: Extent of understanding conveyed about a procedure required as part of a treatment regimen	Teaching: Procedure/ Treatment	Chest Physiotherapy Learning Facilitation Learning Readiness Enhancement
Knowledge: Treatment Regimen Definition: Extent of understanding conveyed about a specific treatment regimen		
Nutritional Status Definition: Extent to which nutrients are available to meet metabolic needs	Nutritional Counseling	Enteral Tube Feeding Nutrition Management Nutrition Therapy Nutritional Monitoring Teaching: Prescribed Diet Weight Gain Assistance Weight Management
Respiratory Status: Gas Exchange Definition: Alveolar exchange of carbon dioxide and oxygen to maintain arterial blood gas concentrations	Oxygen Therapy Phlebotomy: Arterial Blood Sample	Bedside Laboratory Testing Chest Physiotherapy Cough Enhancement
Respiratory Status: Ventilation Definition: Movement of air in and out of the lungs	Airway Management Ventilation Assistance	Airway Suctioning Aspiration Precautions Chest Physiotherapy Cough Enhancement Positioning Respiratory Monitoring
Self-Care Status Definition: Ability to perform personal care activities and instrumental activities of daily living (IADLs)	Self-Care Assistance	Self-Care Assistance: Bathing/Hygiene Self-Care Assistance: Dressing/Grooming Self-Care Assistance: Feeding Self-Care Assistance: IADL Self-Care Assistance: Toileting Self-Care Assistance: Transfer

NOC-NIC LINKAGES FOR CHRONIC OBSTRUCTIVE PULMONARY DISEASE (COPD)			
Outcome	**Major Interventions**	**Suggested Interventions**	
Self-Care: Non-Parenteral Medication Definition: Ability to administer oral and topical medications to meet therapeutic goals independently with or without assistive device	Teaching: Prescribed Medication	Medication Administration: Inhalation Medication Administration: Oral Medication Management	Medication Reconciliation Teaching: Procedure/Treatment
Smoking Cessation Behavior Definition: Personal actions to eliminate tobacco use	Smoking Cessation Assistance	Health Education Risk Identification	Teaching: Disease Process

PART III - C

Colon and Rectal Cancer

Colorectal cancer is any cancer that originates in the colon or the rectum. Most of these cancers start as a polyp, which is an abnormal growth of tissue that begins in the intestinal lining and grows into the center of the colon or rectum. Over time the polyp can become cancerous, growing through some or all of the layers of the intestine or rectum. Staging of the cancer depends to a great degree on how deep the cancer has spread into these layers. In the majority of cases, colorectal cancers develop slowly over many years and early identification and removal of polyps is the focus of treatment (American Cancer Society, 2010).

PREVALENCE, MORTALITY, AND COST

In 2009 the American Cancer Society estimated that there were 106,100 new cases of colon cancer, 40,870 new cases of rectal cancer, and 49,920 deaths from colorectal cancer. The likelihood of an individual developing colorectal cancer is 1 in 19 (American Cancer Society, 2010). According to data from 2002 to 2006 the median age at diagnosis for cancer of the colon and rectum was 71 years (National Cancer Institute, 2009). It is considered the third most common cancer in men and women in the United States, excluding skin cancers. Over the last 15 years the death rate from this type of cancer has been decreasing. Because of the current emphasis on colorectal screening at age 50, polyps can be found and removed before they become cancerous (American Cancer Society, 2010). As a result of the usual age of onset of colorectal cancer, Medicare and Medicaid are the primary payers of cancer care. The cost of colon cancer is usually lower than the cost of rectal cancer. In a recent study of patients age 66 and older diagnosed with colon cancer, data were collected between 1997 and 2000 from the Michigan Tumor Registry. The mean total colon cancer cost for the

first year per Medicare patient was $29,196. Patients with more comorbid conditions had higher costs than patients with fewer comorbidities (Luo, Bradley, Dahman, & Gardiner, 2009).

RISK FACTORS

Risk factors for developing colon cancer have been identified through research. Age is an important risk factor, as the chance of developing the disease increases with age. Nine of 10 people diagnosed with colorectal cancer are older than 50. Another risk factor is a personal history of polyps or colorectal cancer. Individuals who have a history of colorectal cancer are more likely to have new cancers develop in other areas of the colon or rectum. The risk is increased if the person was diagnosed with the first colorectal cancer at a young age (before the usual age of 50). Patients with conditions such as inflammatory bowel disease, ulcerative colitis, and Crohn's disease have an increased risk of developing this cancer and should have more frequent screening. A family history of colorectal cancer also increases the risk of developing colon cancer (i.e., parents, brothers, sisters, or children). This risk is increased if the relative developed the disease at an early age. In addition, African Americans and Jews of Eastern European descent (Ashkenazi Jews) have a higher colorectal cancer risk (American Cancer Society, 2010).

Personal behaviors can also impact a person's risk for developing colorectal cancer. Lifestyle choices such as diet, weight, and exercise are some of the strongest predictors of colon cancer when compared with risk factors for other cancers. Diets high in red meats (such as beef, lamb, and liver) and processed meats (such as hot dogs, bologna, and lunch meat) can increase the risk of colorectal cancer. Frying, broiling, or grilling foods at high temperatures can create chemicals that are associated with an increased risk of cancer. In contrast, diets high in vegetables and fruits have been associated with lower risk. Exercising and maintaining a healthy weight can help reduce a person's risk. Individuals who are very overweight have an increased risk for developing and dying from colorectal cancer. Higher risk is also associated with smoking, heavy use of alcohol, and type 2 diabetes (American Cancer Society, 2010).

COURSE OF THE DISEASE

Colorectal cancer can develop anywhere in the lower gastrointestinal tract. Symptoms of the disease vary by location of the cancer. Patients with lesions in the ascending colon tend to experience dull abdominal pain and black, tarry stools. Patients with lesions of the descending colon experience abdominal cramping, narrowing of the diameter of the stool, constipation, abdominal distention, bloating, and bright red blood in the stool. Lesions in the rectal area cause symptoms of rectal pain and straining to pass stool, blood in the stool, feelings of incomplete evacuation, and episodes of diarrhea alternating with constipation. Pain is a late sign of cancer of the colon. Malignant colorectal tumors develop from benign adenomas in the mucosal and submucosal layers of the walls of the intestine. These are commonly called polyps and can be removed and examined to determine the tissue type. Adenocarcinoma accounts for nearly 95% of cases. The incidence of this cancer varies by location in the colon: ascending colon (22%), transverse colon (11%), descending colon (6%), sigmoid colon (33%), and rectal area (27%). If not treated, the cancer can spread to other organs by way of the mesentery lymph nodes or the portal vein leading to the liver (Timby & Smith, 2007).

Colonoscopy can be the first treatment option for very early staged cancer where the polyp is removed using a flexible scope. This is the same procedure used to detect polyps in at-risk individuals. Early stage cancers that are only on the surface of the colon lining can be removed along with a small amount of nearby tissue. For a polypectomy, the cancer is excised across the base of the polyp's stalk, the area that looks like the stem of a mushroom. Treatment of more advanced colorectal cancer focuses on surgery, radiation therapy, chemotherapy, and other targeted treatments. Two or more treatment options may be recommended depending on the stage of the cancer. For early stages of colon cancer, surgery is often the best option as a segment of the colon can be removed and the intestine can be reconnected. This is called a colectomy or segmental resection of the colon. Sometimes a short-term colostomy is performed to allow the colon to rest. For rectal cancers surgery is usually the main treatment, with procedures focusing on lower anterior resections, proctectomy with coloanal anastomosis, or abdominal-perineal resection. Radiation may be used when the cancer has attached to an internal organ or the lining of the abdomen. Radiation is used to destroy cancer cells still present after surgery but is seldom used to treat cancer that has spread to other organs. Radiation is also used to treat metastatic colon cancer in patients with rectal cancer.

Chemotherapy is sometimes used before surgery to decrease the size of the tumor; it also can be used after surgery to improve the survival rate or increase time of survival for patients with some stages of colorectal cancer (American Cancer Society, 2010). 5-Fluorouracil (5FU) and leucovorin have been used for more than 40 years as the main chemotherapy drugs for persons with later stage colon cancer (Vega-Stromberg, 2005). This combination has demonstrated a survival rate of 35% at 5 years (Abbruzzese, 2004). New drugs such as capecitabine, irinotecan, and oxaliplatin are showing increased survival rates (Vega-Stromberg, 2005). A final treatment option is the use of targeted therapies that attack parts of the cell. These drugs affect only the cancer cells and thus provide fewer side effects than chemotherapy. Monoclonal antibodies have been developed and approved for use along with chemotherapy (American Cancer Society, 2010). New target agents such as bevacizumab and cetuximab are also showing positive benefits in patients with colon cancer (Vega-Stromberg, 2005).

USE OF NOC AND NIC FOR PATIENTS WITH COLON AND RECTAL CANCER

Two linkage examples of NOC and NIC are provided for this clinical condition. The first focuses on providing outcomes and interventions for patients at high risk for colorectal cancer who require early or more frequent screening than the general population. The second set of linkages is for the patient who has a confirmed diagnosis of colorectal cancer. These outcomes and interventions cover a wide range of interventions provided to patients based on

PART III - C

their medical treatments. Although not all patients will require monitoring of all the identified outcomes, they may be helpful for selecting outcomes to fit the patient's situation. Clinical assessment and reasoning by the nurse will be essential to providing quality care. Many of the outcomes are the same both for high-risk patients and for colorectal cancer diagnosed patients, with differences noted in the interventions.

REFERENCES

Abbruzzese, J. (2004). An annual review of gastrointestinal cancers. *Oncology News International, 13*(3), Suppl. 1.

American Cancer Society. (2010). *Overview of colon and rectal cancer.* <http://www.cancer.org/docroot/CRI/CRI_2_1x.asp?dt=10> Accessed 31.03.10.

Luo, Z., Bradley, C. J., Dahman, B. A., & Gardiner, J. C. (2009). Colon cancer treatment costs for Medicare and dually eligible beneficiaries. *Health Care Financing Review, 31*(1), 35–51.

National Cancer Institute. (2009). *Surveillance, epidemiology and end results: Cancer.* <http://seer.cancer.gov/statfacts/html/colorect.html> Accessed 31.03.10.

Timby, B. K., & Smith, N. E. (2007). *Introductory medical-surgical nursing* (9th ed.). Philadelphia: Lippincott Williams & Wilkins.

Vega-Stromberg, T. (2005). Advances in colon cancer chemotherapy: Nursing implications. *Home Healthcare Nurse, 23*(3), 155–166.

NOC-NIC LINKAGES FOR COLORECTAL CANCER, RISK FOR		
Outcome	**Major Interventions**	**Suggested Interventions**
Acceptance: Health Status Definition: Reconciliation to significant change in health circumstances	Coping Enhancement Self-Esteem Enhancement	Active Listening Anticipatory Guidance Counseling Emotional Support Grief Work Facilitation Hope Inspiration Mood Management Presence	Self-Awareness Enhancement Spiritual Support Support Group Support System Enhancement Truth Telling Values Clarification
Anxiety Level Definition: Severity of manifested apprehension, tension, or uneasiness arising from an unidentifiable source	Anxiety Reduction Calming Technique	Active Listening Anger Control Assistance Coping Enhancement Crisis Intervention Decision-Making Support Dementia Management Dementia Management: Bathing	Distraction Medication Administration Music Therapy Relaxation Therapy Security Enhancement Vital Signs Monitoring
Bowel Elimination Definition: Formation and evacuation of stool	Bowel Management Bowel Training Constipation/Impaction Management	Anxiety Reduction Bowel Irrigation Exercise Therapy: Ambulation Flatulence Reduction Fluid Management Medication Administration Medication Administration: Oral	Medication Administration: Rectal Medication Management Nausea Management Nutrition Management Nutritional Counseling Pain Management Vomiting Management

PART III - C

NOC-NIC LINKAGES FOR COLORECTAL CANCER, RISK FOR

Outcome	Major Interventions	Suggested Interventions	
Compliance Behavior Definition: Personal actions to promote wellness, recovery, and rehabilitation recommended by a health professional	Mutual Goal Setting Patient Contracting	Behavior Modification Case Management Coping Enhancement Counseling Culture Brokerage Decision-Making Support Health System Guidance Learning Readiness Enhancement Self-Modification Assistance Self-Responsibility Facilitation	Support Group Teaching: Disease Process Teaching: Individual Teaching: Prescribed Activity/Exercise Teaching: Prescribed Diet Teaching: Prescribed Medication Teaching: Procedure/ Treatment Values Clarification
Health Promoting Behavior Definition: Personal actions to sustain or increase wellness	Health Education Self-Modification Assistance	Coping Enhancement Exercise Promotion Health Screening Nutritional Counseling Risk Identification Self-Awareness Enhancement Smoking Cessation Assistance	Substance Use Prevention Support Group Support System Enhancement Weight Management
Knowledge: Cancer Threat Reduction Definition: Extent of understanding conveyed about causes, prevention, and early detection of cancer	Health Screening Risk Identification	Breast Examination Genetic Counseling Nutritional Counseling Oral Health Maintenance Skin Surveillance	Smoking Cessation Assistance Teaching: Disease Process Teaching: Safe Sex
Knowledge: Disease Process Definition: Extent of understanding conveyed about a specific disease process and prevention of complications	Teaching: Disease Process	Allergy Management Asthma Management Discharge Planning Health System Guidance Risk Identification	Teaching: Group Teaching: Individual Teaching: Procedure/ Treatment
Knowledge: Health Behavior Definition: Extent of understanding conveyed about the promotion and protection of health	Health Education Teaching: Individual	Active Listening Anxiety Reduction Learning Facilitation Learning Readiness Enhancement Teaching: Prescribed Activity/Exercise	Teaching: Prescribed Diet Teaching: Prescribed Medication Teaching: Procedure/ Treatment

Continued

PART III - C

NOC-NIC LINKAGES FOR COLORECTAL CANCER, RISK FOR		
Outcome	**Major Interventions**	**Suggested Interventions**
Knowledge: Treatment Regimen Definition: Extent of understanding conveyed about a specific treatment regimen	Teaching: Disease Process Teaching: Procedure/ Treatment	Allergy Management Asthma Management Health System Guidance Medication Management Nutritional Counseling	Teaching: Group Teaching: Prescribed Activity/Exercise Teaching: Prescribed Diet Teaching: Prescribed Medication
Knowledge: Weight Management Definition: Extent of understanding conveyed about the promotion and mainte-nance of optimal body weight and fat percent-age congruent with height, frame, gender, and age	Nutritional Counseling Weight Management	Behavior Modification Exercise Promotion Health System Guidance Medication Management	Teaching: Group Weight Gain Assistance Weight Reduction Assistance
Participation in Health Care Decisions Definition: Personal involvement in selecting and evaluating health care options to achieve desired outcome	Decision-Making Support Self-Responsibility Facilitation	Assertiveness Training Behavior Modification Coping Enhancement Discharge Planning Health Literacy Enhancement	Health System Guidance Mutual Goal Setting Self-Efficacy Enhancement
Post-Procedure Recovery Definition: Extent to which an individ-ual returns to baseline function following a procedure(s) requiring anesthesia or sedation	Vital Signs Monitoring	Analgesic Administration Bowel Management Fluid Management Infection Protection	Nausea Management Nutritional Monitoring Positioning Respiratory Monitoring
Risk Control Definition: Personal actions to prevent, eliminate, or reduce modifiable health threats	Risk Identification	Behavior Modification Breast Examination Environmental Management: Safety Health Education Health Screening	Immunization/Vaccination Management Infection Control Self-Efficacy Enhancement
Risk Detection Definition: Personal actions to identify personal health threats	Health Screening Risk Identification Risk Identification: Childbearing Family	Environmental Management: Safety Environmental Management: Violence Prevention Genetic Counseling	Immunization/Vaccination Management Smoking Cessation Assistance Substance Use Prevention

NOC-NIC LINKAGES FOR COLORECTAL CANCER		
Outcome	**Major Interventions**	**Suggested Interventions**
Acceptance: Health Status Definition: Reconciliation to significant change in health circumstances	Coping Enhancement Self-Esteem Enhancement	Active Listening Anticipatory Guidance Counseling Emotional Support Grief Work Facilitation Hope Inspiration Mood Management Presence	Self-Awareness Enhancement Spiritual Support Support Group Support System Enhancement Truth Telling Values Clarification
Anxiety Level Definition: Severity of manifested apprehension, tension, or uneasiness arising from an unidentifiable source	Anxiety Reduction Calming Technique	Active Listening Anger Control Assistance Coping Enhancement Crisis Intervention Decision-Making Support Dementia Management Dementia Management: Bathing	Distraction Medication Administration Music Therapy Relaxation Therapy Security Enhancement Vital Signs Monitoring
Bowel Continence Definition: Control of passage of stool from the bowel	Bowel Management Diarrhea Management	Bowel Incontinence Care Bowel Incontinence Care: Encopresis Fluid Management Medication Management	Medication Prescribing Nutrition Management Self-Care Assistance: Toileting
Bowel Elimination Definition: Formation and evacuation of stool	Bowel Management Bowel Training Constipation/ Impaction Management	Anxiety Reduction Bowel Irrigation Exercise Therapy: Ambulation Flatulence Reduction Fluid Management Medication Administration Medication Administration: Oral	Medication Administration: Rectal Medication Management Nausea Management Nutrition Management Nutritional Counseling Pain Management Vomiting Management
Compliance Behavior Definition: Personal actions to promote wellness, recovery, and rehabilitation recommended by a health professional	Mutual Goal Setting Patient Contracting	Behavior Modification Case Management Coping Enhancement Counseling Culture Brokerage Decision-Making Support Discharge Planning Health System Guidance Learning Readiness Enhancement Self-Modification Assistance Self-Responsibility Facilitation Support Group	Teaching: Disease Process Teaching: Individual Teaching: Prescribed Activity/Exercise Teaching: Prescribed Diet Teaching: Prescribed Medication Teaching: Procedure/Treatment Teaching: Psychomotor Skill Values Clarification

PART III - C

Continued

PART III - C

NOC-NIC LINKAGES FOR COLORECTAL CANCER

Outcome	Major Interventions	Suggested Interventions	
Compliance Behavior: Prescribed Diet Definition: Personal actions to follow food and fluid intake recommended by a health professional for a specific health condition	Nutritional Counseling Teaching: Prescribed Diet	Behavior Modification Culture Brokerage Health System Guidance Learning Readiness Enhancement Nutritional Monitoring	Self-Efficacy Enhancement Self-Responsibility Facilitation Support System Enhancement
Compliance Behavior: Prescribed Medication Definition: Personal actions to administer medication safely to meet therapeutic goals as recommended by a health professional	Teaching: Prescribed Medication	Learning Readiness Enhancement Medication Administration Medication Administration: Intramuscular (IM) Medication Administration: Intravenous (IV) Medication Administration: Skin	Medication Administration: Subcutaneous Medication Management Self-Efficacy Enhancement Self-Responsibility Facilitation Teaching: Psychomotor Skill
Coping Definition: Personal actions to manage stressors that tax an individual's resources	Anxiety Reduction Coping Enhancement	Anticipatory Guidance Behavior Modification Genetic Counseling Grief Work Facilitation Guilt Work Facilitation Meditation Facilitation Preparatory Sensory Information	Recreation Therapy Relaxation Therapy Reminiscence Therapy Self-Awareness Enhancement Spiritual Support Support Group
Depression Level Definition: Severity of melancholic mood and loss of interest in life events	Hope Inspiration Mood Management	Animal-Assisted Therapy Anxiety Reduction Dying Care Emotional Support Grief Work Facilitation Medication Management	Music Therapy Reminiscence Therapy Sleep Enhancement Spiritual Support Support System Enhancement
Depression Self-Control Definition: Personal actions to minimize melancholy and maintain interest in life events	Mood Management Resiliency Promotion Self-Modification Assistance	Animal-Assisted Therapy Art Therapy Behavior Modification Coping Enhancement Emotional Support Energy Management Exercise Promotion Grief Work Facilitation Guilt Work Facilitation Hope Inspiration Music Therapy	Mutual Goal Setting Patient Contracting Presence Recreation Therapy Self-Awareness Enhancement Socialization Enhancement Therapeutic Play Therapy Group

NOC-NIC LINKAGES FOR COLORECTAL CANCER		
Outcome	**Major Interventions**	**Suggested Interventions**
Discomfort Level Definition: Severity of observed or reported mental or physical discomfort	Medication Management Pain Management	Analgesic Administration Anxiety Reduction Bathing Biofeedback Bowel Management Calming Technique Coping Enhancement Cutaneous Stimulation Distraction Emotional Support Energy Management Environmental Management: Comfort Flatulence Reduction Guided Imagery Heat/Cold Application Humor Hypnosis Massage Medication Administration Medication Administration: Intramuscular (IM)　　　Medication Administration: Intravenous (IV) Medication Administration: Oral Medication Prescribing Meditation Facilitation Music Therapy Nausea Management Positioning Presence Relaxation Therapy Sedation Management Sleep Enhancement Splinting Therapeutic Touch Transcutaneous Electrical Nerve Stimulation (TENS) Vomiting Management
Endurance Definition: Capacity to sustain activity	Energy Management	Electrolyte Monitoring Exercise Promotion Exercise Promotion: Strength Training Medication Management　　　Nutrition Management Sleep Enhancement Teaching: Prescribed Activity/Exercise
Fatigue Level Definition: Severity of observed or reported prolonged generalized fatigue	Energy Management Fall Prevention	Anxiety Reduction Environmental Management Laboratory Data Interpretation Medication Management Mood Management Nutritional Monitoring　　　Pain Management Self-Care Assistance Self-Care Assistance: IADL Sleep Enhancement Surveillance
Health Promoting Behavior Definition: Personal actions to sustain or increase wellness	Health Education Self-Modification Assistance	Coping Enhancement Exercise Promotion Health Screening Nutritional Counseling Risk Identification Self-Awareness Enhancement Smoking Cessation Assistance　　　Substance Use Prevention Support Group Support System Enhancement Weight Management

PART III - C

Continued

NOC-NIC LINKAGES FOR COLORECTAL CANCER

Outcome	Major Interventions	Suggested Interventions	
Health Seeking Behavior Definition: Personal actions to promote optimal wellness, recovery, and rehabilitation	Health Education Values Clarification	Bibliotherapy Culture Brokerage Health System Guidance Learning Facilitation Learning Readiness Enhancement Mutual Goal Setting Patient Contracting Self-Efficacy Enhancement Self-Modification Assistance Self-Responsibility Facilitation	Smoking Cessation Assistance Support Group Teaching: Disease Process Teaching: Prescribed Activity/Exercise Teaching: Prescribed Diet Teaching: Prescribed Medication Teaching: Procedure/ Treatment Weight Management
Hope Definition: Optimism that is personally satisfying and life-supporting	Hope Inspiration Spiritual Support	Anxiety Reduction Coping Enhancement Decision-Making Support Dying Care	Emotional Support Grief Work Facilitation Presence Touch
Knowledge: Cancer Management Definition: Extent of understanding conveyed about cause, type, progress, symptoms, and treatment of cancer	Teaching: Disease Process Teaching: Procedure/ Treatment	Anticipatory Guidance Chemotherapy Management Coping Enhancement Energy Management Financial Resource Assistance Health System Guidance Medication Management	Nausea Management Pain Management Radiation Therapy Management Risk Identification Support Group Teaching: Individual Vomiting Management
Knowledge: Diet Definition: Extent of understanding conveyed about recommended diet	Nutritional Counseling Teaching: Prescribed Diet	Chemotherapy Management Eating Disorders Management	Self-Modification Assistance Teaching: Group Weight Management
Knowledge: Disease Process Definition: Extent of understanding conveyed about a specific disease process and prevention of complications	Teaching: Disease Process	Allergy Management Discharge Planning Health System Guidance Risk Identification Teaching: Group	Teaching: Individual Teaching: Procedure/ Treatment

NOC-NIC LINKAGES FOR COLORECTAL CANCER		
Outcome	**Major Interventions**	**Suggested Interventions**
Knowledge: Energy Conservation Definition: Extent of understanding conveyed about energy conservation techniques	Energy Management Teaching: Prescribed Activity/Exercise	Body Mechanics Promotion Cardiac Care: Rehabilitative — Health Education Teaching: Group
Knowledge: Health Behavior Definition: Extent of understanding conveyed about the promotion and protection of health	Health Education Teaching: Individual	Active Listening Anxiety Reduction Learning Facilitation Learning Readiness Enhancement Teaching: Prescribed Activity/Exercise — Teaching: Prescribed Diet Teaching: Prescribed Medication Teaching: Procedure/ Treatment
Knowledge: Medication Definition: Extent of understanding conveyed about the safe use of medication	Teaching: Prescribed Medication	Allergy Management Analgesic Administration — Immunization/ Vaccination Management
Knowledge: Ostomy Care Definition: Extent of understanding conveyed about maintenance of an ostomy for elimination	Ostomy Care	Medication Administration: Skin Skin Care: Topical Treatments Skin Surveillance — Teaching: Prescribed Diet Teaching: Procedure/ Treatment Teaching: Psychomotor Skill
Knowledge: Pain Management Definition: Extent of understanding conveyed about causes, symptoms, and treatment of pain	Pain Management Teaching: Prescribed Medication	Analgesic Administration Aromatherapy Health System Guidance Heat/Cold Application Medication Reconciliation Patient-Controlled Analgesia (PCA) Assistance Progressive Muscle Relaxation — Relaxation Therapy Self-Hypnosis Facilitation Support Group Teaching: Prescribed Activity/Exercise Transcutaneous Electrical Nerve Stimulation (TENS)
Knowledge: Treatment Regimen Definition: Extent of understanding conveyed about a specific treatment regimen	Teaching: Disease Process Teaching: Procedure/ Treatment	Allergy Management Health System Guidance Medication Management Nutritional Counseling Teaching: Group Teaching: Prescribed Activity/Exercise — Teaching: Prescribed Diet Teaching: Prescribed Medication

PART III - C

Continued

NOC-NIC LINKAGES FOR COLORECTAL CANCER

Outcome	Major Interventions	Suggested Interventions	
Knowledge: Weight Management Definition: Extent of understanding conveyed about the promotion and mainte-nance of optimal body weight and fat percentage congruent with height, frame, gender, and age	Nutritional Counseling Weight Management	Behavior Modification Exercise Promotion Health System Guidance Medication Management	Teaching: Group Weight Gain Assistance Weight Reduction Assistance
Nausea & Vomiting Severity Definition: Severity of nausea, retching, and vomiting symptoms	Nausea Management Surveillance Vomiting Management	Diet Staging Electrolyte Monitoring Enteral Tube Feeding Environmental Management Fluid/Electrolyte Management Fluid Management	Fluid Monitoring Medication Administration Nutrition Management Nutritional Monitoring Total Parenteral Nutrition (TPN) Administration
Ostomy Self-Care Definition: Personal actions to maintain ostomy for elimination	Diarrhea Management Ostomy Care	Bowel Management Fluid Management Fluid Resuscitation Nutrition Management Skin Care: Topical Treatments	Skin Surveillance Teaching: Individual Teaching: Psychomotor Skill Wound Care
Pain Level Definition: Severity of observed or reported pain	Pain Management Surveillance	Active Listening Analgesic Administration Anxiety Reduction Emotional Support	Massage Positioning Therapeutic Touch Vital Signs Monitoring
Participation in Health Care Decisions Definition: Personal involvement in selecting and evaluat-ing health care options to achieve desired outcome	Coping Enhancement Decision-Making Support Self-Responsibility Facilitation	Assertiveness Training Behavior Modification Discharge Planning Health Literacy Enhancement	Health System Guidance Mutual Goal Setting Self-Efficacy Enhancement
Personal Health Status Definition: Overall physical, psychological, social, and spiritual function-ing of an adult 18 years or older	Medication Management Surveillance Vital Signs Monitoring	Circulatory Precautions Energy Management Exercise Promotion Infection Protection Neurological Monitoring Nutrition Management Nutritional Monitoring Pain Management	Peripheral Sensation Management Respiratory Monitoring Self-Care Assistance Self-Care Assistance: IADL Weight Management

NOC-NIC LINKAGES FOR COLORECTAL CANCER		
Outcome	**Major Interventions**	**Suggested Interventions**
Personal Resiliency Definition: Positive adaptation and function of an individual following significant adversity or crisis	Resiliency Promotion	Conflict Mediation Coping Enhancement Decision-Making Support Emotional Support Mood Management Risk Identification Role Enhancement Self-Efficacy Enhancement	Self-Esteem Enhancement Self-Responsibility Facilitation Substance Use Prevention Support Group
Post-Procedure Recovery Definition: Extent to which an individual returns to baseline function following a procedure(s) requiring anesthesia or sedation	Energy Management Pain Management	Analgesic Administration Bed Rest Care Bowel Management Cough Enhancement Fluid Management Incision Site Care Infection Protection Nausea Management Nutritional Monitoring Oral Health Maintenance Positioning Respiratory Monitoring	Self-Care Assistance Self-Efficacy Enhancement Sleep Enhancement Temperature Regulation Urinary Elimination Management Vital Signs Monitoring Wound Care: Closed Drainage
Risk Control Definition: Personal actions to prevent, eliminate, or reduce modifiable health threats	Risk Identification	Behavior Modification Breast Examination Environmental Management: Safety Health Education Health Screening	Immunization/Vaccination Management Infection Control Self-Efficacy Enhancement
Risk Detection Definition: Personal actions to identify personal health threats	Health Screening Risk Identification Risk Identification: Childbearing Family	Environmental Management: Safety Environmental Management: Violence Prevention Genetic Counseling	Immunization/Vaccination Management Smoking Cessation Assistance Substance Use Prevention
Tissue Integrity: Skin & Mucous Membranes Definition: Structural intactness and normal physiological function of skin and mucous membranes	Wound Care	Bleeding Precautions Chemotherapy Management Fluid Management Infection Control Infection Protection Medication Management	Nutrition Management Oral Health Maintenance Oral Health Promotion Radiation Therapy Management

Continued

PART III - C

NOC-NIC LINKAGES FOR COLORECTAL CANCER		
Outcome	**Major Interventions**	**Suggested Interventions**
Treatment Behavior: Illness or Injury Definition: Personal actions to palliate or eliminate pathology	Self-Responsibility Facilitation Teaching: Disease Process Teaching: Procedure/ Treatment	Behavior Modification Coping Enhancement Discharge Planning Emotional Support Family Involvement Promotion Learning Facilitation Mutual Goal Setting Support Group Support System Enhancement	Teaching: Individual Teaching: Prescribed Activity/Exercise Teaching: Prescribed Diet Teaching: Prescribed Medication Teaching: Psychomotor Skill Telephone Consultation Telephone Follow-Up

Depression is the oldest and most common psychiatric condition (Stuart, 2009) and debilitating illness associated with significant distress, changes of social and occupational functioning, and increased risks for mortality and other medical disorders (Blazer, 2005). Major or significant depression is more than the occasional sadness, unhappiness, or "blues" that most people experience and recover from quickly. Depression contributes to extraordinary personal and family suffering and societal burdens, such as increased use of social and medical services and rising health care costs for its treatment and lost productivity attributable to absenteeism from work (Nathan & Gorman, 2007).

PREVALENCE, MORTALITY, AND COST

The rates of depression have risen remarkably over the past 10 years in the United States with increases in prevalence being noted in most sociodemographic subgroups of the population (Compton, Conway, Stinson, & Grant, 2006). In the United States major depression affects approximately 6.7% of the population (14.8 million individuals) each year. It is the leading cause of disability for young adults between the ages of 15 and 44 (National Institute of Mental Health, 2008). An estimated 121 million individuals of all ages and both genders are affected by depression each year. According to the *Diagnostic and Statistical Manual of Mental Disorders (DSM-IV-TR)* of the American Psychiatric Association (2000), the probability during one's lifetime of developing a major depressive disorder (MDD) is 5% to 12% for males and 10% to 25% for females. Up to 15% of those with MDD die by suicide (Berger, 2010).

The World Health Organization (WHO) lists depression as the number one psychiatric cause of disability in the world and it is projected to be the second highest cause of disability among all diseases

by 2020. It is the fourth leading contributor to the global burden of disease as measured by disability-adjusted life-years—the sum of years of potential life lost attributable to premature mortality and the years of productive life lost attributable to disability. Currently, depression is the second highest cause of disability-adjusted life-years in males and females between the ages of 15 and 44, and by the year 2020 it is expected to reach this rank for the overall population (WHO, 2010).

Major depression is an illness that can affect anyone, making no distinction regarding race, ethnicity, or income level. The yearly incidence of a major depressive episode is 1.59%, with 1.89% of women and 1.10% of men likely to experience this disease each year (Sadock & Sadock, 2007). Depression is nearly a universal observation, independent of country or culture. Depression is more common in older persons than it is in the general population. There are various reported prevalence rates from 25% to 50%, although it is unclear if this high prevalence rate is exclusively from major depressive disorder. Depression in the elderly is correlated with low socioeconomic status, loss of a spouse, concurrent physical illness, and social isolation. Some studies have shown that depression in the elderly is underdiagnosed and undertreated by general practitioners (Sadock & Sadock, 2007). This situation could be caused by an acceptance of depressive symptoms in the elderly, and the tendency of the elderly to present with more somatic complaints (Sadock & Sadock, 2007).

SYMPTOMS OF THE DISEASE

Culture can shape the experience and communication of symptoms of depression. Misdiagnosis can be avoided by being alert to ethnic and cultural specificity in the presenting complaints. In many cultures, depression may be experienced largely in somatic terms, rather than sadness or guilt. Some examples are complaints of "nerves" and headaches in Latino and Mediterranean cultures, and complaints of weakness, tiredness, or "imbalance" in Chinese and Asian cultures (American Psychiatric Association [APA], 2000, p. 353).

The term "depression" is most often used to identify a complex pattern of negative feelings, cognitions, and behaviors. Beck and Alford (2009) define depression in terms of the following attributes: (1) a specific alteration in mood: sadness, loneliness, apathy; (2) a negative self-concept associated with self-reproach and self-blame; (3) regressive and self-punitive wishes: desires to escape, hide, or die; (4) vegetative changes: anorexia, insomnia, loss of libido; and (5) change in activity level: retardation or agitation. Because there is no current NANDA-I diagnosis for depression, the *DSM-IV-TR* diagnostic manual for psychiatric disorders can be used to identify the major symptoms. Major depression is defined as depressed mood or loss of interest or pleasure in activities. These symptoms need to occur for at least a 2-week period before a diagnosis of major depression can be assigned. The essential feature of a major depressive episode "is a period of at least 2 weeks during which there is either depressed mood or the loss of interest or pleasure in nearly all activities" (APA, 2000, p. 349). In addition to this feature, the individual must also experience at least four additional symptoms, including changes in weight or appetite, sleep, and psychomotor activity; decreased energy; feelings of worthlessness or guilt; difficulty thinking, concentrating, or making decisions; or recurrent thoughts of death or suicidal ideation, plans, or attempts (APA, 2000, p. 349).

USE OF NOC AND NIC FOR PATIENTS WITH DEPRESSION

Fortunately, major depression is a treatable disorder with a good prognosis. Numerous nursing interventions are appropriate for the treatment of major depression, allowing the patient and clinician to choose a treatment approach that is most fitting to the patient's situation. In addition to the outcomes suggested in the generic care plan, the following outcomes might also be considered: *Body Image, Loneliness Severity, Mood Equilibrium, Postpartum Maternal Health Behavior, Psychosocial Adjustment: Life Change,* and *Social Support.* Outcomes and interventions may vary with the severity and chronicity of the symptoms.

REFERENCES

American Psychiatric Association. (2000). *Diagnostic and statistical manual of mental disorders (DSM-IV-TR).* Washington, DC: Author.

Beck, A. T., & Alford, B. A. (2009). *Depression: Causes and treatment* (2nd ed.). Philadelphia: University of Pennsylvania Press.

Berger, P. K. (2010). *Major depression.* <www.nlm.nih.gov/medlineplus/ency/article/000945.htm> Accessed 04.04.10.

Blazer, D. G. (2005). *The age of melancholy: Major depression and its social origins.* New York: Routledge.

Compton, W. M., Conway, K. P., Stinson, F. S., & Grant, B. F. (2006). Changes in the prevalence of major depression and comorbid substance use disorders in the United States between 1991-1992 and 2001-2002. *American Journal of Psychiatry, 163*(12), 2141.

Nathan, P. E., & Gorman, J. M. (Eds.), (2007). *A guide to treatments that work* (3rd ed.). New York: Oxford University Press.

National Institute of Mental Health. (2008). *The numbers count: Mental disorders in America.* <http://www.nimh.nih.gov/health/publications/the-numbers-count-mental-disorders-in-America> Accessed 08.03.10.

Sadock, B. J., & Sadock, V. A. (2007). *Kaplan & Sadock's synopsis of psychiatry: Behavioral sciences/clinical psychiatry* (10th ed.). Philadelphia: Lippincott, Williams, & Wilkins.

Stuart, G. W. (2009). *Principles and practice of psychiatric nursing* (9th ed.). St. Louis: Mosby Elsevier.

World Health Organization. (2010). *Depression: What is depression?* <http://www.who.int/mental_health/management/depression/definition/en/index.html> Accessed 03.08.10.

NOC-NIC LINKAGES FOR DEPRESSION		
Outcome	**Major Interventions**	**Suggested Interventions**
Appetite Definition: Desire to eat when ill or receiving treatment	Nutrition Management	Diet Staging Fluid Monitoring	Nutritional Monitoring
Cognition Definition: Ability to execute complex mental processes	Cognitive Restructuring	Cognitive Stimulation Mood Management	
Coping Definition: Personal actions to manage stressors that tax an individual's resources	Coping Enhancement	Decision-Making Support Emotional Support Resiliency Promotion	Support System Enhancement Therapy Group
Depression Level Definition: Severity of melancholic mood and loss of interest in life events	Mood Management Coping Enhancement Self-Esteem Enhancement	Active Listening Counseling Emotional Support Forgiveness Facilitation	Guilt Work Facilitation Medication Administration Therapy Group
Depression Self-Control Definition: Personal actions to minimize melancholy and maintain interest in life events	Mood Management Resiliency Promotion Self-Modification Assistance	Animal-Assisted Therapy Art Therapy Behavior Modification Coping Enhancement Emotional Support Energy Management Exercise Promotion Grief Work Facilitation Grief Work Facilitation: Perinatal Death Guilt Work Facilitation	Journaling Hope Inspiration Music Therapy Presence Recreation Therapy Self-Awareness Enhancement Self-Esteem Enhancement Socialization Enhancement Therapeutic Play Therapy Group
Grief Resolution Definition: Adjustment to actual or impending loss	Grief Work Facilitation	Active Listening Coping Enhancement	Emotional Support Hope Inspiration
Hope Definition: Optimism that is personally satisfying and life-supporting	Hope Inspiration	Coping Enhancement Spiritual Growth	Support Group
Knowledge: Depression Management Definition: Extent of understanding conveyed about depression and interrelationships among causes, effects, and treatments	Teaching: Disease Process Teaching: Prescribed Medication	Learning Facilitation Health System Guidance Journaling Medication Management	Mood Management Substance Use Prevention Support Group

PART III - D

Continued

NOC-NIC LINKAGES FOR DEPRESSION

Outcome	Major Interventions	Suggested Interventions	
Knowledge: Medication Definition: Extent of understanding conveyed about the safe use of medication	Teaching: Prescribed Medication	Learning Facilitation	
Psychomotor Energy Definition: Personal drive and energy to maintain activities of daily living, nutrition, and personal safety	Mood Management	Counseling Grief Work Facilitation Guilt Work Facilitation Hope Inspiration Medication Management	Self-Esteem Enhancement Self-Responsibility Facilitation Therapy Group
Self-Care Status Definition: Ability to perform personal care activities and instrumental activities of daily living	Self-Care Assistance	Self-Care Assistance: Bathing/Hygiene Self-Care Assistance: Dressing/Grooming	
Self-Esteem Definition: Personal judgment of self-worth	Self-Awareness Enhancement Self-Esteem Enhancement	Art Therapy Body Image Enhancement Emotional Support	Journaling Music Therapy Spiritual Support
Sleep Definition: Natural periodic suspension of consciousness during which the body is restored	Sleep Enhancement	Massage Music Therapy	Relaxation Therapy
Social Involvement Definition: Social interactions with persons, groups, or organizations	Behavior Modification: Social Skills Socialization Enhancement	Recreation Therapy Role Enhancement Support System Enhancement	Therapeutic Play Visitation Facilitation
Suicide Self-Restraint Definition: Personal actions to refrain from gestures and attempts at killing self	Behavior Modification Suicide Prevention	Coping Enhancement Emotional Support Environmental Management: Safety Hope Inspiration Mood Management	Patient Contracting Support Group Support System Enhancement Surveillance

Diabetes Mellitus

Diabetes mellitus is a chronic metabolic disease characterized by high blood sugar (glucose) levels that result from defects in insulin secretion by the beta cells of the islets of Langerhans in the pancreas or from impaired insulin action, or both. Insulin controls the blood glucose levels by regulating the production and storage of glucose (Smeltzer, Bare, Hinkle, & Cheever, 2008). With the exception of pancreatic transplantation (with which there has been some success), currently diabetes is controlled, not cured.

PREVALENCE, MORTALITY, AND COST

Diabetes is the third leading cause of death in the United States following heart disease and cancer, and its prevalence has been increasing for several decades. In 2007 in the United States, 23.5 million people, or 10.7% of all people age 20 or older, had diabetes, including 12 million men and 11.5 million women. Of persons age 60 and older, 12.2 million (or 23.1% of those in this age group) have the disease (National Institute of Diabetes and Digestive and Kidney Diseases [NIDDK], 2008). Globally, the prevalence of diabetes is staggering. The prevalence is expected to continue to increase because of the aging of the population, the sedentary lifestyle of many persons, and the genetic characteristics of the disease.

Direct medical and indirect expenditures attributable to diabetes in 2007 were estimated at $174 billion. Direct medical expenditures alone totaled $116 billion and comprised $27 billion for diabetes care, $58 billion for chronic complications attributable to diabetes, and $31 billion for excess prevalence of general medical conditions (Dall et al., 2008).

RISK FACTORS

The exact cause of type 1 diabetes is not known, but genetics, viruses, and autoimmune problems seem to play a role. In type 1 diabetes the immune system has a tendency to generate antibodies and inflammatory cells that attack the beta cells of the pancreas (Mathur, 2008). This autoimmune disorder is believed, in part, to be genetically inherited. Currently, there is no known way to prevent type 1 diabetes and no effective screening test for people who do not have symptoms (Wexler, 2009).

There are a number of risk factors for type 2 diabetes, some of which can be controlled. Some of the factors that cannot be controlled include age older than 45 years, parents or siblings with diabetes, and ethnicity, with African Americans, Native Americans, Asians, and Hispanic Americans having a higher incidence of type 2 diabetes. There are a number of risk factors that can be controlled by the individual, including heart disease, high blood cholesterol level, obesity, sedentary lifestyle, and inadequate exercise. A recent study found that patients participating in an intensive program that promoted lifestyle changes to achieve a weight loss ≥7% of initial body weight and consistent, moderate intensity physical exercise had a 58% lower incidence of type 2 diabetes than those receiving instruction and a placebo medication. Of particular importance was the fact that these findings occurred in both genders and across all ethnic groups (Diabetes Prevention Program Research Group, 2002).

COURSE OF THE DISEASE

A certain amount of glucose normally circulates in the blood. The level of glucose in the blood of persons who do not have diabetes is controlled within a range of approximately 90 to 150 mg/dl by insulin, although the blood glucose level varies throughout the day depending mainly upon the amount of food ingested and the amount of exercise in which a person engages. The normal range of a fasting blood glucose level (no food or drink other than water for at least 8 hours) is less than 100 mg/dl.

In diabetes the blood glucose level is elevated and can be associated with increased fat breakdown, the production of ketone bodies, and metabolic acidosis (Smeltzer et al., 2008). There are several types of diabetes, including type 1, type 2, gestational, and elevated glucose levels associated with other conditions. The disease has been traditionally classified as type 1, insulin-dependent; or type 2, non–insulin-dependent, but classification is now known to be more complex with the presence of several mixed types of diabetes. The inability of cells to use insulin properly and efficiently leads to hyperglycemia, usually called type 2 diabetes; it affects mostly the cells of muscle and fat tissues and results in a condition known as insulin resistance (Saltiel & Olefsky, 1996). The absolute lack of insulin production by beta cells in the pancreas is the main disorder in type 1 diabetes.

There are many serious secondary effects of diabetes that occur over time. Diabetes can lead to blindness, kidney failure, and nerve damage attributable to injury to small blood vessels (microvascular disease); in addition, diabetes is an important contributor to accelerated hardening and narrowing of the arteries (atherosclerosis), leading to strokes (clots or hemorrhaging in vessels in the brain), coronary disease, and other large blood vessel diseases (macrovascular disease) (Perkins, Aiello, & Krolewski, 2009).

Treatment for diabetes includes injection of insulin or oral medications that stimulate insulin secretion by the pancreas, as well as adherence to a specific controlled diet and exercise regimen (NIDDK, 2008). Individuals with type 1 diabetes will need to receive insulin for their lifetime unless a surgical pancreatic transplant is successful. The goals for treatment of individuals with type 2 diabetes are to maintain beta cell function and to sustain normal blood glucose levels (Campbell, 2009).

USE OF NOC AND NIC FOR PATIENTS WITH DIABETES MELLITUS

Nurses have a substantial role in assisting individuals and their families with the management of diabetes to prevent secondary effects and maintain quality of life.

Smeltzer and colleagues (2008) identify the following five components of diabetes management: nutritional management, exercise, monitoring, pharmacological therapy, and education. The nurse has a primary role or shares a collaborative role with other health professionals in all of these areas. The following generic plan of care does not include the care of acute episodes for which the patient might be hospitalized or the care of the patient with life-altering complications. There are other outcomes that might be selected, for example: *Acceptance: Health Status; Compliance Behavior: Prescribed Diet; Compliance Behavior: Prescribed Medication; Coping; Family Normalization; Health Beliefs: Perceived Ability to Perform; Physical Fitness;* and *Weight Loss Behavior.* The outcome *Prenatal Health Behavior* should be considered for the pregnant woman with diabetes mellitus.

REFERENCES

Campbell, K. (2009). Type 2 diabetes: Where we are today: An overview of disease burden, current treatments, and treatment strategies. *Journal of the American Pharmacists Association,* 49(Suppl. 1), S3–S9.

Dall, T., Mann, S. E., Zhang, Y., Martin, J., Chen, Y., & Hogan, P. (2008). Economic costs of diabetes in the U.S. in 2007. *Diabetes Care, 31*(3), 596–615.

Diabetes Prevention Program Research Group. (2002). Reduction in the incidence of type 2 diabetes with lifestyle intervention or metformin. *New England Journal of Medicine, 346*(6), 393–403.

Mathur, R. (2008). *Diabetes mellitus.* <http://www.medicinenet.com/diabetes_mellitus/page2.htm> Accessed 27.03.10.

National Institute of Diabetes and Digestive and Kidney Diseases (NIDDK). (2008). *National diabetes statistics, 2007* (NIH Publication No. 08-3892). Bethesda, MD: National Diabetes Information Clearinghouse.

Perkins, B. A., Aiello, L. P., & Krolewski, A. S. (2009). Diabetes complications and the renin-angiotensin system. *New England Journal of Medicine, 361*(1), 83–85.

Saltiel, A. R., & Olefsky, J. M. (1996). Insulin resistance and type II diabetes. *Diabetes, 45*(12), 1661–1669.

Smeltzer, S. C., Bare, B. G., Hinkle, J. L., & Cheever, K. H. (2008). *Brunner and Suddarth's textbook of medical-surgical nursing* (11th ed., pp. 1376–1436). Philadelphia: Lippincott Williams & Wilkins.

Wexler, D. (2009). *Type 1 diabetes.* <http://www.nlm.nih.gov/medlineplus/ency/article/000305.htm> Accessed 06.04.10.

NOC-NIC LINKAGES FOR DIABETES MELLITUS			
Outcome	**Major Interventions**	**Suggested Interventions**	
Blood Glucose Level			
Definition: Extent to which glucose levels in plasma and urine are maintained in normal range	Bedside Laboratory Testing	Capillary Blood Sample Hyperglycemia Management Hypoglycemia Management	Laboratory Data Interpretation Teaching: Prescribed Medication Teaching: Psychomotor Skill
Compliance Behavior			
Definition: Personal actions to promote wellness, recovery, and rehabilitation recommended by a health professional	Self-Efficacy Enhancement Self-Responsibility Facilitation	Anticipatory Guidance Coping Enhancement Culture Brokerage Health System Guidance	Learning Readiness Enhancement Self-Modification Assistance
Diabetes Self-Management			
Definition: Personal actions to manage diabetes mellitus, its treatment, and prevent disease progression	Self-Efficacy Enhancement Self-Responsibility Facilitation	Exercise Promotion Hyperglycemia Management Hypoglycemia Management Infection Control Medication Administration: Subcutaneous	Medication Administration: Oral Medication Management Nutritional Management Self-Modification Assistance
Fluid Balance			
Definition: Water balance in the intracellular and extracellular compartments of the body	Fluid Management	Fluid/Electrolyte Management Fluid Monitoring	Surveillance Vital Signs Monitoring
Kidney Function			
Definition: Filtration of blood and elimination of metabolic waste products through the formation of urine	Laboratory Data Interpretation Surveillance	Acid-Base Management Bedside Laboratory Testing Dialysis Access Maintenance Electrolyte Monitoring Fluid Monitoring Hemodialysis Therapy	Peritoneal Dialysis Therapy Specimen Management Urinary Elimination Management Weight Management
Knowledge: Diabetes Management			
Definition: Extent of understanding conveyed about diabetes mellitus, its treatment, and the prevention of complications	Teaching: Disease Process Teaching: Prescribed Diet Teaching: Prescribed Medication	Nutritional Counseling Teaching: Prescribed Activity/Exercise Teaching: Foot Care	Teaching: Procedure/ Treatment Teaching: Psychomotor Skill

PART III - D

Continued

NOC-NIC LINKAGES FOR DIABETES MELLITUS		
Outcome	**Major Interventions**	**Suggested Interventions**
Medication Response Definition: Therapeutic and adverse effects of prescribed medication	Teaching: Prescribed Medication	Bedside Laboratory Testing Hypoglycemia Management	Medication Management Surveillance
Nutritional Status Definition: Extent to which nutrients are available to meet metabolic needs	Nutritional Counseling Nutritional Monitoring	Fluid Management Nutrition Management	Weight Reduction Assistance Weight Management

Heart Failure

Heart failure (HF) is defined as the impaired capacity of the right or left ventricle of the heart to fill with or eject blood to sustain body metabolism (Hunt et al., 2001). This means that the heart is working inefficiently and pumping too weakly. Depending on the side of the heart affected, this causes fluid accumulation in the lungs and/or other organs. Heart failure may also be referred to as congestive heart failure (CHF) (Smeltzer, Bare, Hinkle, & Cheever, 2008). The condition may be acute or chronic in nature and has been classified as systolic or diastolic heart failure, depending on the presenting symptoms.

PREVALENCE, MORTALITY, AND COST

Heart failure is more prevalent among African Americans, Hispanics, and American Indians than among whites but there is no difference in rates of diagnosis between men and women. Of the patients diagnosed with HF, 75% to 85% are older than 65 years (U.S. News & World Report, 2006). The American Heart Association estimates that 5.7 million Americans are living with heart failure, and 670,000 new cases are diagnosed each year. Approximately 25% to 35% of persons with HF die within 12 months following hospital admission and 80% of men and 70% of women younger than age 65 die within 8 years of being diagnosed (Lloyd-Jones et al., 2009). In industrialized countries, hospitalizations for HF have doubled since 1990 (Moser & Mann, 2002). In 2009 approximately 75% of the more than $37 billion annual expenditure for HF in the United States was due to hospitalizations (Lloyd-Jones et al., 2009). Both direct and indirect costs for the treatment of HF in the United States in 2010 are estimated to be over $39.2 billion. These data are based on heart failure as the primary diagnosis; therefore this value is probably underestimated (Lloyd-Jones et al., 2010).

RISK FACTORS

Causes of HF identified by the American Heart Association are coronary artery disease, past heart attack (myocardial infarction), hypertension, abnormal heart valves, heart muscle disease or inflammation, congenital heart disease, severe lung disease, diabetes, severe anemia, hyperthyroidism, and abnormal heart rhythms (Lloyd-Jones et al., 2009). HF also may occur after toxic exposure to alcohol or cocaine.

COURSE OF THE DISEASE

Signs and symptoms of HF are many, varied, and somewhat vague in nature and may result in patients seeking treatment long after the onset of symptoms. Common symptoms are shortness of breath (dyspnea) while exercising, climbing stairs, or after eating; a general state of exercise intolerance; fluid retention and edema, especially in the ankles, legs, and abdomen; weight gain; fatigue; weakness, because major organs have poor blood circulation; dizziness or confusion caused by inadequate blood flow to the brain; nausea, bloating, and loss of appetite; and rapid or irregular heartbeat and palpitations (Smeltzer, Bare, Hinkle, & Cheever, 2008). These signs and symptoms usually produce impaired function and quality of life. Persons with preexisting hypertension, coronary artery disease, and/or diabetes are at increased risk, making HF a prevalent disease of older persons (Lloyd-Jones et al., 2009). In 2001 the American Heart Association and the American College of Cardiology identified four specific stages of HF. Stage A is present when the patient has no diagnosis or symptoms of HF but has a high risk. Stage B is present when the patient is diagnosed as having an ejection fraction less than 40% but has no past symptoms. The ejection fraction is a measure of the amount of blood pumped out of the left ventricle, with a normal measurement being 55% or higher. Stage C heart failure occurs when the patient is diagnosed with HF and with past or current symptoms, including shortness of breath, fatigue, and reduced exercise tolerance. Stage D is diagnosed when the patient has advanced symptoms of HF after receiving optimal medical care (Diepenbrock, 2008).

Treatment focuses on significantly improving symptoms because in most cases damage to the heart is irreversible. In some patients the underlying cause can be treated, such as tachycardia. Prescribing appropriate medications, following a specific diet, and managing fluid intake can lessen the burden of the presenting symptoms. Many patients, however, continue to experience dyspnea on exertion and generalized fatigue that impacts both work and interpersonal relationships (Goodlin, 2009). In many cases treatments focus on lifestyle changes and medications but trans-catheter interventions, medical devices, and surgery may also be considered based on the patient's condition. These treatments often increase the patient's life expectancy and quality of life. Research has shown that comprehensive discharge planning improves HF self-management and reduces the number of hospital readmissions (Phillips et al., 2004). Nurses are major contributors to discharge planning for these patients (Raman, DeVine, & Lau, 2008), although evidence describing the contribution of nurses is limited (Coster & Norman, 2009). This lack of evidence regarding nursing's contribution to discharge planning for HF patients underscores the need for the use of standardized nursing nomenclatures in hospital electronic care planning and documentation systems.

USE OF NOC AND NIC FOR PATIENTS WITH HEART FAILURE

To assist with the development and use of standardized nursing languages in hospital electronic systems, and to provide some decision support for evidence-based nursing practices, the following linkages between Nursing Interventions Classification (NIC) interventions and Nursing Outcomes Classification (NOC) outcomes are provided. These reflect the complexity of care needed by patients with HF depending on the stage of their illness. Careful selection of outcomes should be made by nurses to maximize the care provided to patients with HF. As the disease progresses, care needs to be modified to address evolving problems encountered by patients with HF. Specific knowledge outcomes (for example, for diet medications and activity) may need to be applied if the patient is having particular difficulty incorporating knowledge about one of these areas to his or her management of HF.

REFERENCES

Coster, S., & Norman, I. (2009). Cochrane reviews of educational and self-management interventions to guide nursing practice: A review. *International Journal of Nursing Studies, 46*(4), 508–528.

Diepenbrock, N. H. (2008). *Quick reference to critical care* (3rd ed.). Philadelphia: Lippincott Williams & Wilkins.

Goodlin, S. J. (2009). Palliative care in congestive heart failure. *Journal of the American College of Cardiology, 54*(5), 386–396.

Hunt, S. A., Baker, D. W., Chin, M. H., Feldman, A. M., Francis, G. S., Ganiats, T. G., et al. (2001). ACC/AHA guidelines for the evaluation and management of chronic heart failure in the adult: Executive summary. *Circulation, 104*(24), 2996–3007.

Lloyd-Jones, D., Adams, R. J., Brown, T. M., Carnethon, M., Dai, S., De Simone, G., et al. (2010). Heart disease and stroke statistics 2010 update. A report from the American Heart Association. *Circulation, 121*(17), e46–e215.

Lloyd-Jones, D., Adams, R., Carnethon, M., De Simone, G., Ferguson, T. B., Flegal, K., et al. (2009). Heart disease and stroke statistics-2009 update: A report for the American Heart Association Statistics Committee and Stroke Statistics Subcommittee. *Circulation, 119*(3), e21–e181.

Moser, D. K., & Mann, D. L. (2002). Improving outcomes in heart failure: It's not unusual beyond usual care. *Circulation, 105*(24), 2810–2812.

Phillips, C. O., Wright, S. M., Kern, D. E., Singa, R. M., Shepperd, S., & Rubin, H. R. (2004). Comprehensive discharge planning with post discharge support for older patients with congestive heart failure. *The Journal of the American Medical Association, 291*(11), 1358–1367.

Raman, G., DeVine, D., & Lau, J. (2008). *Technology assessment, non-pharmacological interventions for post-discharge care in heart failure.* Rockville, MD: Agency for Healthcare Research and Quality.

Smeltzer, S. C., Bare, B. G., Hinkle, J. L., & Cheever, K. H. (2008). *Brunner and Suddarth's textbook of medical-surgical nursing* (11th ed., pp. 946–965). Philadelphia: Lippincott Williams & Wilkins.

U.S. New & World Report, 2006, p. 318.

Outcome	Major Interventions	Suggested Interventions	

NOC-NIC LINKAGES FOR HEART FAILURE

Acceptance: Health Status

Definition:
Reconciliation to significant change in health circumstances

Coping Enhancement
Self-Esteem Enhancement

Active Listening
Anticipatory Guidance
Counseling
Emotional Support
Grief Work Facilitation
Hope Inspiration
Mood Management
Presence

Self-Awareness Enhancement
Spiritual Support
Support Group
Support System Enhancement
Truth Telling
Values Clarification

Adaptation to Physical Disability

Definition:
Adaptive response to a significant functional challenge due to a physical disability

Behavior Modification
Coping Enhancement

Anger Control Assistance
Anticipatory Guidance
Anxiety Reduction
Behavior Management: Self-Harm
Body Image Enhancement
Counseling
Decision-Making Support

Emotional Support
Security Enhancement
Self-Care Assistance
Self-Care Assistance: IADL
Sleep Enhancement
Substance Use Prevention
Support Group

Cardiac Pump Effectiveness

Definition:
Adequacy of blood volume ejected from the left ventricle to support systemic perfusion pressure

Cardiac Care
Cardiac Care: Acute
Shock Management: Cardiac

Acid-Base Management
Acid-Base Monitoring
Airway Management
Cardiac Care: Rehabilitative
Cardiac Precautions
Code Management
Dysrhythmia Management
Electrolyte Management
Electrolyte Monitoring
Energy Management
Fluid/Electrolyte Management
Fluid Management
Fluid Monitoring
Hemodynamic Regulation
Intravenous (IV) Insertion
Intravenous (IV) Therapy

Invasive Hemodynamic Monitoring
Medication Administration
Medication Management
Pacemaker Management: Permanent
Pacemaker Management: Temporary
Phlebotomy: Arterial Blood Sample
Phlebotomy: Cannulated Vessel
Phlebotomy: Venous Blood Sample
Resuscitation
Resuscitation: Neonate
Vital Signs Monitoring

Cardiac Disease Self-Management

Definition:
Personal actions to manage heart disease, its treatment, and prevent disease progression

Teaching: Disease Process
Teaching: Prescribed Activity/Exercise
Teaching: Prescribed Diet
Teaching: Prescribed Medication

Cardiac Care: Rehabilitative
Cardiac Precautions
Energy Management
Exercise Promotion
Immunization/Vaccination Management
Medication Management
Nutrition Management

Self-Efficacy Enhancement
Self-Modification Assistance
Sexual Counseling
Smoking Cessation Assistance
Vital Signs Monitoring
Weight Management

Continued

PART III - H

NOC-NIC LINKAGES FOR HEART FAILURE		
Outcome	**Major Interventions**	**Suggested Interventions**
Circulation Status Definition: Unobstructed, unidi-rectional blood flow at an appropriate pressure through large vessels of the systemic and pul-monary circuits	Circulatory Care: Arterial Insufficiency Circulatory Care: Mechanical Assist Device Circulatory Care: Venous Insufficiency	Bedside Laboratory Testing Circulatory Precautions Fluid Monitoring Fluid Resuscitation Hemodynamic Regulation Hypervolemia Manage-ment Hypovolemia Manage-ment Intravenous (IV) Insertion Intravenous (IV) Therapy Invasive Hemodynamic Monitoring Laboratory Data Interpretation Lower Extremity Monitoring Medication Management Peripherally Inserted Central (PIC) Catheter Care Pneumatic Tourniquet Precautions Shock Management: Vasogenic Shock Prevention Surveillance Vital Signs Monitoring
Compliance Behavior Definition: Personal actions to promote wellness, recovery, and rehabilitation recommended by a health professional	Mutual Goal Setting Patient Contracting	Behavior Modification Case Management Coping Enhancement Counseling Culture Brokerage Decision-Making Support Discharge Planning Health System Guidance Learning Readiness Enhancement Self-Modification Assistance Self-Responsibility Facilitation Support Group Teaching: Disease Process Teaching: Individual Teaching: Prescribed Activity/Exercise Teaching: Prescribed Diet Teaching: Prescribed Medication Teaching: Procedure/Treatment Teaching: Psychomotor Skill Values Clarification
Compliance Behavior: Prescribed Diet Definition: Personal actions to follow food and fluid intake recom-mended by a health professional for a specific health condition	Nutritional Counseling Teaching: Prescribed Diet	Behavior Modification Culture Brokerage Health System Guidance Learning Readiness Enhancement Nutritional Monitoring Self-Efficacy Enhancement Self-Responsibility Facilitation Support System Enhancement
Compliance Behavior: Prescribed Medication Definition: Personal actions to administer medica-tion safely to meet therapeutic goals as recommended by a health professional	Teaching: Prescribed Medication	Learning Readiness Enhancement Medication Administration Medication Administra-tion: Intramuscular (IM) Medication Administra-tion: Intravenous (IV) Medication Administration: Skin Medication Administra-tion: Subcutaneous Medication Management Self-Efficacy Enhancement Self-Responsibility Facilitation Teaching: Psychomotor Skill

NOC-NIC LINKAGES FOR HEART FAILURE

Outcome	Major Interventions	Suggested Interventions	
Depression Level			
Definition: Severity of melancholic mood and loss of interest in life events	Hope Inspiration Mood Management	Animal-Assisted Therapy Anxiety Reduction Dying Care Emotional Support Grief Work Facilitation Medication Management	Music Therapy Reminiscence Therapy Sleep Enhancement Spiritual Support Support System Enhancement
Depression Self-Control			
Definition: Personal actions to minimize melancholy and maintain interest in life events	Mood Management Resiliency Promotion Self-Modification Assistance	Animal-Assisted Therapy Art Therapy Behavior Modification Coping Enhancement Emotional Support Energy Management Exercise Promotion Grief Work Facilitation Guilt Work Facilitation Hope Inspiration Music Therapy	Mutual Goal Setting Patient Contracting Presence Recreation Therapy Self-Awareness Enhancement Socialization Enhancement Therapeutic Play Therapy Group
Endurance			
Definition: Capacity to sustain activity	Energy Management	Electrolyte Monitoring Exercise Promotion Exercise Promotion: Strength Training Medication Management	Nutrition Management Sleep Enhancement Teaching: Prescribed Activity/Exercise
Fatigue Level			
Definition: Severity of observed or reported prolonged generalized fatigue	Energy Management Fall Prevention	Anxiety Reduction Environmental Management Laboratory Data Interpretation Medication Management Mood Management Nutritional Monitoring	Pain Management Self-Care Assistance Self-Care Assistance: IADL Sleep Enhancement Surveillance
Fluid Balance			
Definition: Water balance in the intracellular and extracellular compartments of the body	Fluid Management	Fluid/Electrolyte Management Fluid Monitoring	Vital Signs Monitoring Weight Management
Fluid Overload Severity			
Definition: Severity of excess fluids in the intracellular and extracellular compartments of the body	Fluid/Electrolyte Management Hypervolemia Management	Anxiety Reduction Cerebral Edema Management Electrolyte Management Electrolyte Monitoring Fluid Management Fluid Monitoring Medication Administration	Medication Management Neurological Monitoring Respiratory Monitoring Skin Surveillance Temperature Regulation Urinary Elimination Management Vital Signs Monitoring

Continued

PART III - H

NOC-NIC LINKAGES FOR HEART FAILURE		
Outcome	**Major Interventions**	**Suggested Interventions**
Health Promoting Behavior Definition: Personal actions to sustain or increase wellness	Health Education Self-Modification Assistance	Coping Enhancement Exercise Promotion Health Screening Nutritional Counseling Risk Identification Self-Awareness Enhancement	Smoking Cessation Assistance Substance Use Prevention Support Group Support System Enhancement Weight Management
Knowledge: Cardiac Disease Management Definition: Extent of understanding conveyed about heart disease, its treatment, and the prevention of complications	Cardiac Precautions Teaching: Disease Process	Anxiety Reduction Cardiac Care: Rehabilitative Culture Brokerage Energy Management Family Involvement Promotion Health System Guidance Nutritional Counseling Relaxation Therapy Resiliency Promotion Risk Identification Sexual Counseling	Smoking Cessation Assistance Support Group Teaching: Prescribed Activity/Exercise Teaching: Prescribed Diet Teaching: Prescribed Medication Teaching: Procedure/Treatment Weight Management Weight Reduction Assistance
Knowledge: Diet Definition: Extent of understanding conveyed about recommended diet	Nutritional Counseling Teaching: Prescribed Diet	Self-Modification Assistance	Teaching: Group Weight Management
Knowledge: Energy Conservation Definition: Extent of understanding conveyed about energy conservation techniques	Energy Management Teaching: Prescribed Activity/Exercise	Body Mechanics Promotion Cardiac Care: Rehabilitative	Health Education Teaching: Group
Knowledge: Medication Definition: Extent of understanding conveyed about the safe use of medication	Teaching: Prescribed Medication	Analgesic Administration	Immunization/Vaccination Management
Knowledge: Prescribed Activity Definition: Extent of understanding conveyed about prescribed activity and exercise	Teaching: Prescribed Activity/Exercise	Energy Management Exercise Promotion Exercise Therapy: Ambulation	Exercise Therapy: Muscle Control Teaching: Group

NOC-NIC LINKAGES FOR HEART FAILURE		
Outcome	**Major Interventions**	**Suggested Interventions**

Knowledge: Treatment Regimen

Definition:
Extent of understanding conveyed about a specific treatment regimen

Teaching: Disease Process Teaching: Procedure/Treatment	Health System Guidance Medication Management Nutritional Counseling Teaching: Group	Teaching: Prescribed Activity/Exercise Teaching: Prescribed Diet Teaching: Prescribed Medication

Knowledge: Weight Management

Definition:
Extent of understanding conveyed about the promotion and maintenance of optimal body weight and fat percentage congruent with height, frame, gender, and age

Nutritional Counseling Weight Management	Behavior Modification Exercise Promotion Health System Guidance Medication Management	Teaching: Group Weight Gain Assistance Weight Reduction Assistance

Pain Level

Definition:
Severity of observed or reported pain

Pain Management Surveillance	Active Listening Analgesic Administration Anxiety Reduction Emotional Support	Massage Positioning Therapeutic Touch Vital Signs Monitoring

Participation in Health Care Decisions

Definition:
Personal involvement in selecting and evaluating health care options to achieve desired outcome

Coping Enhancement Decision-Making Support Self-Responsibility Facilitation	Assertiveness Training Behavior Modification Discharge Planning Health Literacy Enhancement	Health System Guidance Mutual Goal Setting Self-Efficacy Enhancement

Personal Health Status

Definition:
Overall physical, psychological, social, and spiritual functioning of an adult 18 years or older

Medication Management Surveillance Vital Signs Monitoring	Circulatory Precautions Energy Management Exercise Promotion Infection Protection Neurological Monitoring Nutrition Management Nutritional Monitoring	Pain Management Peripheral Sensation Management Respiratory Monitoring Self-Care Assistance Self-Care Assistance: IADL Weight Management

Psychosocial Adjustment: Life Change

Definition:
Adaptive psychosocial response of an individual to a significant life change

Anticipatory Guidance Coping Enhancement	Decision-Making Support Emotional Support Mood Management Mutual Goal Setting Relocation Stress Reduction Reminiscence Therapy Role Enhancement Security Enhancement	Self-Esteem Enhancement Sleep Enhancement Socialization Enhancement Substance Use Prevention Support Group Support System Enhancement

PART III - H

Continued

NOC-NIC LINKAGES FOR HEART FAILURE		
Outcome	**Major Interventions**	**Suggested Interventions**
Respiratory Status Definition: Movement of air in and out of the lungs and exchange of carbon dioxide and oxygen at the alveolar level	Respiratory Monitoring Ventilation Assistance	Airway Management Anxiety Reduction Aspiration Precautions Chest Physiotherapy Cough Enhancement	Energy Management Mechanical Ventilation Management: Noninvasive Oxygen Therapy
Tissue Perfusion: Abdominal Organs Definition: Adequacy of blood flow through the small vessels of the abdominal viscera to maintain organ function	Circulatory Care: Arterial Insufficiency Circulatory Care: Venous Insufficiency	Acid-Base Management Acid-Base Management: Metabolic Acidosis Acid-Base Management: Metabolic Alkalosis Acid-Base Monitoring Bedside Laboratory Testing Bleeding Precautions Electrolyte Management Electrolyte Monitoring Emergency Care Fluid Management	Fluid Monitoring Hypovolemia Management Intravenous (IV) Insertion Intravenous (IV) Therapy Laboratory Data Interpretation Nausea Management Pain Management Shock Prevention Surveillance Vital Signs Monitoring
Tissue Perfusion: Cardiac Definition: Adequacy of blood flow through the coronary vasculature to maintain heart function	Circulatory Care: Arterial Insufficiency Shock Management: Cardiac	Anxiety Reduction Cardiac Care: Acute Circulatory Care: Venous Insufficiency Code Management Dysrhythmia Management Electrolyte Management Fluid Management Fluid Monitoring Invasive Hemodynamic Monitoring Medication Management	Nausea Management Oxygen Therapy Pacemaker Management: Temporary Pain Management Shock Management: Vasogenic Shock Management: Volume Surveillance Vital Signs Monitoring
Tissue Perfusion: Peripheral Definition: Adequacy of blood flow through the small vessels of the extremities to maintain tissue function	Circulatory Care: Venous Insufficiency Embolus Care: Peripheral Lower Extremity Monitoring	Cardiac Care: Acute Circulatory Care: Arterial Insufficiency Circulatory Care: Mechanical Assist Device Circulatory Precautions Fluid Management Fluid Monitoring Fluid Resuscitation Hemodynamic Regulation Hypovolemia Management Intravenous (IV) Insertion	Intravenous (IV) Therapy Pain Management Pneumatic Tourniquet Precautions Resuscitation Resuscitation: Neonate Shock Prevention Skin Care: Topical Treatments Skin Surveillance Surveillance Vital Signs Monitoring

NOC-NIC LINKAGES FOR HEART FAILURE		
Outcome	**Major Interventions**	**Suggested Interventions**
Treatment Behavior: Illness Or Injury Definition: Personal actions to palliate or eliminate pathology	Self-Responsibility Facilitation Teaching: Disease Process Teaching: Procedure/ Treatment	Behavior Modification Coping Enhancement Discharge Planning Emotional Support Family Involvement Promotion Learning Facilitation Mutual Goal Setting Support Group Support System Enhancement	Teaching: Individual Teaching: Prescribed Activity/Exercise Teaching: Prescribed Diet Teaching: Prescribed Medication Teaching: Psychomotor Skill Telephone Consultation Telephone Follow-Up
Vital Signs Definition: Extent to which temperature, pulse, respiration, and blood pressure are within normal range	Hemodynamic Regulation Vital Signs Monitoring	Acid-Base Management Anxiety Reduction Blood Products Administration Cardiac Care Dysrhythmia Management Electrolyte Management Emergency Care Fluid Management Fluid Monitoring Fluid Resuscitation Hypovolemia Management	Intravenous (IV) Therapy Medication Administration Medication Management Medication Prescribing Oxygen Therapy Resuscitation Shock Management Shock Prevention Surveillance

Hypertension

Blood pressure (BP) is a measure of the pressure of blood against the walls of the blood vessels. Blood pressure depends physiologically on the amount of blood the heart pumps and the amount of resistance to blood flow in the arteries (Mayo Clinic Staff, 2008; Smeltzer, Bare, Hinkle, & Cheever, 2008). High blood pressure (HBP) is defined in the following ways: having a systolic blood pressure (SBP) $\geq$140 mm Hg or a diastolic blood pressure (DBP) $\geq$90 mm Hg; taking an antihypertensive medication; having been informed at least twice by a health care professional that one has high blood pressure (Lloyd-Jones et al., 2010). In addition, the latest blood pressure guidelines for adults presented by the Joint National Committee on Prevention, Detection, Evaluation, and Treatment of High Blood Pressure (JNC, 2004) are as follows:

Blood Pressure

Classification	SBP (mm Hg)	DBP (mm Hg)
Normal	<120	<80
Prehypertension	120-139	80-89
Stage 1 hypertension	140-159	90-99
Stage 2 hypertension	$\geq$160	$\geq$100

The guidelines presented by the JNC (2004) state that prehypertension is not a disease category, but a label selected to identify persons at high risk for developing hypertension. The guidelines further note that individuals with prehypertension who also have diabetes or kidney disease should be considered for appropriate medication therapy, if lifestyle modifications are **not** successful in reducing their BP to 130/80 mm Hg or less. For persons with prehypertension and no other adverse health conditions, the goal is to adopt lifestyle changes that lower their BP measurements to within normal levels. All persons classified with either stage 1 hypertension or stage 2 hypertension should be treated and have a therapeutic goal of achieving a BP of <140/90 mm Hg (JNC, 2004).

There are two types of high blood pressure (HBP): primary (essential) hypertension and secondary hypertension (Timby & Smith, 2007). Essential hypertension is an elevated systemic arterial pressure for which there is no known cause, representing approximately 95% of cases (Timby & Smith, 2007). Secondary hypertension is defined as an elevated BP that is the result of or secondary to another disorder (Timby & Smith, 2007). Various conditions and medications that can lead to this type of hypertension include kidney abnormalities, tumors of the adrenal gland, certain congenital heart defects, birth control pills, cold remedies, over-the-counter pain relievers, and illegal drugs, such as cocaine and amphetamines (Mayo Clinic Staff, 2008). Two articles discuss "white-coat" hypertension, a reference to the HBP resulting from the anxiousness individuals experience while visiting health care professionals (i.e., "white coats") (Hajjar, Kotchen, & Kotchen, 2006; Timby & Smith, 2007). When the BP is measured after the individual leaves the facility, the reading falls into the range of normal.

PREVALENCE, MORTALITY, AND COST

Hypertension is a worldwide health challenge due to its high incidence and accompanying risks for comorbid diseases, namely, cardiovascular and kidney disease (Kearney, Whelton, Reynolds, Muntner, Whelton, & He, 2005). Ezzati and colleagues (2002) state that hypertension is the leading factor in mortality and ranked third for disability-adjusted life-years. Responding to the need for information on the prevalence of hypertension worldwide, Kearney and associates (2005) reviewed studies that reported data on the prevalence of hypertension in representative samples of world populations.

They concluded "the estimated total number of adults with hypertension in 2000 was 972 million, 333 million in economically developed countries and 639 million in economically developing countries" (Kearney et al., 2005, p. 217). Further, their work projected that the number of persons with hypertension will increase by 60% to a total of 1.56 billion by 2025.

According to Lloyd-Jones and colleagues (2010) one in three adults in the United States has HBP and the incidence continues to rise. They noted that from 1996 to 2006, the death rate due to HBP increased to 19.5% as compared to the rate of 17.5% projected by Xu and colleagues (2009). Using National Center for Health Statistics, Lloyd-Jones and colleagues (2010) stated that the number of deaths in this time period actually rose 48.1%. It is striking that there were obvious racial differences in the death rate resulting from HBP. The death rates were 15.6 per million for white males, 51.1 per million for black males, 14.3 per million for white females, and 37.7 per million for black females (Lloyd-Jones et al., 2010). The costs associated with hypertension are staggering as well. According to the JNC (2004), the estimated direct and indirect costs for hypertension are projected to be $76.6 billion for 2010.

RISK FACTORS

There are a number of risk factors identified for hypertension that fall within the categories of being in the individual's control as well as being outside of the individual's control. Numerous risk factors have been suggested, including age, gender, genetic disposition, family history of hypertension, race, lower education and socioeconomic status, obesity, certain chronic conditions, lack of physical activity, alcohol use, tobacco use, stress, sodium intake, potassium intake, and insufficient levels of vitamin D (Hajjar, Kotchen, & Kotchen, 2006; JNC, 2004; Kearney et al., 2005; Lloyd-Jones et al., 2010; Mayo Clinic Staff, 2008). Not only do these risks exist for hypertension but also there is a definite relationship between BP and the risk of cardiovascular disease (Kearney et al., 2005). As reported by the Joint National Committee on Prevention, Detection, Evaluation, and Treatment of High Blood Pressure (2004, p. 12), " . . . the higher the BP, the greater the chance of heart attack, HF [heart failure], stroke, and kidney disease."

COURSE OF THE DISEASE

It is generally understood that most persons with hypertension have no signs or symptoms. Thus it is referred to as the "silent killer" (Timby & Smith, 2007). Although Mayo Clinic Staff (2008) state that some individuals do experience dull headaches, dizzy spells, or more nosebleeds than normal in the early stages of hypertension, these symptoms do not usually occur until the hypertension is at advanced levels. As reported by Timby and Smith (2007), the most significant finding indicating hypertension is an elevated systolic or diastolic BP measurement. In addition, individuals may be overweight (JNC, 2004).

USE OF NOC AND NIC FOR PATIENTS WITH HYPERTENSION

Nursing care may vary depending on the type of the hypertension and the point at which the hypertension is diagnosed. Although there are established interventions for the nursing treatment of hypertension that will facilitate lowering of the patient's blood pressure without resorting to medication therapies, some pharmacological intervention may be necessary at various times in the course of the condition. The following plan of care focuses on the goal of controlling hypertension without the need for drug therapy. A number of the nursing interventions implemented focus on teaching nonpharmacological approaches as well as techniques for self-management. These interventions also serve to reinforce the importance of family and peer support in disease management.

REFERENCES

Ezzati, M., Lopez, A. D., Rodgers, A., Vander Hoorn, S., & Murray, C. J. (2002). Selected major risk factors and global and regional burden of disease. *Lancet, 360*(9343), 1347–1360.

Hajjar, I., Kotchen, J. M., Kotchen, T. A. (2006). Hypertension: Trends in prevalence, incidence, and control. *Annual Review of Public Health, 27*, 465–490.

Joint National Committee on Prevention, Detection, Evaluation, and Treatment of High Blood Pressure (JNC). (2004). *The seventh report of the Joint National Committee on Prevention, Detection, Evaluation, and Treatment of High Blood Pressure* (NIH Publication No. 04-5230). Bethesda, MD: National Heart, Lung, and Blood Institute.

Kearney, P. M., Whelton, B. S., Reynolds, K., Muntner, P., Whelton, P. K., & He, J. (2005). Global burden of hypertension: Analysis of worldwide data. *Lancet, 365*(9455), 217–223.

Lloyd-Jones, D., Adams, R. J., Brown, T. M., Carnethon, M., Dai, S., De Simone, G., et al. (2010). Heart disease and stroke statistics 2010 update. A report from the American Heart Association. *Circulation, 121*, e46–e215.

Mayo Clinic Staff. (2008). *High blood pressure (hypertension).* <http://www.mayoclinic.com/health/high-blood-pressure/DS00100/DSECTION=symptoms> Accessed 25.03.10.

Smeltzer, S. C., Bare, B. G., Hinkle, J. L., & Cheever, K.H. (2008). *Brunner and Suddarth's textbook of medical-surgical nursing* (11th ed.). Philadelphia: Lippincott Williams & Wilkins.

Timby, B. K., & Smith, N. E. (2007). *Introductory medical-surgical nursing* (9th ed.). Philadelphia: Lippincott Williams & Wilkins.

Xu, J., Kochanek, K. D., Tejada-Vera, B. (2009). Deaths: Preliminary data for 2007. *National Vital Statistics Reports; 58*(1), 1–52.

NOC-NIC LINKAGES FOR HYPERTENSION

Outcome	Major Interventions	Suggested Interventions
Compliance Behavior: Prescribed Diet Definition: Personal actions to follow food and fluid intake recommended by a health professional for a specific health condition	Nutritional Counseling Teaching: Prescribed Diet	Nutritional Monitoring
Knowledge: Diet Definition: Extent of understanding conveyed about recommended diet	Nutritional Counseling Teaching: Prescribed Diet	Nutritional Monitoring Self-Efficacy Enhancement Teaching: Individual · Weight Reduction Assistance
Knowledge: Hypertension Management Definition: Extent of understanding conveyed about high blood pressure, its treatment, and the prevention of complications	Teaching: Disease Process Teaching: Prescribed Diet Teaching: Procedure/ Treatment	Exercise Promotion Health System Guidance · Smoking Cessation Assistance Vital Signs Monitoring
Knowledge: Medication Definition: Extent of understanding conveyed about the safe use of medication	Teaching: Prescribed Medication	Learning Facilitation Learning Readiness Enhancement · Self-Responsibility Facilitation Teaching: Individual
Knowledge: Weight Management Definition: Extent of understanding conveyed about the promotion and maintenance of optimal body weight and fat percentage congruent with height, frame, gender, and age	Nutritional Counseling Weight Management	Behavior Modification Exercise Promotion Teaching: Group · Weight Reduction Assistance
Medication Response Definition: Therapeutic and adverse effects of prescribed medication	Medication Reconciliation Surveillance	Medication Management Teaching: Prescribed Medication

PART III - H

	NOC-NIC LINKAGES FOR HYPERTENSION		
Outcome	**Major Interventions**	**Suggested Interventions**	
Smoking Cessation Behavior			
Definition: Personal actions to eliminate tobacco use	Counseling Self-Responsibility Facilitation Smoking Cessation Assistance	Coping Enhancement Self-Efficacy Enhancement	Self-Modification Assistance
Stress Level			
Definition: Severity of manifested physical or mental tension resulting from factors that alter an existing equilibrium	Anxiety Reduction Meditation Facilitation Relaxation Therapy	Distraction	Self-Hypnosis Facilitation
Weight Loss Behavior			
Definition: Personal actions to lose weight through diet, exercise, and behavior modification	Exercise Promotion Nutritional Monitoring Weight Reduction Assistance	Mutual Goal Setting Nutrition Management	Self-Awareness Enhancement Support Group

PART III - H

Pneumonia

Pneumonia is an inflammation of one or both of the lungs caused by a microbial agent, such as bacteria, viruses, or fungi. The alveoli become inflamed and may fill with fluid or pus, causing symptoms such as a productive cough, fever, chills, and dyspnea. The most widely used classification of pneumonia is based on the setting in which the pneumonia is acquired. Community-acquired pneumonia (CAP) occurs outside of hospitals and other health care settings; hospital-acquired pneumonia (HAP), often referred to as nosocomial, tends to be more serious because the patient is already ill; health care–associated pneumonia can be acquired in nursing homes, dialysis centers, and outpatient clinics (National Heart Lung and Blood Institute [NHLBI], 2008). Other types of pneumonia include aspiration pneumonia, which can occur after inhalation of food, drink, saliva, or emesis. This can cause pus to accumulate in the lung and the formation of a cavity or lung abscess. Atypical pneumonia is readily passed from person to person and includes *Legionella, Mycoplasma,* and *Chlamydia* bacterial forms of pneumonias. Pneumonia can vary from mild to severe; it is often more serious for infants, young children, older adults, and people with chronic health problems and/or compromised immune systems.

PREVALENCE, MORTALITY, AND COST

Approximately 4 million Americans are affected with CAP each year, with minorities 3 to 10 times more likely to be infected and the elderly 60% more likely to be infected than the general population (Stanton, 2002). Hospital-acquired pneumonia is not a reportable disease, but available data indicate that between 5 and 10 cases occur per 1000 hospital admissions and the incidence increases by 6 to 20 times in patients on ventilators. About 25% of intensive care unit (ICU) infections are due to HAP and approximately 50% of the antibiotics prescribed are for treatment of HAP (American Thoracic Society, 2005).

Mortality figures vary with the type of pneumonia, patient age, and other factors. The National Center for Vital Statistics reported influenza and pneumonia as the eighth leading cause of death in 2006 (American Lung Association, 2007). The number of deaths in 2006 was 55,477, or 18.5 per 100,000 population (Centers for Disease Control and Prevention, 2009). The mortality rate each year for low-risk patients treated at home is less than 1% and the rate for more serious cases treated in a hospital is between 2% and 30% (Stanton, 2002). In 2006, 1.2 million people were hospitalized with pneumonia, with an average length of stay of 5.1 days (Centers for Disease Control and Prevention, 2009). Globally, pneumonia kills 4 million people every year—half of the deaths among children younger than 5 years of age; this is greater than the number of deaths from any other infectious agent (Centers for Disease Control and Prevention, 2009).

Direct costs for pneumonia and influenza in 2005 were determined to be about $34.2 billion (American Lung Association, 2007). It is estimated that approximately $10 billion per year is spent on caring for patients with CAP and the costs for antimicrobial therapy for CAP outpatients is approximately $100 billion per year (Stanton, 2002). It is estimated that HAP increases hospital stay by 7 to 9 days per patient and produces an excess cost of $40,000 per patient (American Thoracic Society, 2005).

RISK FACTORS

Factors associated with an increased risk of pneumonia (Mayo Clinic Staff, 2009; Smeltzer, Bare, Hinkle, & Cheever, 2008):

1. Age—Persons 65 years or older and very young children.

2. Ethnicity—Native Alaskans and certain Native American tribes.
3. Immune deficiency diseases and chronic diseases, such as cardiovascular disease, diabetes, emphysema, and other lung diseases.
4. Smoking and alcohol abuse—Smoking decreases ciliary action and allows secretions to pool in the lungs; chronic alcohol abuse interferes with the action of white blood cells that fight infection.
5. Hospitalization in an intensive care unit, particularly if placed on a ventilator—the normal defenses of the upper respiratory tract are bypassed, coughing is prevented, and aspiration can occur.
6. Using inhaled corticosteroids for more than 24 weeks for chronic obstructive lung disease (COPD) or other chronic lung conditions.
7. Exposure to certain chemicals and air pollutants, especially those found in agriculture, construction, or around certain industrial chemicals or animals.
8. Surgery or a serious injury that makes coughing and clearing the lungs more difficult.

Vaccines are available to prevent pneumococcal pneumonia and influenza, and should be administered if the person is in a high-risk group. The pneumococcal vaccine is effective for at least 5 years. The *Haemophilus influenzae* type b (Hib) vaccine should be given to all children younger than 5 years to prevent pneumonia and meningitis. Other steps to prevent pneumonia include performing proper handwashing, refraining from smoking, avoiding pollutants, and maintaining a strong immune system by ensuring adequate rest, exercise, and nutrition (NHLBI, 2008).

COURSE OF THE DISEASE

Symptoms of pneumonia can vary from mild to severe and can include (1) fever, (2) shaking chills, (3) productive cough, (4) shortness of breath with exertion, and (5) chest pain with breathing or coughing. Infants may not show any of these signs, but may vomit and appear restless and lethargic. If the immune system is suppressed the symptoms may be milder and not indicative of the seriousness of the infection.

Medical treatment depends on the cause and severity of the infection as well as the patient's age and overall state of health. Many people with mild symptoms can be treated at home. The goals of treatment are to eliminate the infection and prevent complications (NHLBI, 2008). Bacterial and mycoplasmal pneumonias are treated with antibiotics, and fungal pneumonia is treated with antifungal medication. Viral pneumonia is treated with rest and fluids; however, if the condition is severe, antiviral medication may be administered. If the infection is severe and/or the patient has other health problems, the patient may require treatment in a hospital setting with intravenous medications and, if needed, oxygen (Mayo Clinic Staff, 2009). Complications of pneumonia can be life-threatening, particularly bacteremia. Other serious complications include the development of a lung abscess or pleural effusion.

USE OF NOC AND NIC FOR PATIENTS WITH PNEUMONIA

Nursing has a major role in ensuring the patient is complying with the medication regimen, especially if being treated at home. Monitoring patient status and symptoms is important to detect if the infection is worsening or the patient is not responding to medication. The following should be monitored: changes in temperature and pulse; amount, odor, and color of secretions; frequency and severity of cough; degree of shortness of breath; and changes in lung sounds with auscultation (Smeltzer, Bare, Hinkle, & Cheever, 2008). Helping the patient remain comfortable, at home or in the hospital is often a nursing responsibility. The patient will need assistance to cope with the fever, cough, and generalized aches and pains that can accompany pneumonia. It may take time for the patient to recover from pneumonia; some may experience fatigue for 1 month or longer following the infection.

REFERENCES

American Lung Association. (2007). *Pneumonia fact sheet.* <http://www.lungusa.org/lung-disease/pneumonia/pneumonia-influenza/resources/pneumonia-fact-sheet.html> Accessed 04.05.10.

American Thoracic Society. (2005). Guidelines for the management of adults with hospital-acquired, ventilator-associated, and healthcare-associated pneumonia. *American Journal of Respiratory and Critical Care Medicine, 171*(4), 388–416.

Centers for Disease Control and Prevention. (2009). *Pneumonia can be prevented – vaccines can help.* <http://www.cdc.gov/Features/Pneumonia> Accessed 07.04.10.

Mayo Clinic Staff. (2009). *Pneumonia: Risk factors.* <http://www.mayoclinic.com/health/pneumonia/DS00135> Accessed 07.04.10.

National Heart Lung and Blood Institute [NHLBI]. (2008). *What is pneumonia?* <http://www.nhlbi.nih.gov/health/dci/Diseases/pnu/pnu_whatis.html> Accessed 29.03.10.

Smeltzer, S. C., Bare, B. G., Hinkle, J. L., & Cheever, K. H. (2008). *Brunner and Suddarth's textbook of medical-surgical nursing* (11th ed., pp. 1020–1033). Philadelphia: Lippincott Williams & Wilkins.

Stanton, MW. (2002). *Improving treatment decisions for patients with community-acquired pneumonia* [AHRQ Pub. No. 02-0033]. Rockville, MD: Agency for Healthcare Research and Quality.

NOC-NIC LINKAGES FOR PNEUMONIA

Outcome	Major Interventions	Suggested Interventions	
Activity Tolerance Definition: Physiologic response to energy-consuming movements with daily activities	Teaching: Prescribed Activity/Exercise	Energy Management	Smoking Cessation Assistance
Comfort Status: Physical Definition: Physical ease related to bodily sensations and homeostatic mechanisms	Environmental Management: Comfort	Energy Management Fever Treatment	Massage Positioning
Fatigue Level Definition: Severity of observed or reported prolonged generalized fatigue	Sleep Enhancement	Energy Management Medication Management	Massage Positioning
Hydration Definition: Adequate water in the intracellular and extra-cellular compartments of the body	Fluid Monitoring	Fever Treatment Fluid Management Intravenous (IV) Therapy	Temperature Regulation Vomiting Management
Infection Severity Definition: Severity of infection and associated symptoms **Infection Severity: Newborn** Definition: Severity of infection and associated symptoms during the first 28 days of life	Infection Protection Medication Administration	Fever Treatment Fluid Management Medication Administration: Inhalation	Medication Administration: Intravenous (IV) Medication Administration: Oral
Knowledge: Disease Process Definition: Extent of understanding conveyed about a specific disease process and prevention of complications	Teaching: Disease Process	Discharge Planning Medication Management	Risk Identification Teaching: Individual

NOC-NIC LINKAGES FOR PNEUMONIA		
Outcome	**Major Interventions**	**Suggested Interventions**
Knowledge: Medication Definition: Extent of understanding conveyed about the safe use of medication	Teaching: Prescribed Medication	Discharge Planning Immunization/Vaccination Management Medication Management Teaching: Individual
Knowledge: Treatment Regimen Definition: Extent of understanding conveyed about a specific treatment regimen	Teaching: Procedure/Treatment	Energy Management Teaching: Prescribed Activity/Exercise Teaching: Individual
Respiratory Status: Gas Exchange Definition: Alveolar exchange of carbon dioxide and oxygen to maintain arterial blood gas concentrations	Oxygen Therapy	Anxiety Reduction Bedside Laboratory Testing Chest Physiotherapy Cough Enhancement Respiratory Monitoring
Respiratory Status: Ventilation Definition: Movement of air in and out of the lungs	Airway Management	Airway Suctioning Anxiety Reduction Chest Physiotherapy Cough Enhancement Fluid Management Positioning Respiratory Monitoring Smoking Cessation Assistance
Symptom Control Definition: Personal actions to minimize perceived adverse changes in physical and emotional functioning	Cough Enhancement Fever Treatment	Anxiety Reduction Chest Physiotherapy Energy Management Environmental Management: Comfort Massage Medication Administration Nausea Management Nutritional Monitoring Pain Management Sleep Enhancement Vomiting Management
Thermoregulation Definition: Balance among heat production, heat gain, and heat loss	Fever Treatment Temperature Regulation	Fluid Management Fluid Monitoring Infection Protection Medication Administration
Thermoregulation: Newborn Definition: Balance among heat production, heat gain, and heat loss during the first 28 days of life		
Vital Signs Definition: Extent to which temperature, pulse, respiration, and blood pressure are within normal range	Vital Signs Monitoring	Respiratory Monitoring Surveillance

PART III - P

Stroke

A general definition of a stroke according to *Mosby's Dictionary of Medicine, Nursing and Health Professions* (2009) is an abnormal condition in a localized area of the brain attributable to inadequate blood flow. There are two major types of stroke—hemorrhagic and ischemic. Approximately 15% to 20% of strokes are hemorrhagic, divided between subarachnoid hemorrhage and primary intracerebral hemorrhage. The majority of strokes (approximately 80%) are ischemic in nature. When the condition is rapidly reversed with treatment, the event is referred to as a transient ischemic attack (Curioni, Cunha, Veras, & André, 2009). Regardless of the type of stroke, there is a well-established relationship with hypertension (Alter, Friday, Lai, O'Connell, & Sobel, 1994; Balu, 2009; Li, Engström, Hedblad, Berglund, & Janzon, 2005). In addition, clinical trials have shown the beneficial effect of pharmacological antihypertensive therapy on decreasing the incidence of stroke (Aronow & Frishman, 2004).

PREVALENCE, MORTALITY, AND COST

According to the World Health Organization, 15 million people worldwide will suffer a stroke annually, of which 5 million will die and another 5 million will be permanently disabled (Mackay & Mensah, 2004). The estimates in the United States are that 795,000 persons will suffer a stroke annually. Someone dies in the United States every 3 to 4 minutes from a stroke. It is also a chief cause of serious, long-term disability in all of the persons affected (Lloyd-Jones et al., 2010). These statistics make stroke the third leading cause of death in the United States (Heron et al., 2009) and the second leading cause of death in the world (World Health Organization, 2008).

Gender and race impact the incidence and prevalence of strokes in populations of the world. Generally, the overall prevalence of stroke among American Indian/Alaska native (6.0%), multiracial persons (4.6%), and blacks (4.0%) was higher than the prevalence among whites (2.3%). At the same time, the prevalence for Asian/Pacific Islanders and Hispanics was similar to that of the white population. With regard to gender, more men than women have a stroke, but there is a higher mortality among women (Lloyd-Jones et al., 2010). The high mortality is largely due to the greater number of elderly women in proportion to the male population. In 2010 the estimated direct and indirect costs of stroke are projected to be $73.7 billion. Seventy percent of the first year post stroke costs are from inpatient hospital stays (Lloyd-Jones et al., 2010).

RISK FACTORS

With limited options available for treating patients once a stroke has occurred, knowledge and recognition of risk factors are critical to reducing the devastating effects of a stroke. Goldstein and colleagues (2001) classified risk factors for a stroke as nonmodifiable, modifiable, or potentially modifiable. The factors identified as nonmodifiable are age, gender, race or ethnicity, and family history. The modifiable factors include hypertension, smoking, diabetes, high cholesterol level, atrial fibrillation, and other cardiac diseases. The final group referred to by Goldstein and colleagues (2001) as potentially modifiable relates to conditions that appear to be risk factors but for which there is no substantial base of evidence as yet to confirm the relationship. These conditions include obesity, alcohol and drug abuse, lack of physical activity, use of oral contraceptives and hormone replacement. It is noted that appropriate control of known risk factors does reduce the incidence of the occurrence (Curioni, Cunha, Veras, & André, 2009).

COURSE OF THE DISEASE

The course, signs, and symptoms of the disease are dependent on the region of the brain affected and the speed with which treatment occurs. A stroke may include the following: sudden numbness and tingling of the face or extremities, weakness or paralysis of one side of the body, sudden changes in vision, difficulty walking or standing, difficulty with speaking or comprehension, confusion, and severe headache (Mayo Clinic Staff, 2008; Smeltzer, Bare, Hinkle, & Cheever, 2008). Prompt treatment improves chances of survival and increases the degree of recovery that may be expected.

Stroke is a leading cause of serious, long-term disability in the United States. However, about two thirds of stroke survivors will have disabilities ranging from moderate to severe. According to the National Stroke Association 10% of stroke victims recover almost completely, 25% recover with minor impairments, 40% experience moderate to severe impairments requiring special care, and 10% necessitate care in a nursing home or other type of long-term care facility (National Stroke Association, 2009).

Treatment of the stroke is dependent upon the cause of the stroke. Ischemic strokes are treated with thrombolytic therapy and continuous monitoring during the first 24 hours (Smeltzer et al., 2008). Treatment for hemorrhagic stroke varies with the type of stroke, but the goals of medical treatment are the same for all types of stroke: (1) to allow the brain to recover, (2) to prevent a second bleed, and (3) to treat complications (Smeltzer et al., 2008). With both types of stroke, rehabilitation will follow recovery from the acute phase and will be dependent on the degree of functional loss the person has experienced.

USE OF NOC AND NIC FOR PATIENTS WITH STROKE

Nursing care goals and interventions will vary as the patient moves from the acute phase to recovery and intensive rehabilitation. However, the need to sustain adequate cerebral perfusion, prevent complications, and maintain patient function will be important in all phases of care. The care plan that follows is for the acute phase of care up to recovery. This generic care plan does not include outcomes and interventions for complications or impending death.

REFERENCES

Alter, M., Friday, G., Lai, S. M., O'Connell, J., & Sobel, E. (1994). Hypertension and risk of stroke recurrence. *Stroke, 25*(8), 1605–1610.

Aronow, W. S., & Frishman, W. H. (2004). Treatment of hypertension and prevention of ischemic stroke. *Current Cardiology Reports, 6*(2), 124–129.

Balu, S. (2009). Estimated annual direct expenditures in the United States as a result of inappropriate hypertension treatment according to national treatment guidelines. *Clinical Therapeutic, 31*(7), 1581–1594.

Curioni, C., Cunha, C. B., Veras, R. P., & André, C. (2009). The decline in mortality from circulatory diseases in Brazil. *Revista Panamericana de Salud Pública/Pan American Journal of Public Health, 25*(1), 9–15.

Goldstein, L. B., Adams, R. Becker, K., Furberg, C. D., Gorelick, P. B., Hademenos, G., et al. (2001). Primary prevention of ischemic stroke: A statement for healthcare professionals from the Stroke Council of the American Heart Association. *Stroke, 32*(1), 280–299.

Heron, M., Hoyert, D. L., Murphy, S. L., Xu, J., Kochanek, K. D., & Tejada-Vera, B. (2009). Deaths: Final Data for 2006. *National Vital Statistics Reports, 57*(14), 1–135.

Li, C., Engström, G., Hedblad, B., Berglund, G., & Janzon, L. (2005). Blood pressure control and risk of stroke: A population-based prospective cohort study. *Stroke, 36*(4), 725–730.

Lloyd-Jones, D., Adams, R. J., Brown, T. M., Carnethon, M., Dai, S., De Simone, G., et al. (2010). Heart disease and stroke statistics 2010 update. A report from the American Heart Association. *Circulation, 121*, e46–e215.

Mackay, J., & Mensah, G. (Eds.), (2004). *The atlas of heart disease and stroke.* Geneva, Switzerland: World Health Organization.

Mayo Clinic Staff. (2008). *Stroke: Symptoms.* <http://www.mayoclinic.com/health/stroke/DS00150/DSECTION=symptoms> Accessed 25.03.10.

Mosby's dictionary of medicine, nursing and health professions (8th ed.). (2009). St. Louis: Mosby Elsevier.

National Stroke Association. (2009). *Rehabilitation therapy.* <http://www.stroke.org/site/PageServer?pagename=REHABT> Accessed 05.04.10.

Smeltzer, S. C., Bare, B. G., Hinkle, J. L., & Cheever, K. H. (2008). *Brunner and Suddarth's textbook of medical-surgical nursing* (11th ed., pp. 2207–2210). Philadelphia: Lippincott Williams & Wilkins.

World Health Organization. (2008). *The top ten causes of death.* <http://www.who.int/mediacentre/factsheets/fs310/en/index.html> Accessed 05.04.10.

NOC-NIC LINKAGES FOR STROKE

Outcome	Major Interventions	Suggested Interventions	
Bowel Continence Definition: Control of passage of stool from the bowel	Bowel Management Self-Care Assistance: Toileting	Bathing Constipation/Impaction Management Flatulence Reduction Fluid Management	Medication Administration: Oral Medication Administration: Rectal Surveillance: Skin
Cognition Definition: Ability to execute complex mental processes	Cerebral Edema Management Cerebral Perfusion Promotion Neurologic Monitoring	Anxiety Reduction Delirium Management Fall Prevention	Memory Training Reality Orientation
Comfort Status Definition: Overall physical, psychospiritual, sociocultural, and environmental ease and safety of an individual	Environmental Management: Comfort Pain Management	Anxiety Reduction Bed Rest Care Emotional Support Energy Management Grief Work Facilitation Hope Inspiration Massage	Mood Management Patient Rights Protection Positioning Relaxation Therapy Spiritual Support Visitation Facilitation
Communication Definition: Reception, interpretation, and expression of spoken, written, and non-verbal messages	Communication Enhancement: Speech Deficit	Active Listening Anxiety Reduction	Patient Rights Protection Referral
Mobility Definition: Ability to move purposefully in own environment independently with or without assistive device	Exercise Therapy: Ambulation Exercise Therapy: Balance Positioning	Bed Rest Care Exercise Therapy: Joint Mobility Exercise Therapy: Muscle Control	Environmental Management: Safety Fall Prevention
Nutritional Status Definition: Extent to which nutrients are available to meet metabolic needs	Nutrition Management Nutritional Monitoring Self-Care Assistance: Feeding	Enteral Tube Feeding Fluid Management Fluid Monitoring	Intravenous (IV) Therapy
Self-Care: Activities of Daily Living (ADL) Definition: Ability to perform the most basic physical tasks and personal care activities independently with or without assistive device	Self-Care Assistance	Self-Care Assistance: Bathing/Hygiene Self-Care Assistance: Dressing/Grooming Self-Care Assistance: Feeding	Self-Care Assistance: Toileting Self-Care Assistance: Transfer

NOC-NIC LINKAGES FOR STROKE		
Outcome	**Major Interventions**	**Suggested Interventions**
Swallowing Status Definition: Safe passage of fluids and/or solids from the mouth to the stomach	Swallowing Therapy	Aspiration Precautions Referral Positioning Surveillance
Tissue Integrity: Skin and Mucous Membranes Definition: Structural intactness and normal physiological function of skin and mucous membranes	Positioning Pressure Management Skin Surveillance	Bathing Fluid Management Bed Rest Care
Urinary Continence Definition: Control of elimination of urine from the bladder	Urinary Incontinence Care	Bathing Surveillance: Skin Fluid Management Urinary Catheterization Perineal Care Prompted Voiding

Total Joint Replacement: Hip/Knee

Joint replacement surgery is used to alleviate pain and improve mobility in patients with severe destructive changes of the joints (Bongartz et al., 2008). Although total joint replacement can be used with any joint, this description will focus on the most common joints replaced—the hip (THR) and the knee (TKR). Most artificial joints (prostheses) consist of metal alloys, high-grade plastics, and polymeric materials. Technological advances have provided for an increased range of motion, enhanced stability, and very low wear. Minimally invasive surgery has allowed for more rapid healing with accelerated discharge and rehabilitation (Learmonth, Young, & Rorabeck, 2007). Total joint replacement has been an orthopedic success story, providing pain relief and return of function and allowing individuals to live fuller, active lives (American Academy of Orthopaedic Surgeons [AAOS], 2007).

PREVALENCE, MORTALITY, AND COST

More than 780,000 joint replacement procedures were performed in the United States in 2006 (AAOS, 2009). The number of surgeries has increased steadily since the first total hip replacement prosthesis was developed in 1938 (Learmonth, Young, & Rorabeck, 2007). There was a 53% increase in knee replacements and a 37% increase in hip replacements between 2000 and 2004 (Kim, 2008). There has also been a change in age distribution, with the highest number of procedures in persons 65 to 84 years of age. The proportion of surgeries is slightly higher among women—around the mid-50th percentile for women for THR and mid-50th to high-60th percentile for TKR (Kim, 2008). A cross-sectional study of Medicare recipients who had elective THR and TKR surgery in 2005 showed that rural beneficiaries were 27% more likely to have surgery than urban beneficiaries (Francis, Scaife, Zahnd, Cook, & Schneeweiss, 2009).

There has been a significant increase in the number of TKR procedures performed for osteoarthritis and a slight reduction in the number performed for rheumatoid arthritis between 1971-1975 and 2000-2003. The cost for THR in 2004 was approximately $8.3 billion and for TKR was approximately $14.6 billion, for a total of $22.9 billion for 657,000 procedures in 2004 (Kim, 2008). Based on the current increase in procedures and accounting for inflation, the national bill for hospital charges for hip/knee replacements could be nearly $80.2 billion in the year 2015 (Kim, 2008). Many of these procedures are paid for by Medicare because of patient age; based on the projected increases, the national bill for these procedures will continue to escalate.

According to a study published in the January 2010 issue of *The Journal of Bone and Joint Surgery,* postoperative mortality following hip/knee replacement was estimated to be 0.12% for the first 26 days. After 26 days the risk was negligible (Lie et al., 2010). The primary risk factors were found to be male gender and age older than 70 years. This suggests that previous studies indicating postoperative mortality exists for 60 or 90 days may no longer be accurate.

RISK FACTORS

Joint degeneration causing pain and disability is the reason for most total joint replacements. Degeneration in the knee and hip is most frequently associated with osteoarthritis, although other conditions, such as severe hemophilia with frequent joint bleeds, can cause joint degeneration. Trauma and congenital deformities can also be reasons for joint replacement. For the person with osteoarthritis, a sedentary lifestyle places the person at greater risk for joint degeneration; a balanced fitness program that includes walking, swimming, cycling, and stretching exercises is important (AAOS, 2009). Exercises that place excessive stress on the joints should be avoided. For the person with hemophilia, immediate treatment of a joint bleed with factor replacement has caused a decrease in the number of persons who reach an advanced stage of joint degeneration (Dodson & Roher, n.d.).

INDICATIONS FOR SURGERY AND POSTOPERATIVE COURSE

The indications for joint replacement surgery are severe pain and disability. The pain may be so severe that a person avoids using the joint, thereby weakening the muscles around the joint and making it more difficult to move the joint (AAOS, 2007).

Materials used for joint replacement are biocompatible and resistant to corrosion and wear, and they have properties that duplicate those of the joint they are replacing (for example, strength and flexibility) (AAOS, 2007). The joint can be either fully or partially cemented in place; alternatively, some procedures use no cement at all. If the joint is cemented in place, weight can be placed on the joint immediately, resulting in a faster rehabilitation; however, not all persons are candidates for this type of replacement and the possibility exists that the joint can loosen. If the joint is not cemented in place, the joint is designed to promote bone growth around the surface of the implant; because of this healing time and rehabilitation time are longer.

Depending upon the patient age, the length of surgery, and the type of anesthetic agent, immediate postoperative care can include attention to (1) maintaining cardiovascular stability, (2) preventing bleeding and shock, (3) relieving pain and anxiety, and (4) controlling nausea and vomiting (Smeltzer, Bare, Hinkle & Cheever, 2008). Possible complications that can occur include infection, blood clots, and loosening of the prosthesis (AAOS, 2007). Computer-assisted surgery, which is being used more frequently, may reduce the rate of complications, particularly dislocations (Learmonth et al., 2007).

USE OF NOC AND NIC FOR TOTAL JOINT REPLACEMENT: HIP/KNEE

The nurse must be aware of and monitor for the complications previously mentioned. Among the most serious complications is joint infection. Prosthetic joint infection often requires removal of the prosthesis followed by administration of prolonged intravenous antibiotic therapy; this complication has a death rate of 2.7% to 18% (Bongartz et al., 2008). The nurse is responsible for or collaborates with others in providing patient education in preparation for discharge home. The following generic care plan will be limited primarily to those areas of postoperative care of primary importance for joint replacement surgery, and postoperative care important for all surgical patients will be considered as it relates to the outcome *Post-Procedure Recovery*.

REFERENCES

American Academy of Orthopaedic Surgeons (AAOS). (2007). *Total joint replacement.* <http:// www.orthoinfo.aaos.org/ topic.cfm?topic=A00233> Accessed 30.02.10.

American Academy of Orthopaedic Surgeons (AAOS). (2009). *Exercise and bone and joint conditions.* <www.orthoinfo.aaos. org/topic.cfm?topic=A00100> Accessed 31.03.10.

Bongartz, T., Halligan, C. S., Osmon, D. R., Reinalda, M. S., Bamlet, W. R., Crowson, C. S., et al. (2008). Incidence and risk factors of prosthetic joint infection after total hip or knee replacement in patients with rheumatoid arthritis. *Arthritis & Rheumatism (Arthritis Care & Research), 59*(12), 1713–1720.

Dodson, S. R., & Roher, S. M. (n.d.). *Joint replacement.* <http:// www.haemophilia.org.za/Joint2.htm> Accessed 26.03.10.

Francis, M. L., Scaife, S. L., Zahnd, W. E., Cook, E. F., & Schneeweiss, S. (2009). Joint replacement surgeries among Medicare beneficiaries in rural compared with urban areas. *Arthritis & Rheumatism, 60*(12), 3554–3562.

Kim, S. (2008). Changes in surgical loads and economic burden of hip and knee replacements in the US: 1997–2004. *Arthritis & Rheumatism (Arthritis Care & Research), 59*(4), 481–488.

Learmonth, I. D., Young, C., & Rorabeck, C. (2007). The operation of the century: Total hip replacement. *Lancet, 370*(9597), 1508–1509.

Lie, S. A., Pratt, N., Ryan, P., Engesaeter, L. B., Havelin, L. I., Furnes, O., & Graves, S. (2010). Duration of the increase in early postoperative mortality after elective hip and knee replacement. *The Journal of Bone & Joint Surgery, 92*(1), 58–63.

Smeltzer, S. C., Bare, B. G., Hinkle, J. L., & Cheever, K. H. (2008). *Brunner and Suddarth's textbook of medical-surgical nursing* (11th ed., pp. 424–546). Philadelphia: Lippincott Williams & Wilkins.

PART III - T

PART III - T

NOC-NIC LINKAGES FOR TOTAL JOINT REPLACEMENT: HIP/KNEE		
Outcome	**Major Interventions**	**Suggested Interventions**
Ambulation Definition: Ability to walk from place to place independently with or without assistive device	Exercise Therapy: Ambulation	Body Mechanics Promotion Energy Management Exercise Therapy: Balance	Fall Prevention Teaching: Prescribed Activity/Exercise
Discharge Readiness: Independent Living Definition: Readiness of a patient to relocate from a health care institution to living independently	Discharge Planning Health System Guidance	Pain Management Exercise Therapy: Joint Mobility Self-Efficacy Enhancement Support System Enhancement	Teaching: Prescribed Activity/Exercise Teaching: Procedure/ Treatment Thrombolytic Therapy Management
Discharge Readiness: Supported Living Definition: Readiness of a patient to relocate from a health care institution to a lower level of supported living	Discharge Planning Health System Guidance	Exercise Therapy: Joint Mobility Pain Management Relocation Stress Reduction Support System Enhancement	Teaching: Prescribed Activity/Exercise Thrombolytic Therapy Management
Joint Movement: Hip Definition: Active range of motion of the hip with self-initiated movement	Exercise Therapy: Joint Mobility	Energy Management Pain Management	Teaching: Prescribed Activity/Exercise
Joint Movement: Knee Definition: Active range of motion of the knee with self-initiated movement			
Knowledge: Fall Prevention Definition: Extent of understanding conveyed about prevention of falls	Teaching: Individual	Environmental Management: Safety Fall Prevention	Self-Responsibility Facilitation
Knowledge: Prescribed Activity Definition: Extent of understanding conveyed about prescribed activity and exercise	Teaching: Prescribed Activity/Exercise	Exercise Promotion Exercise Therapy: Ambulation	Self-Efficacy Enhancement Self-Responsibility Facilitation

NOC-NIC LINKAGES FOR TOTAL JOINT REPLACEMENT: HIP/KNEE			
Outcome	**Major Interventions**	**Suggested Interventions**	
Mobility			
Definition: Ability to move purposefully in own environment independently with or without assistive device	Energy Management Exercise Promotion	Environmental Management: Safety Exercise Promotion: Strength Training Exercise Therapy: Ambulation	Exercise Therapy: Joint Mobility Fall Prevention
Pain Level			
Definition: Severity of observed or reported pain	Pain Management	Analgesic Administration Anxiety Reduction Energy Management Positioning	Relaxation Therapy Transcutaneous Electrical Nerve Stimulation (TENS) Vital Signs Monitoring
Post-Procedure Recovery			
Definition: Extent to which an individual returns to baseline function following a procedure(s) requiring anesthesia or sedation	Incision Site Care Pain Management	Energy Management Environmental Management: Comfort Fluid Management Infection Control Nausea Management	Respiratory Monitoring Self-Care Assistance Sleep Enhancement Temperature Regulation Urinary Elimination Management
Self-Care: Activities of Daily Living (ADL)			
Definition: Ability to perform the most basic physical tasks and personal care activities independently with or without assistive device	Self-Care Assistance	Home Maintenance Assistance	Support System Enhancement
Wound Healing: Primary Intention			
Definition: Extent of regeneration of cells and tissue following intentional closure	Incision Site Care	Circulatory Precautions Infection Control Medication Administration	Nutrition Management Skin Surveillance Wound Care: Closed Drainage

PART III - T

NOC Outcome Labels and Definitions

NOC Outcome Label		Definition
2500	Abuse Cessation	Evidence that the victim is no longer hurt or exploited
2501	Abuse Protection	Protection of self and/or dependent others from abuse
2514	Abuse Recovery	Extent of healing following physical or psychological abuse that may include sexual or financial exploitation
2502	Abuse Recovery: Emotional	Extent of healing of psychological injuries due to abuse
2503	Abuse Recovery: Financial	Extent of control of monetary and legal matters following financial exploitation
2504	Abuse Recovery: Physical	Extent of healing of physical injuries due to abuse
2505	Abuse Recovery: Sexual	Extent of healing of physical and psychological injuries due to sexual abuse or exploitation
1400	Abusive Behavior Self-Restraint	Self-restraint of abusive and neglectful behaviors toward others
1300	Acceptance: Health Status	Reconciliation to significant change in health circumstances
0005	Activity Tolerance	Physiologic response to energy-consuming movements with daily activities
0916	Acute Confusion Level	Severity of disturbance in consciousness and cognition that develops over a short period of time
1308	Adaptation to Physical Disability	Adaptive response to a significant functional challenge due to a physical disability
1600	Adherence Behavior	Self-initiated actions to promote optimal wellness, recovery, and rehabilitation
1621	Adherence Behavior: Healthy Diet	Personal actions to monitor and optimize a healthy and nutritional dietary regimen
1401	Aggression Self-Control	Self-restraint of assaultive, combative, or destructive behaviors toward others
1214	Agitation Level	Severity of disruptive physiological and behavioral manifestations of stress or biochemical triggers
1629	Alcohol Abuse Cessation Behavior	Personal actions to eliminate alcohol use that poses a threat to health
0705	Allergic Response: Localized	Severity of localized hypersensitive immune response to a specific environmental (exogenous) antigen
0706	Allergic Response: Systemic	Severity of systemic hypersensitive immune response to a specific environmental (exogenous) antigen
0200	Ambulation	Ability to walk from place to place independently with or without assistive device
0201	Ambulation: Wheelchair	Ability to move from place to place in a wheelchair
1211	Anxiety Level	Severity of manifested apprehension, tension, or uneasiness arising from an unidentifiable source

NOC Outcome Label		Definition
1402	Anxiety Self-Control	Personal actions to eliminate or reduce feelings of apprehension, tension, or uneasiness from an unidentifiable source
1014	Appetite	Desire to eat when ill or receiving treatment
1918	Aspiration Prevention	Personal actions to prevent the passage of fluid and solid particles into the lung
0704	Asthma Self-Management	Personal actions to prevent or reverse inflammatory condition resulting in bronchial constriction of the airways
0202	Balance	Ability to maintain body equilibrium
0409	Blood Coagulation	Extent to which blood clots within normal period of time
2300	Blood Glucose Level	Extent to which glucose levels in plasma and urine are maintained in normal range
0413	Blood Loss Severity	Severity of internal or external bleeding/hemorrhage
0700	Blood Transfusion Reaction	Severity of complications with blood transfusion reaction
1200	Body Image	Perception of own appearance and body functions
1616	Body Mechanics Performance	Personal actions to maintain proper body alignment and to prevent muscular skeletal strain
0203	Body Positioning: Self-Initiated	Ability to change own body position independently with or without assistive device
1104	Bone Healing	Extent of regeneration of cells and tissues following bone injury
0500	Bowel Continence	Control of passage of stool from the bowel
0501	Bowel Elimination	Formation and evacuation of stool
1000	Breastfeeding Establishment: Infant	Infant attachment to and sucking from the mother's breast for nourishment during the first 3 weeks of breastfeeding
1001	Breastfeeding Establishment: Maternal	Maternal establishment of proper attachment of an infant to and sucking from the breast for nourishment during the first 3 weeks of breastfeeding
1002	Breastfeeding Maintenance	Continuation of breastfeeding from establishment to weaning for nourishment of an infant/toddler
1003	Breastfeeding Weaning	Progressive discontinuation of breastfeeding of an infant/toddler
1106	Burn Healing	Extent of healing of a burn site
1107	Burn Recovery	Extent of overall physical and psychological healing following major burn injury
1617	Cardiac Disease Self-Management	Personal actions to manage heart disease, its treatment, and prevent disease progression
0400	Cardiac Pump Effectiveness	Adequacy of blood volume ejected from the left ventricle to support systemic perfusion pressure
0414	Cardiopulmonary Status	Adequacy of blood volume ejected from the ventricles and exchange of carbon dioxide and oxygen at the alveolar level
2200	Caregiver Adaptation to Patient Institutionalization	Adaptive response of family caregiver when the care recipient is moved to an institution
2506	Caregiver Emotional Health	Emotional well-being of a family care provider while caring for a family member
2202	Caregiver Home Care Readiness	Preparedness of a caregiver to assume responsibility for the health care of a family member in the home
2203	Caregiver Lifestyle Disruption	Severity of disturbances in the lifestyle of a family member due to caregiving

Continued

PART IV - NOC

NOC Outcome Label		Definition
2204	Caregiver-Patient Relationship	Positive interactions and connections between the caregiver and care recipient
2205	Caregiver Performance: Direct Care	Provision by family care provider of appropriate personal and health care for a family member
2206	Caregiver Performance: Indirect Care	Arrangement and oversight by family care provider of appropriate care for a family member
2507	Caregiver Physical Health	Physical well-being of a family care provider while caring for a family member
2210	Caregiver Role Endurance	Factors that promote family care provider's capacity to sustain caregiving over an extended period of time
2208	Caregiver Stressors	Severity of biopsychosocial pressure on a family care provider caring for another over an extended period of time
2508	Caregiver Well-Being	Extent of positive perception of primary care provider's health status
1301	Child Adaptation to Hospitalization	Adaptive response of a child from 3 years through 17 years of age to hospitalization
0120	Child Development: 1 Month	Milestones of physical, cognitive, and psychosocial progression by 1 month of age
0100	Child Development: 2 Months	Milestones of physical, cognitive, and psychosocial progression by 2 months of age
0101	Child Development: 4 Months	Milestones of physical, cognitive, and psychosocial progression by 4 months of age
0102	Child Development: 6 Months	Milestones of physical, cognitive, and psychosocial progression by 6 months of age
0103	Child Development: 12 Months	Milestones of physical, cognitive, and psychosocial progression by 12 months of age
0104	Child Development: 2 Years	Milestones of physical, cognitive, and psychosocial progression by 2 years of age
0105	Child Development: 3 Years	Milestones of physical, cognitive, and psychosocial progression by 3 years of age
0106	Child Development: 4 Years	Milestones of physical, cognitive, and psychosocial progression by 4 years of age
0107	Child Development: 5 Years	Milestones of physical, cognitive, and psychosocial progression by 5 years of age
0108	Child Development: Middle Childhood	Milestones of physical, cognitive, and psychosocial progression from 6 years through 11 years of age
0109	Child Development: Adolescence	Milestones of physical, cognitive, and psychosocial progression from 12 years through 17 years of age
0401	Circulation Status	Unobstructed, unidirectional blood flow at an appropriate pressure through large vessels of the systemic and pulmonary circuits
3014	Client Satisfaction	Extent of positive perception of care provided by nursing staff
3000	Client Satisfaction: Access to Care Resources	Extent of positive perception of access to nursing staff, supplies, and equipment needed for care
3001	Client Satisfaction: Caring	Extent of positive perception of nursing staff's concern for the client
3015	Client Satisfaction: Case Management	Extent of positive perception of case management services
3002	Client Satisfaction: Communication	Extent of positive perception of information exchanged between client and nursing staff

NOC Outcome Label	Definition
3003 Client Satisfaction: Continuity of Care	Extent of positive perception of coordination of care as the client moves from one care setting to another
3004 Client Satisfaction: Cultural Needs Fulfillment	Extent of positive perception of integration of cultural beliefs, values, and social structures into nursing care
3005 Client Satisfaction: Functional Assistance	Extent of positive perception of nursing assistance to achieve mobility and self-care
3016 Client Satisfaction: Pain Management	Extent of positive perception of nursing care to relieve pain
3006 Client Satisfaction: Physical Care	Extent of positive perception of nursing care to maintain body functions and cleanliness
3007 Client Satisfaction: Physical Environment	Extent of positive perception of living environment, treatment environment, equipment, and supplies in acute or long term care settings
3008 Client Satisfaction: Protection of Rights	Extent of positive perception of protection of a client's legal and moral rights provided by nursing staff
3009 Client Satisfaction: Psychological Care	Extent of positive perception of nursing assistance to cope with emotional issues and perform mental activities
3010 Client Satisfaction: Safety	Extent of positive perception of procedures, information, and nursing care to prevent harm or injury
3011 Client Satisfaction: Symptom Control	Extent of positive perception of nursing care to relieve symptoms of illness
3012 Client Satisfaction: Teaching	Extent of positive perception of instruction provided by nursing staff to improve knowledge, understanding, and participation in care
3013 Client Satisfaction: Technical Aspects of Care	Extent of positive perception of nursing staff's knowledge and expertise used in providing care
0900 Cognition	Ability to execute complex mental processes
0901 Cognitive Orientation	Ability to identify person, place, and time accurately
2008 Comfort Status	Overall physical, psychospiritual, sociocultural, and environmental ease and safety of an individual
2009 Comfort Status: Environment	Environmental ease, comfort, and safety of surroundings
2010 Comfort Status: Physical	Physical ease related to bodily sensations and homeostatic mechanisms
2011 Comfort Status: Psychospiritual	Psychospiritual ease related to self-concept, emotional well-being, source of inspiration, and meaning and purpose in one's life
2012 Comfort Status: Sociocultural	Social ease related to interpersonal, family, and societal relationships within a cultural context
2007 Comfortable Death	Physical, psychospiritual, sociocultural, and environmental ease with the impending end of life
0902 Communication	Reception, interpretation, and expression of spoken, written, and non-verbal messages
0903 Communication: Expressive	Expression of meaningful verbal and/or non-verbal messages
0904 Communication: Receptive	Reception and interpretation of verbal and/or non-verbal messages
2700 Community Competence	Capacity of a community to collectively problem solve to achieve community goals
2804 Community Disaster Readiness	Community preparedness to respond to a natural or man-made calamitous event

Continued

NOC Outcome Label		Definition
2806	Community Disaster Response	Community response following a natural or man-made calamitous event
2701	Community Health Status	General state of well-being of a community or population
2800	Community Health Status: Immunity	Resistance of community members to the invasion and spread of an infectious agent that could threaten public health
2801	Community Risk Control: Chronic Disease	Community actions to reduce the risk of chronic diseases and related complications
2802	Community Risk Control: Communicable Disease	Community actions to eliminate or reduce the spread of infectious agents that threaten public health
2803	Community Risk Control: Lead Exposure	Community actions to reduce lead exposure and poisoning
2805	Community Risk Control: Violence	Community actions to eliminate or reduce intentional violent acts resulting in serious physical or psychological harm
2702	Community Violence Level	Incidence of violent acts compared with local, state, or national values
1601	Compliance Behavior	Personal actions to promote wellness, recovery, and rehabilitation recommended by a health professional
1622	Compliance Behavior: Prescribed Diet	Personal actions to follow food and fluid intake recommended by a health professional for a specific health condition
1623	Compliance Behavior: Prescribed Medication	Personal actions to administer medication safely to meet therapeutic goals as recommended by a health professional
0905	Concentration	Ability to focus on a specific stimulus
0212	Coordinated Movement	Ability of muscles to work together voluntarily for purposeful movement
1302	Coping	Personal actions to manage stressors that tax an individual's resources
0906	Decision-Making	Ability to make judgments and choose between two or more alternatives
1208	Depression Level	Severity of melancholic mood and loss of interest in life events
1409	Depression Self-Control	Personal actions to minimize melancholy and maintain interest in life events
0121	Development: Late Adulthood	Cognitive, psychosocial, and moral progression from 65 years of age and older
0122	Development: Middle Adulthood	Cognitive, psychosocial, and moral progression from 40 through 64 years of age
0123	Development: Young Adulthood	Cognitive, psychosocial, and moral progression from 18 through 39 years of age
1619	Diabetes Self-Management	Personal actions to manage diabetes mellitus, its treatment, and prevent disease progression
1307	Dignified Life Closure	Personal actions to maintain control during approaching end of life
0311	Discharge Readiness: Independent Living	Readiness of a patient to relocate from a health care institution to living independently
0312	Discharge Readiness: Supported Living	Readiness of a patient to relocate from a health care institution to a lower level of supported living

NOC Outcome Label		Definition
2109	Discomfort Level	Severity of observed or reported mental or physical discomfort
1403	Distorted Thought Self-Control	Self-restraint of disruptions in perception, thought processes, and thought content
1630	Drug Abuse Cessation Behavior	Personal actions to eliminate drug use that poses a threat to health
0600	Electrolyte & Acid/Base Balance	Balance of the electrolytes and non-electrolytes in the intracellular and extracellular compartments of the body
1919	Elopement Occurrence	Number of times in the past 24 hours/1 week/1 month (select one) that an individual with a cognitive impairment escapes a secure area
1920	Elopement Propensity Risk	The propensity of an individual with cognitive impairment to escape a secure area
0001	Endurance	Capacity to sustain activity
0002	Energy Conservation	Personal actions to manage energy for initiating and sustaining activity
1909	Fall Prevention Behavior	Personal or family caregiver actions to minimize risk factors that might precipitate falls in the personal environment
1912	Falls Occurrence	Number of times an individual falls
2600	Family Coping	Family actions to manage stressors that tax family resources
2602	Family Functioning	Capacity of the family system to meet the needs of its members during developmental transitions
2606	Family Health Status	Overall health and social competence of family unit
2603	Family Integrity	Family members' behaviors that collectively demonstrate cohesion, strength, and emotional bonding
2604	Family Normalization	Capacity of the family system to develop strategies for optimal functioning when a member has a chronic illness or disability
2605	Family Participation in Professional Care	Family involvement in decision-making, delivery, and evaluation of care provided by health care personnel
2608	Family Resiliency	Positive adaptation and function of the family system following significant adversity or crises
2601	Family Social Climate	Supportive milieu as characterized by family member relationships and goals
2609	Family Support During Treatment	Family presence and emotional support for an individual undergoing treatment
0007	Fatigue Level	Severity of observed or reported prolonged generalized fatigue
1210	Fear Level	Severity of manifested apprehension, tension, or uneasiness arising from an identifiable source
1213	Fear Level: Child	Severity of manifested apprehension, tension, or uneasiness arising from an identifiable source in a child from 1 year through 17 years of age
1404	Fear Self-Control	Personal actions to eliminate or reduce disabling feelings of apprehension, tension, or uneasiness from an identifiable source
0111	Fetal Status: Antepartum	Extent to which fetal signs are within normal limits from conception to the onset of labor
0112	Fetal Status: Intrapartum	Extent to which fetal signs are within normal limits from onset of labor to delivery

Continued

NOC Outcome Label		Definition
0601	Fluid Balance	Water balance in the intracellular and extracellular compartments of the body
0603	Fluid Overload Severity	Severity of excess fluids in the intracellular and extracellular compartments of the body
1015	Gastrointestinal Function	Extent to which foods (ingested or tube-fed) are moved from ingestion to excretion
1304	Grief Resolution	Adjustment to actual or impending loss
0110	Growth	Normal increase in bone size and body weight during growth years
1700	Health Beliefs	Personal convictions that influence health behaviors
1701	Health Beliefs: Perceived Ability to Perform	Personal conviction that one can carry out a given health behavior
1702	Health Beliefs: Perceived Control	Personal conviction that one can influence a health outcome
1703	Health Beliefs: Perceived Resources	Personal conviction that one has adequate means to carry out a health behavior
1704	Health Beliefs: Perceived Threat	Personal conviction that a threatening health problem is serious and has potential negative consequences for lifestyle
1705	Health Orientation	Personal commitment to health behaviors as lifestyle priorities
1602	Health Promoting Behavior	Personal actions to sustain or increase wellness
1603	Health Seeking Behavior	Personal actions to promote optimal wellness, recovery, and rehabilitation
1610	Hearing Compensation Behavior	Personal actions to identify, monitor, and compensate for hearing loss
0918	Heedfulness of Affected Side	Personal actions to acknowledge, protect, and cognitively integrate affected body part(s) into self
1105	Hemodialysis Access	Functionality of a dialysis access site
1201	Hope	Optimism that is personally satisfying and life-supporting
0602	Hydration	Adequate water in the intracellular and extracellular compartments of the body
0915	Hyperactivity Level	Severity of patterns of inattention or impulsivity in a child from 1 year through 17 years of age
1202	Identity	Distinguishes between self and non-self and characterizes one's essence
0204	Immobility Consequences: Physiological	Severity of compromise in physiological functioning due to impaired physical mobility
0205	Immobility Consequences: Psycho-Cognitive	Severity of compromise in psycho-cognitive functioning due to impaired physical mobility
0707	Immune Hypersensitivity Response	Severity of inappropriate immune responses
0702	Immune Status	Natural and acquired appropriately targeted resistance to internal and external antigens
1900	Immunization Behavior	Personal actions to obtain immunization to prevent a communicable disease
1405	Impulse Self-Control	Self-restraint of compulsive or impulsive behaviors
0703	Infection Severity	Severity of infection and associated symptoms
0708	Infection Severity: Newborn	Severity of infection and associated symptoms during the first 28 days of life
0907	Information Processing	Ability to acquire, organize, and use information

NOC Outcome Label		Definition
0206	Joint Movement	Active range of motion of all joints with self-initiated movement
0213	Joint Movement: Ankle	Active range of motion of the ankle with self-initiated movement
0214	Joint Movement: Elbow	Active range of motion of the elbow with self-initiated movement
0215	Joint Movement: Fingers	Active range of motion of the fingers with self-initiated movement
0216	Joint Movement: Hip	Active range of motion of the hip with self-initiated movement
0217	Joint Movement: Knee	Active range of motion of the knee with self-initiated movement
0218	Joint Movement: Neck	Active range of motion of the neck with self-initiated movement
0207	Joint Movement: Passive	Joint movement with assistance
0219	Joint Movement: Shoulder	Active range of motion of the shoulder with self-initiated movement
0220	Joint Movement: Spine	Active range of motion of the spine with self-initiated movement
0221	Joint Movement: Wrist	Active range of motion of the wrist with self-initiated movement
0504	Kidney Function	Filtration of blood and elimination of metabolic waste products through the formation of urine
1831	Knowledge: Arthritis Management	Extent of understanding conveyed about arthritis, its treatment, and the prevention of complications
1832	Knowledge: Asthma Management	Extent of understanding conveyed about asthma, its treatment, and the prevention of complications
1827	Knowledge: Body Mechanics	Extent of understanding conveyed about proper body alignment, balance, and coordinated movement
1800	Knowledge: Breastfeeding	Extent of understanding conveyed about lactation and nourishment of an infant through breastfeeding
1833	Knowledge: Cancer Management	Extent of understanding conveyed about cause, type, progress, symptoms, and treatment of cancer
1834	Knowledge: Cancer Threat Reduction	Extent of understanding conveyed about causes, prevention, and early detection of cancer
1830	Knowledge: Cardiac Disease Management	Extent of understanding conveyed about heart disease, its treatment, and the prevention of complications
1801	Knowledge: Child Physical Safety	Extent of understanding conveyed about safely caring for a child from 1 year through 17 years of age
1821	Knowledge: Conception Prevention	Extent of understanding conveyed about prevention of unintended pregnancy
1835	Knowledge: Congestive Heart Failure Management	Extent of understanding conveyed about heart failure, its treatment, and the prevention of exacerbations
1836	Knowledge: Depression Management	Extent of understanding conveyed about depression and interrelationships among causes, effects, and treatments
1820	Knowledge: Diabetes Management	Extent of understanding conveyed about diabetes mellitus, its treatment, and the prevention of complications
1802	Knowledge: Diet	Extent of understanding conveyed about recommended diet
1803	Knowledge: Disease Process	Extent of understanding conveyed about a specific disease process and prevention of complications

Continued

PART IV - NOC

NOC Outcome Label		Definition
1804	Knowledge: Energy Conservation	Extent of understanding conveyed about energy conservation techniques
1828	Knowledge: Fall Prevention	Extent of understanding conveyed about prevention of falls
1816	Knowledge: Fertility Promotion	Extent of understanding conveyed about fertility testing and the conditions that affect conception
1805	Knowledge: Health Behavior	Extent of understanding conveyed about the promotion and protection of health
1823	Knowledge: Health Promotion	Extent of understanding conveyed about information needed to obtain and maintain optimal health
1806	Knowledge: Health Resources	Extent of understanding conveyed about relevant health care resources
1837	Knowledge: Hypertension Management	Extent of understanding conveyed about high blood pressure, its treatment, and the prevention of complications
1824	Knowledge: Illness Care	Extent of understanding conveyed about illness-related information needed to achieve and maintain optimal health
1819	Knowledge: Infant Care	Extent of understanding conveyed about caring for a baby from birth to first birthday
1842	Knowledge: Infection Management	Extent of understanding conveyed about infection, its treatment, and the prevention of complications
1817	Knowledge: Labor & Delivery	Extent of understanding conveyed about labor and vaginal delivery
1808	Knowledge: Medication	Extent of understanding conveyed about the safe use of medication
1838	Knowledge: Multiple Sclerosis Management	Extent of understanding conveyed about multiple sclerosis, its treatment, and the prevention of relapses or exacerbations
1829	Knowledge: Ostomy Care	Extent of understanding conveyed about maintenance of an ostomy for elimination
1843	Knowledge: Pain Management	Extent of understanding conveyed about causes, symptoms, and treatment of pain
1826	Knowledge: Parenting	Extent of understanding conveyed about provision of a nurturing and constructive environment for a child from 1 year through 17 years of age
1809	Knowledge: Personal Safety	Extent of understanding conveyed about prevention of unintentional injuries
1818	Knowledge: Postpartum Maternal Health	Extent of understanding conveyed about maternal health in the period following birth of an infant
1822	Knowledge: Preconception Maternal Health	Extent of understanding conveyed about maternal health prior to conception to ensure a healthy pregnancy
1810	Knowledge: Pregnancy	Extent of understanding conveyed about promotion of a healthy pregnancy and prevention of complications
1839	Knowledge: Pregnancy & Postpartum Sexual Functioning	Extent of understanding conveyed about sexual function during pregnancy and postpartum
1811	Knowledge: Prescribed Activity	Extent of understanding conveyed about prescribed activity and exercise
1840	Knowledge: Preterm Infant Care	Extent of understanding conveyed about the care of a premature infant born 24 to 37 weeks (term) gestation
1815	Knowledge: Sexual Functioning	Extent of understanding conveyed about sexual development and responsible sexual practices

NOC Outcome Label — Definition

	NOC Outcome Label	Definition
1812	Knowledge: Substance Use Control	Extent of understanding conveyed about controlling the use of addictive drugs, toxic chemicals, tobacco, or alcohol
1814	Knowledge: Treatment Procedure	Extent of understanding conveyed about a procedure required as part of a treatment regimen
1813	Knowledge: Treatment Regimen	Extent of understanding conveyed about a specific treatment regimen
1841	Knowledge: Weight Management	Extent of understanding conveyed about the promotion and maintenance of optimal body weight and fat percentage congruent with height, frame, gender, and age
1604	Leisure Participation	Use of relaxing, interesting, and enjoyable activities to promote well-being
1203	Loneliness Severity	Severity of emotional, social, or existential isolation response
2509	Maternal Status: Antepartum	Extent to which maternal well-being is within normal limits from conception to the onset of labor
2510	Maternal Status: Intrapartum	Extent to which maternal well-being is within normal limits from onset of labor to delivery
2511	Maternal Status: Postpartum	Extent to which maternal well-being is within normal limits from delivery of placenta to completion of involution
0411	Mechanical Ventilation Response: Adult	Alveolar exchange and tissue perfusion are supported by mechanical ventilation
0412	Mechanical Ventilation Weaning Response: Adult	Respiratory and psychological adjustment to progressive removal of mechanical ventilation
2301	Medication Response	Therapeutic and adverse effects of prescribed medication
0908	Memory	Ability to cognitively retrieve and report previously stored information
0208	Mobility	Ability to move purposefully in own environment independently with or without assistive device
1204	Mood Equilibrium	Appropriate adjustment of prevailing emotional tone in response to circumstances
1209	Motivation	Inner urge that moves or prompts an individual to positive action(s)
1631	Multiple Sclerosis Self-Management	Personal actions to manage multiple sclerosis and prevent disease progression
1618	Nausea & Vomiting Control	Personal actions to control nausea, retching, and vomiting symptoms
2106	Nausea & Vomiting: Disruptive Effects	Severity of observed or reported disruptive effects of nausea, retching, and vomiting on daily functioning
2107	Nausea & Vomiting Severity	Severity of nausea, retching, and vomiting symptoms
2513	Neglect Cessation	Evidence that the victim is no longer receiving substandard care
2512	Neglect Recovery	Extent of physical, emotional, and spiritual healing following the cessation of substandard care
0909	Neurological Status	Ability of the peripheral and central nervous systems to receive, process, and respond to internal and external stimuli
0910	Neurological Status: Autonomic	Ability of the autonomic nervous system to coordinate visceral and homeostatic functions
0911	Neurological Status: Central Motor Control	Ability of the central nervous system to coordinate skeletal muscle activity for body movement
0912	Neurological Status: Consciousness	Arousal, orientation, and attention to the environment

Continued

NOC Outcome Label		Definition
0913	Neurological Status: Cranial Sensory/Motor Function	Ability of the cranial nerves to convey sensory and motor impulses
0917	Neurological Status: Peripheral	Ability of the peripheral nervous system to transmit impulses to and from the central nervous system
0914	Neurological Status: Spinal Sensory/Motor Function	Ability of the spinal nerves to convey sensory and motor impulses
0118	Newborn Adaptation	Adaptive response to the extrauterine environment by a physiologically mature newborn during the first 28 days
1004	Nutritional Status	Extent to which nutrients are available to meet metabolic needs
1005	Nutritional Status: Biochemical Measures	Body fluid components and chemical indices of nutritional status
1007	Nutritional Status: Energy	Extent to which nutrients and oxygen provide cellular energy
1008	Nutritional Status: Food & Fluid Intake	Amount of food and fluid taken into the body over a 24-hour period
1009	Nutritional Status: Nutrient Intake	Nutrient intake to meet metabolic needs
1100	Oral Hygiene	Condition of the mouth, teeth, gums, and tongue
1615	Ostomy Self-Care	Personal actions to maintain ostomy for elimination
1306	Pain: Adverse Psychological Response	Severity of observed or reported adverse cognitive and emotional responses to physical pain
1605	Pain Control	Personal actions to control pain
2101	Pain: Disruptive Effects	Severity of observed or reported disruptive effects of chronic pain on daily functioning
2102	Pain Level	Severity of observed or reported pain
1500	Parent-Infant Attachment	Parent and infant behaviors that demonstrate anenduring affectionate bond
2902	Parenting: Adolescent Physical Safety	Parental actions to prevent physical injury in an adolescent from 12 years through 17 years of age
2901	Parenting: Early/Middle Childhood Physical Safety	Parental actions to avoid physical injury of a child from 3 years through 11 years of age
2900	Parenting: Infant/Toddler Physical Safety	Parental actions to avoid physical injury of a child from birth through 2 years of age
2211	Parenting Performance	Parental actions to provide a child with a nurturing and constructive physical, emotional, and social environment
1901	Parenting: Psychosocial Safety	Parental actions to protect a child from social contacts that might cause harm or injury
1606	Participation in Health Care Decisions	Personal involvement in selecting and evaluating health care options to achieve desired outcome
1614	Personal Autonomy	Personal actions of a competent individual to exercise governance in life decisions
2006	Personal Health Status	Overall physical, psychological, social, and spiritual functioning of an adult 18 years or older
1309	Personal Resiliency	Positive adaptation and function of an individual following significant adversity or crisis
1911	Personal Safety Behavior	Personal actions that prevent physical injury to self
2002	Personal Well-Being	Extent of positive perception of one's health status
0113	Physical Aging	Normal physical changes that occur with the natural aging process
2004	Physical Fitness	Performance of physical activities with vigor

NOC Outcome Label

Definition

1913	Physical Injury Severity	Severity of injuries from accidents and trauma
0114	Physical Maturation: Female	Normal physical changes in the female that occur with the transition from childhood to adulthood
0115	Physical Maturation: Male	Normal physical changes in the male that occur with the transition from childhood to adulthood
0116	Play Participation	Use of activities by a child from 1 year through 11 years of age to promote enjoyment, entertainment, and development
1624	Postpartum Maternal Health Behavior	Personal actions to promote health of a mother in the period following birth of infant
2303	Post-Procedure Recovery	Extent to which an individual returns to baseline function following a procedure(s) requiring anesthesia or sedation
1607	Prenatal Health Behavior	Personal actions to promote a healthy pregnancy and a healthy newborn
1921	Pre-Procedure Readiness	Readiness of a patient to safely undergo a procedure requiring anesthesia or sedation
0117	Preterm Infant Organization	Extrauterine integration of physiological and behavioral function by the infant born 24 to 37 (term) weeks gestation
0006	Psychomotor Energy	Personal drive and energy to maintain activities of daily living, nutrition, and personal safety
1305	Psychosocial Adjustment: Life Change	Adaptive psychosocial response of an individual to a significant life change
2000	Quality of Life	Extent of positive perception of current life circumstances
0415	Respiratory Status	Movement of air in and out of the lungs and exchange of carbon dioxide and oxygen at the alveolar level
0410	Respiratory Status: Airway Patency	Open, clear tracheobronchial passages for air exchange
0402	Respiratory Status: Gas Exchange	Alveolar exchange of carbon dioxide and oxygen to maintain arterial blood gas concentrations
0403	Respiratory Status: Ventilation	Movement of air in and out of the lungs
0003	Rest	Quantity and pattern of diminished activity for mental and physical rejuvenation
1902	Risk Control	Personal actions to prevent, eliminate, or reduce modifiable health threats
1903	Risk Control: Alcohol Use	Personal actions to prevent, eliminate, or reduce alcohol use that poses a threat to health
1917	Risk Control: Cancer	Personal actions to detect or reduce the threat of cancer
1914	Risk Control: Cardiovascular Health	Personal actions to eliminate or reduce threats to cardiovascular health
1904	Risk Control: Drug Use	Personal actions to prevent, eliminate, or reduce drug use that poses a threat to health
1915	Risk Control: Hearing Impairment	Personal actions to prevent, eliminate, or reduce threats to hearing function
1922	Risk Control: Hyperthermia	Personal actions to prevent, detect, or reduce the threat of high body temperature
1923	Risk Control: Hypothermia	Personal actions to prevent, detect, or reduce the threat of low body temperature
1924	Risk Control: Infectious Process	Personal actions to prevent, eliminate, or reduce the threat of infection

Continued

NOC Outcome Label		Definition
1905	Risk Control: Sexually Transmitted Diseases (STD)	Personal actions to prevent, eliminate, or reduce behaviors associated with sexually transmitted disease
1925	Risk Control: Sun Exposure	Personal actions to prevent or reduce threats to the skin and eyes from sun exposure
1906	Risk Control: Tobacco Use	Personal actions to prevent tobacco use
1907	Risk Control: Unintended Pregnancy	Personal actions to prevent or reduce the possibility of unintended pregnancy
1916	Risk Control: Visual Impairment	Personal actions to prevent, eliminate, or reduce threats to visual function
1908	Risk Detection	Personal actions to identify personal health threats
1501	Role Performance	Congruence of an individual's role behavior with role expectations
1910	Safe Home Environment	Physical arrangements to minimize environmental factors that might cause physical harm or injury in the home
1926	Safe Wandering	Safe, socially acceptable moving about without apparent purpose in an individual with cognitive impairment
1620	Seizure Control	Personal actions to reduce or minimize the occurrence of seizure episodes
0313	Self-Care Status	Ability to perform basic personal care activities and instrumental activities of daily living
0300	Self-Care: Activities of Daily Living (ADL)	Ability to perform the most basic physical tasks and personal care activities independently with or without assistive device
0301	Self-Care: Bathing	Ability to cleanse own body independently with or without assistive device
0302	Self-Care: Dressing	Ability to dress self independently with or without assistive device
0303	Self-Care: Eating	Ability to prepare and ingest food and fluid independently with or without assistive device
0305	Self-Care: Hygiene	Ability to maintain own personal cleanliness and kempt appearance independently with or without assistive device
0306	Self-Care: Instrumental Activities of Daily Living (IADL)	Ability to perform activities needed to function in the home or community independently with or without assistive device
0307	Self-Care: Non-Parenteral Medication	Ability to administer oral and topical medications to meet therapeutic goals independently with or without assistive device
0308	Self-Care: Oral Hygiene	Ability to care for own mouth and teeth independently with or without assistive device
0309	Self-Care: Parenteral Medication	Ability to administer parenteral medications to meet therapeutic goals independently with or without assistive device
0310	Self-Care: Toileting	Ability to toilet self independently with or without assistive device
1613	Self-Direction of Care	Care recipient actions taken to direct others who assist with or perform physical tasks and personal health care
1205	Self-Esteem	Personal judgment of self-worth

NOC Outcome Label		Definition
1406	Self-Mutilation Restraint	Personal actions to refrain from intentional self-inflicted injury (nonlethal)
2405	Sensory Function	Extent to which an individual correctly senses skin stimulation, sounds, proprioception, taste and smell, and visual images
2400	Sensory Function: Cutaneous	Extent to which stimulation of the skin is correctly sensed
2401	Sensory Function: Hearing	Extent to which sounds are correctly sensed
2402	Sensory Function: Proprioception	Extent to which the position and movement of the head and body are correctly sensed
2403	Sensory Function: Taste & Smell	Extent to which chemicals inhaled or dissolved in saliva are correctly sensed
2404	Sensory Function: Vision	Extent to which visual images are correctly sensed
0119	Sexual Functioning	Integration of physical, socioemotional, and intellectual aspects of sexual expression and performance
1207	Sexual Identity	Acknowledgment and acceptance of own sexual identity
0211	Skeletal Function	Ability of the bones to support the body and facilitate movement
0004	Sleep	Natural periodic suspension of consciousness during which the body is restored
1625	Smoking Cessation Behavior	Personal actions to eliminate tobacco use
1502	Social Interaction Skills	Personal behaviors that promote effective relationships
1503	Social Involvement	Social interactions with persons, groups, or organizations
1504	Social Support	Reliable assistance from others
2001	Spiritual Health	Connectedness with self, others, higher power, all life, nature, and the universe that transcends and empowers the self
1212	Stress Level	Severity of manifested physical or mental tension resulting from factors that alter an existing equilibrium
2005	Student Health Status	Physical, cognitive, emotional, and social status of a school-age child
1407	Substance Addiction Consequences	Severity of change in health status and social functioning due to substance addiction
2108	Substance Withdrawal Severity	Severity of physical and psychological signs or symptoms caused by withdrawal from addictive drugs, toxic chemicals, tobacco, or alcohol
2003	Suffering Severity	Severity of anguish associated with a distressing symptom, injury, or loss that has potential long-term effects
1408	Suicide Self-Restraint	Personal actions to refrain from gestures and attempts at killing self
1010	Swallowing Status	Safe passage of fluids and/or solids from the mouth to the stomach
1011	Swallowing Status: Esophageal Phase	Safe passage of fluids and/or solids from the pharynx to the stomach
1012	Swallowing Status: Oral Phase	Preparation, containment, and posterior movement of fluids and/or solids in the mouth
1013	Swallowing Status: Pharyngeal Phase	Safe passage of fluids and/or solids from the mouth to the esophagus
1608	Symptom Control	Personal actions to minimize perceived adverse changes in physical and emotional functioning

Continued

PART IV - NOC

NOC Outcome Label		Definition
2103	Symptom Severity	Severity of perceived adverse changes in physical, emotional, and social functioning
2104	Symptom Severity: Perimenopause	Severity of symptoms caused by declining hormonal levels
2105	Symptom Severity: Premenstrual Syndrome (PMS)	Severity of symptoms caused by cyclic hormonal fluctuations
2302	Systemic Toxin Clearance: Dialysis	Clearance of toxins from the body with peritoneal dialysis or hemodialysis
0800	Thermoregulation	Balance among heat production, heat gain, and heat loss
0801	Thermoregulation: Newborn	Balance among heat production, heat gain, and heat loss during the first 28 days of life
1101	Tissue Integrity: Skin & Mucous Membranes	Structural intactness and normal physiological function of skin and mucous membranes
0404	Tissue Perfusion: Abdominal Organs	Adequacy of blood flow through the small vessels of the abdominal viscera to maintain organ function
0405	Tissue Perfusion: Cardiac	Adequacy of blood flow through the coronary vasculature to maintain heart function
0416	Tissue Perfusion: Cellular	Adequacy of blood flow through the vasculature to maintain function at the cellular level
0406	Tissue Perfusion: Cerebral	Adequacy of blood flow through the cerebral vasculature to maintain brain function
0407	Tissue Perfusion: Peripheral	Adequacy of blood flow through the small vessels of the extremities to maintain tissue function
0408	Tissue Perfusion: Pulmonary	Adequacy of blood flow through pulmonary vasculature to perfuse alveoli/capillary unit
0210	Transfer Performance	Ability to change body location independently with or without assistive device
1609	Treatment Behavior: Illness or Injury	Personal actions to palliate or eliminate pathology
0502	Urinary Continence	Control of elimination of urine from the bladder
0503	Urinary Elimination	Collection and discharge of urine
1611	Vision Compensation Behavior	Personal actions to compensate for visual impairment
0802	Vital Signs	Extent to which temperature, pulse, respiration, and blood pressure are within normal range
1006	Weight: Body Mass	Extent to which body weight, muscle, and fat are congruent to height, frame, gender, and age
1626	Weight Gain Behavior	Personal actions to gain weight following voluntary or involuntary significant weight loss
1627	Weight Loss Behavior	Personal actions to lose weight through diet, exercise, and behavior modification
1628	Weight Maintenance Behavior	Personal actions to maintain optimum body weight
1206	Will to Live	Desire, determination, and effort to survive
1102	Wound Healing: Primary Intention	Extent of regeneration of cells and tissue following intentional closure
1103	Wound Healing: Secondary Intention	Extent of regeneration of cells and tissue in an open wound

NIC Intervention Labels and Definitions

NIC Intervention Label		Definition
6400	Abuse Protection Support	Identification of high-risk dependent relationships and actions to prevent further infliction of physical or emotional harm
6402	Abuse Protection Support: Child	Identification of high-risk, dependent child relationships and actions to prevent possible or further infliction of physical, sexual, or emotional harm or neglect of basic necessities of life
6403	Abuse Protection Support: Domestic Partner	Identification of high-risk, dependent domestic relationships and actions to prevent possible or further infliction of physical, sexual, or emotional harm or exploitation of a domestic partner
6404	Abuse Protection Support: Elder	Identification of high-risk, dependent elder relationships and actions to prevent possible or further infliction of physical, sexual, or emotional harm; neglect of basic necessities of life; or exploitation
6408	Abuse Protection Support: Religious	Identification of high-risk, controlling religious relationships and actions to prevent infliction of physical, sexual, or emotional harm and/or exploitation
1910	Acid-Base Management	Promotion of acid-base balance and prevention of complications resulting from acid-base imbalance
1911	Acid-Base Management: Metabolic Acidosis	Promotion of acid-base balance and prevention of complications resulting from serum HCO_3 levels lower than desired
1912	Acid-Base Management: Metabolic Alkalosis	Promotion of acid-base balance and prevention of complications resulting from serum HCO_3 levels higher than desired
1913	Acid-Base Management: Respiratory Acidosis	Promotion of acid-base balance and prevention of complications resulting from serum PCO_2 levels higher than desired
1914	Acid-Base Management: Respiratory Alkalosis	Promotion of acid-base balance and prevention of complications resulting from serum PCO_2 levels lower than desired
1920	Acid-Base Monitoring	Collection and analysis of patient data to regulate acid-base balance
4920	Active Listening	Attending closely to and attaching significance to a patient's verbal and nonverbal messages
4310	Activity Therapy	Prescription of and assistance with specific physical, cognitive, social, and spiritual activities to increase the range, frequency, or duration of an individual's (or group's) activity

Continued

NIC Intervention Label		Definition
1320	Acupressure	Application of firm, sustained pressure to special points on the body to decrease pain, produce relaxation, and prevent or reduce nausea
7310	Admission Care	Facilitating entry of a patient into a health care facility
3120	Airway Insertion and Stabilization	Insertion or assistance with insertion and stabilization of an artificial airway
3140	Airway Management	Facilitation of patency of air passages
3160	Airway Suctioning	Removal of airway secretions by inserting a suction catheter into the patient's oral airway and/or trachea
6410	Allergy Management	Identification, treatment, and prevention of allergic responses to food, medications, insect bites, contrast material, blood, and other substances
6700	Amnioinfusion	Infusion of fluid into the uterus during labor to relieve umbilical cord compression or to dilute meconium-stained fluid
3420	Amputation Care	Promotion of physical and psychological healing before and after amputation of a body part
2210	Analgesic Administration	Use of pharmacological agents to reduce or eliminate pain
2214	Analgesic Administration: Intraspinal	Administration of pharmacological agents into the epidural or intrathecal space to reduce or eliminate pain
6412	Anaphylaxis Management	Promotion of adequate ventilation and tissue perfusion for an individual with a severe allergic (antigen-antibody) reaction
2840	Anesthesia Administration	Preparation for and administration of anesthetic agents and monitoring of patient responsiveness during administration
4640	Anger Control Assistance	Facilitation of the expression of anger in an adaptive, nonviolent manner
4320	Animal-Assisted Therapy	Purposeful use of animals to provide affection, attention, diversion, and relaxation
5210	Anticipatory Guidance	Preparation of patient for an anticipated developmental and/or situational crisis
5820	Anxiety Reduction	Minimizing apprehension, dread, foreboding, or uneasiness related to an unidentified source of anticipated danger
6420	Area Restriction	Use of least restrictive limitation of patient mobility to a specified area for purposes of safety or behavior management
1330	Aromatherapy	Administration of essential oils through massage, topical ointments or lotions, baths, inhalation, douches, or compresses (hot or cold) to calm and soothe, provide pain relief, and enhance relaxation and comfort
4330	Art Therapy	Facilitation of communication through drawings or other art forms
3180	Artificial Airway Management	Maintenance of endotracheal and tracheostomy tubes and prevention of complications associated with their use
3200	Aspiration Precautions	Prevention or minimization of risk factors in the patient at risk for aspiration
4340	Assertiveness Training	Assistance with the effective expression of feelings, needs, and ideas while respecting the rights of others
3210	Asthma Management	Identification, treatment, and prevention of reactions to inflammation/constriction in the airway passages

NIC Intervention Label | ## Definition

	NIC Intervention Label	Definition
6710	Attachment Promotion	Facilitation of the development of the parent-infant relationship
5840	Autogenic Training	Assisting with self-suggestions about feelings of heaviness and warmth for the purpose of inducing relaxation
2860	Autotransfusion	Collecting and reinfusing blood that has been lost intraoperatively or postoperatively from clean wounds
1610	Bathing	Cleaning of the body for the purposes of relaxation, cleanliness, and healing
0740	Bed Rest Care	Promotion of comfort and safety and prevention of complications for a patient unable to get out of bed
7610	Bedside Laboratory Testing	Performance of laboratory tests at the bedside or point of care
4350	Behavior Management	Helping a patient to manage negative behavior
4352	Behavior Management: Overactivity/Inattention	Provision of a therapeutic milieu that safely accommodates the patient's attention deficit and/or overactivity while promoting optimal function
4354	Behavior Management: Self-Harm	Assisting the patient to decrease or eliminate self-mutilating or self-abusive behaviors
4356	Behavior Management: Sexual	Delineation and prevention of socially unacceptable sexual behaviors
4360	Behavior Modification	Promotion of a behavior change
4362	Behavior Modification: Social Skills	Assisting the patient to develop or improve interpersonal social skills
4680	Bibliotherapy	Therapeutic use of literature to enhance the expression of feelings, active problem solving, coping, or insight
5860	Biofeedback	Assisting the patient to gain voluntary control over physiologic responses using feedback from electronic equipment that monitor physiological processes
8810	Bioterrorism Preparedness	Preparing for an effective response to bioterrorism events or disaster
6720	Birthing	Delivery of a baby
0550	Bladder Irrigation	Instillation of a solution into the bladder to provide cleansing or medication
4010	Bleeding Precautions	Reduction of stimuli that may induce bleeding or hemorrhage in at-risk patients
4020	Bleeding Reduction	Limitation of the loss of blood volume during an episode of bleeding
4021	Bleeding Reduction: Antepartum Uterus	Limitation of the amount of blood loss from the pregnant uterus during third trimester of pregnancy
4022	Bleeding Reduction: Gastrointestinal	Limitation of the amount of blood loss from the upper and lower gastrointestinal tract and related complications
4024	Bleeding Reduction: Nasal	Limitation of the amount of blood loss from the nasal cavity
4026	Bleeding Reduction: Postpartum Uterus	Limitation of the amount of blood loss from the postpartum uterus
4028	Bleeding Reduction: Wound	Limitation of the blood loss from a wound that may be a result of trauma, incisions, or placement of a tube or catheter
4030	Blood Products Administration	Administration of blood or blood products and monitoring of patient's response

Continued

NIC Intervention Label | Definition

NIC Intervention Label	Definition
5220 Body Image Enhancement	Improving a patient's conscious and unconscious perceptions and attitudes toward his/her body
0140 Body Mechanics Promotion	Facilitating the use of posture and movement in daily activities to prevent fatigue and musculoskeletal strain or injury
1052 Bottle Feeding	Preparation and administration of fluids to an infant via a bottle
0410 Bowel Incontinence Care	Promotion of bowel continence and maintenance of perianal skin integrity
0412 Bowel Incontinence Care: Encopresis	Promotion of bowel continence in children
0420 Bowel Irrigation	Instillation of a substance into the lower gastrointestinal tract
0430 Bowel Management	Establishment and maintenance of a regular pattern of bowel elimination
0440 Bowel Training	Assisting the patient to train the bowel to evacuate at specific intervals
6522 Breast Examination	Inspection and palpation of the breasts and related areas
1054 Breastfeeding Assistance	Preparing a new mother to breastfeed her infant
5880 Calming Technique	Reducing anxiety in patient experiencing acute distress
4035 Capillary Blood Sample	Obtaining an arteriovenous sample from a peripheral body site, such as the heel, finger, or other transcutaneous site
4040 Cardiac Care	Limitation of complications resulting from an imbalance between myocardial oxygen supply and demand for a patient with symptoms of impaired cardiac function
4044 Cardiac Care: Acute	Limitation of complications for a patient recently experiencing an episode of an imbalance between myocardial oxygen supply and demand resulting in impaired cardiac function
4046 Cardiac Care: Rehabilitative	Promotion of maximum functional activity level for a patient who has experienced an episode of impaired cardiac function that resulted from an imbalance between myocardial oxygen supply and demand
4050 Cardiac Precautions	Prevention of an acute episode of impaired cardiac function by minimizing myocardial oxygen consumption or increasing myocardial oxygen supply
7040 Caregiver Support	Provision of the necessary information, advocacy, and support to facilitate primary patient care by someone other than a health care professional
7320 Case Management	Coordinating care and advocating for specified individuals and patient populations across settings to reduce cost, reduce resource use, improve quality of health care, and achieve desired outcomes
0762 Cast Care: Maintenance	Care of a cast after the drying period
0764 Cast Care: Wet	Care of a new cast during the drying period
2540 Cerebral Edema Management	Limitation of secondary cerebral injury resulting from swelling of brain tissue
2550 Cerebral Perfusion Promotion	Promotion of adequate perfusion and limitation of complications for a patient experiencing or at risk for inadequate cerebral perfusion

NIC Intervention Label

Definition

6750	Cesarean Section Care	Preparation and support of patient delivering a baby by cesarean section
6430	Chemical Restraint	Administration, monitoring, and discontinuation of psychotropic agents used to control an individual's extreme behavior
2240	Chemotherapy Management	Assisting the patient and family to understand the action and minimize side effects of antineoplastic agents
3230	Chest Physiotherapy	Assisting the patient to move airway secretions from peripheral airways to more central airways for expectoration and/or suctioning
6760	Childbirth Preparation	Providing information and support to facilitate childbirth and to enhance the ability of an individual to develop and perform the parental role
4062	Circulatory Care: Arterial Insufficiency	Promotion of arterial circulation
4064	Circulatory Care: Mechanical Assist Device	Temporary support of the circulation through the use of mechanical devices or pumps
4066	Circulatory Care: Venous Insufficiency	Promotion of venous circulation
4070	Circulatory Precautions	Protection of a localized area with limited perfusion
3000	Circumcision Care	Preprocedural and postprocedural support to males undergoing circumcision
6140	Code Management	Coordination of emergency measures to sustain life
4700	Cognitive Restructuring	Challenging a patient to alter distorted thought patterns and view self and the world more realistically
4720	Cognitive Stimulation	Promotion of awareness and comprehension of surroundings by utilization of planned stimuli
8820	Communicable Disease Management	Working with a community to decrease and manage the incidence and prevalence of contagious diseases in a specific population
4974	Communication Enhancement: Hearing Deficit	Assistance in accepting and learning alternate methods for living with diminished hearing
4976	Communication Enhancement: Speech Deficit	Assistance in accepting and learning alternate methods for living with impaired speech
4978	Communication Enhancement: Visual Deficit	Assistance in accepting and learning alternate methods for living with diminished vision
8840	Community Disaster Preparedness	Preparing for an effective response to a large-scale disaster
8500	Community Health Development	Assisting members of a community to identify a community's health concerns, mobilize resources, and implement solutions
5000	Complex Relationship Building	Establishing a therapeutic relationship with a patient to promote insight and behavioral change
5020	Conflict Mediation	Facilitation of constructive dialogue between opposing parties with a goal of resolving disputes in a mutually acceptable manner
0450	Constipation/Impaction Management	Prevention and alleviation of constipation/impaction
7910	Consultation	Using expert knowledge to work with those who seek help in problem solving to enable individuals, families, groups, or agencies to achieve identified goals

Continued

PART IV - NIC

NIC Intervention Label	Definition
1620 Contact Lens Care	Prevention of eye injury and lens damage by proper use of contact lenses
7620 Controlled Substance Checking	Promoting appropriate use and maintaining security of controlled substances
5230 Coping Enhancement	Assisting a patient to adapt to perceived stressors, changes, or threats which interfere with meeting life demands and roles
7630 Cost Containment	Management and facilitation of efficient and effective use of resources
3250 Cough Enhancement	Promotion of deep inhalation by the patient with subsequent generation of high intrathoracic pressures and compression of underlying lung parenchyma for the forceful expulsion of air
5240 Counseling	Use of an interactive helping process focusing on the needs, problems, or feelings of the patient and significant others to enhance or support coping, problem solving, and interpersonal relationships
6160 Crisis Intervention	Use of short-term counseling to help the patient cope with a crisis and resume a state of functioning comparable to or better than the precrisis state
7640 Critical Path Development	Constructing and using a timed sequence of patient care activities to enhance desired patient outcomes in a cost-efficient manner
7330 Culture Brokerage	The deliberate use of culturally competent strategies to bridge or mediate between the patient's culture and the biomedical health care system
1340 Cutaneous Stimulation	Stimulation of the skin and underlying tissues for the purpose of decreasing undesirable signs and symptoms such as pain, muscle spasm, or inflammation
5250 Decision-Making Support	Providing information and support for a patient who is making a decision regarding health care
4095 Defibrillator Management: External	Care of the patient receiving defibrillation for termination of life-threatening cardiac rhythm disturbances
4096 Defibrillator Management: Internal	Care of the patient receiving permanent detection and termination of life-threatening cardiac rhythm disturbances through the insertion and use of an internal cardiac defibrillator
7650 Delegation	Transfer of responsibility for the performance of patient care while retaining accountability for the outcome
6440 Delirium Management	Provision of a safe and therapeutic environment for the patient who is experiencing an acute confusional state
6450 Delusion Management	Promoting the comfort, safety, and reality orientation of a patient experiencing false, fixed beliefs that have little or no basis in reality
6460 Dementia Management	Provision of a modified environment for the patient who is experiencing a chronic confusional state
6462 Dementia Management: Bathing	Reduction of aggressive behavior during cleaning of the body
7930 Deposition/Testimony	Provision of recorded sworn testimony for legal proceedings based upon knowledge of the case
8250 Developmental Care	Structuring the environment and providing care in response to the behavioral cues and states of the preterm infant

NIC Intervention Label   Definition

8272	Developmental Enhancement: Adolescent	Facilitating optimal physical, cognitive, social, and emotional growth of individuals during the transition from childhood to adulthood
8274	Developmental Enhancement: Child	Facilitating or teaching parents/caregivers to facilitate the optimal gross motor, fine motor, language, cognitive, social, and emotional growth of preschool and school-aged children
4240	Dialysis Access Maintenance	Preservation of vascular (arterial-venous) access sites
0460	Diarrhea Management	Management and alleviation of diarrhea
1020	Diet Staging	Instituting required diet restrictions with subsequent progression of diet as tolerated
7370	Discharge Planning	Preparation for moving a patient from one level of care to another within or outside the current health care agency
5900	Distraction	Purposeful focusing of attention away from undesirable sensations
7920	Documentation	Recording of pertinent patient data in a clinical record
1630	Dressing	Choosing, putting on, and removing clothes for a person who cannot do this for self
5260	Dying Care	Promotion of physical comfort and psychological peace in the final phase of life
2560	Dysreflexia Management	Prevention and elimination of stimuli that cause hyperactive reflexes and inappropriate autonomic responses in a patient with a cervical or high thoracic cord lesion
4090	Dysrhythmia Management	Preventing, recognizing, and facilitating treatment of abnormal cardiac rhythms
1640	Ear Care	Prevention or minimization of threats to ear or hearing
1030	Eating Disorders Management	Prevention and treatment of severe diet restriction and overexercising or binging and purging of food and fluids
2570	Electroconvulsive Therapy (ECT) Management	Assisting with the safe and efficient provision of electroconvulsive therapy in the treatment of psychiatric illness
2000	Electrolyte Management	Promotion of electrolyte balance and prevention of complications resulting from abnormal or undesired serum electrolyte levels
2001	Electrolyte Management: Hypercalcemia	Promotion of calcium balance and prevention of complications resulting from serum calcium levels higher than desired
2002	Electrolyte Management: Hyperkalemia	Promotion of potassium balance and prevention of complications resulting from serum potassium levels higher than desired
2003	Electrolyte Management: Hypermagnesemia	Promotion of magnesium balance and prevention of complications resulting from serum magnesium levels higher than desired
2004	Electrolyte Management: Hypernatremia	Promotion of sodium balance and prevention of complications resulting from serum sodium levels higher than desired
2005	Electrolyte Management: Hyperphosphatemia	Promotion of phosphate balance and prevention of complications resulting from serum phosphate levels higher than desired

PART IV - NIC

Continued

NIC Intervention Label		Definition
2006	Electrolyte Management: Hypocalcemia	Promotion of calcium balance and prevention of complications resulting from serum calcium levels lower than desired
2007	Electrolyte Management: Hypokalemia	Promotion of potassium balance and prevention of complications resulting from serum potassium levels lower than desired
2008	Electrolyte Management: Hypomagnesemia	Promotion of magnesium balance and prevention of complications resulting from serum magnesium levels lower than desired
2009	Electrolyte Management: Hyponatremia	Promotion of sodium balance and prevention of complications resulting from serum sodium levels lower than desired
2010	Electrolyte Management: Hypophosphatemia	Promotion of phosphate balance and prevention of complications resulting from serum phosphate levels lower than desired
2020	Electrolyte Monitoring	Collection and analysis of patient data to regulate electrolyte balance
6771	Electronic Fetal Monitoring: Antepartum	Electronic evaluation of fetal heart rate response to movement, external stimuli, or uterine contractions during antepartal testing
6772	Electronic Fetal Monitoring: Intrapartum	Electronic evaluation of fetal heart rate response to uterine contractions during intrapartal care
6470	Elopement Precautions	Minimizing the risk of a patient leaving a treatment setting without authorization when departure presents a threat to the safety of patient or others
4104	Embolus Care: Peripheral	Limitation of complications for a patient experiencing, or at risk for, occlusion of peripheral circulation
4106	Embolus Care: Pulmonary	Limitation of complications for a patient experiencing, or at risk for, occlusion of pulmonary circulation
4110	Embolus Precautions	Reduction of the risk of an embolus in a patient with thrombi or at risk for thrombus formation
6200	Emergency Care	Providing life-saving measures in life-threatening situations
7660	Emergency Cart Checking	Systematic review and maintenance of the contents of an emergency cart at established time intervals
5270	Emotional Support	Provision of reassurance, acceptance, and encouragement during times of stress
3270	Endotracheal Extubation	Purposeful removal of the endotracheal tube from the nasopharyngeal or oropharyngeal airway
0180	Energy Management	Regulating energy use to treat or prevent fatigue and optimize function
1056	Enteral Tube Feeding	Delivering nutrients and water through a gastrointestinal tube
6480	Environmental Management	Manipulation of the patient's surroundings for therapeutic benefit, sensory appeal, and psychological well-being
6481	Environmental Management: Attachment Process	Manipulation of the patient's surroundings to facilitate the development of the parent-infant relationship
6482	Environmental Management: Comfort	Manipulation of the patient's surroundings for promotion of optimal comfort
6484	Environmental Management: Community	Monitoring and influencing of the physical, social, cultural, economic, and political conditions that affect the health of groups and communities

NIC Intervention Label | Definition

	NIC Intervention Label	Definition
6485	Environmental Management: Home Preparation	Preparing the home for safe and effective delivery of care
6486	Environmental Management: Safety	Monitoring and manipulation of the physical environment to promote safety
6487	Environmental Management: Violence Prevention	Monitoring and manipulation of the physical environment to decrease the potential for violent behavior directed toward self, others, or environment
6489	Environmental Management: Worker Safety	Monitoring and manipulation of the worksite environment to promote safety and health of workers
8880	Environmental Risk Protection	Preventing and detecting disease and injury in populations at risk from environmental hazards
7680	Examination Assistance	Providing assistance to the patient and another health care provider during a procedure or exam
0200	Exercise Promotion	Facilitation of regular physical activity to maintain or advance to a higher level of fitness and health
0201	Exercise Promotion: Strength Training	Facilitating regular resistive muscle training to maintain or increase muscle strength
0202	Exercise Promotion: Stretching	Facilitation of systematic slow-stretch-hold muscle exercises to induce relaxation, to prepare muscles/joints for more vigorous exercise, or to increase or maintain body flexibility
0221	Exercise Therapy: Ambulation	Promotion and assistance with walking to maintain or restore autonomic and voluntary body functions during treatment and recovery from illness or injury
0222	Exercise Therapy: Balance	Use of specific activities, postures, and movements to maintain, enhance, or restore balance
0224	Exercise Therapy: Joint Mobility	Use of active or passive body movement to maintain or restore joint flexibility
0226	Exercise Therapy: Muscle Control	Use of specific activity or exercise protocols to enhance or restore controlled body movement
1650	Eye Care	Prevention or minimization of threats to eye or visual integrity
6490	Fall Prevention	Instituting special precautions with patient at risk for injury from falling
7100	Family Integrity Promotion	Promotion of family cohesion and unity
7104	Family Integrity Promotion: Childbearing Family	Facilitation of the growth of individuals or families who are adding an infant to the family unit
7110	Family Involvement Promotion	Facilitating participation of family members in the emotional and physical care of the patient
7120	Family Mobilization	Utilization of family strengths to influence patient's health in a positive direction
6784	Family Planning: Contraception	Facilitation of pregnancy prevention by providing information about the physiology of reproduction and methods to control conception
6786	Family Planning: Infertility	Management, education, and support of the patient and significant other undergoing evaluation and treatment for infertility
6788	Family Planning: Unplanned Pregnancy	Facilitation of decision-making regarding pregnancy outcome
7170	Family Presence Facilitation	Facilitation of the family's presence in support of an individual undergoing resuscitation and/or invasive procedures

Continued

PART IV · NIC

NIC Intervention Label		Definition
7130	Family Process Maintenance	Minimization of family process disruption effects
7140	Family Support	Promotion of family values, interests, and goals
7150	Family Therapy	Assisting family members to move their family toward a more productive way of living
1050	Feeding	Providing nutritional intake for patient who is unable to feed self
7160	Fertility Preservation	Providing information, counseling, and treatment that facilitate reproductive health and the ability to conceive
3740	Fever Treatment	Management of a patient with hyperpyrexia caused by nonenvironmental factors
7380	Financial Resource Assistance	Assisting an individual/family to secure and manage finances to meet health care needs
6500	Fire-Setting Precautions	Prevention of fire-setting behaviors
6240	First Aid	Providing initial care for a minor injury
8550	Fiscal Resource Management	Procuring and directing the use of financial resources to ensure the development and continuation of programs and services
0470	Flatulence Reduction	Prevention of flatus formation and facilitation of passage of excessive gas
2080	Fluid/Electrolyte Management	Regulation and prevention of complications from altered fluid and/or electrolyte levels
4120	Fluid Management	Promotion of fluid balance and prevention of complications resulting from abnormal or undesired fluid levels
4130	Fluid Monitoring	Collection and analysis of patient data to regulate fluid balance
4140	Fluid Resuscitation	Administering prescribed intravenous fluids rapidly
1660	Foot Care	Cleansing and inspecting the feet for the purposes of relaxation, cleanliness, and healthy skin
7940	Forensic Data Collection	Collection and recording of pertinent patient data for a forensic report
5280	Forgiveness Facilitation	Assisting an individual's willingness to replace feeling of anger and resentment toward another, self, or higher power, with beneficence, empathy, and humility
1080	Gastrointestinal Intubation	Insertion of a tube into the gastrointestinal tract
5242	Genetic Counseling	Use of an interactive helping process focusing on assisting an individual, family, or group, manifesting or at risk for developing or transmitting a birth defect or genetic condition, to cope
5290	Grief Work Facilitation	Assistance with the resolution of a significant loss
5294	Grief Work Facilitation: Perinatal Death	Assistance with the resolution of a perinatal loss
6000	Guided Imagery	Purposeful use of imagination to achieve a particular state, outcome, or action or to direct attention away from undesirable sensations
5300	Guilt Work Facilitation	Helping another to cope with painful feelings of actual or perceived responsibility
1670	Hair Care	Promotion of neat, clean, attractive hair

NIC Intervention Label		Definition
6510	Hallucination Management	Promoting the safety, comfort, and reality orientation of a patient experiencing hallucinations
7960	Health Care Information Exchange	Providing patient care information to other health professionals
5510	Health Education	Developing and providing instruction and learning experiences to facilitate voluntary adaptation of behavior conducive to health in individuals, families, groups, or communities
5515	Health Literacy Enhancement	Assisting individuals with limited ability to obtain, process, and understand information related to health and illness
7970	Health Policy Monitoring	Surveillance and influence of government and organization regulations, rules, and standards that affect nursing systems and practices to ensure quality care of patients
6520	Health Screening	Detecting health risks or problems by means of history, examination, and other procedures
7400	Health System Guidance	Facilitating a patient's location and use of appropriate health services
1380	Heat/Cold Application	Stimulation of the skin and underlying tissues with heat or cold for the purpose of decreasing pain, muscle spasms, or inflammation
3780	Heat Exposure Treatment	Management of patient overcome by heat due to excessive environmental heat exposure
2100	Hemodialysis Therapy	Management of extracorporeal passage of the patient's blood through a dialyzer
4150	Hemodynamic Regulation	Optimization of heart rate, preload, afterload, and contractility
2110	Hemofiltration Therapy	Cleansing of acutely ill patient's blood via a hemofilter controlled by the patient's hydrostatic pressure
4160	Hemorrhage Control	Reduction or elimination of rapid and excessive blood loss
6800	High-Risk Pregnancy Care	Identification and management of a high-risk pregnancy to promote healthy outcomes for mother and baby
7180	Home Maintenance Assistance	Helping the patient/family to maintain the home as a clean, safe, and pleasant place to live
5310	Hope Inspiration	Enhancing the belief in one's capacity to initiate and sustain actions
2280	Hormone Replacement Therapy	Facilitation of safe and effective use of hormone replacement therapy
5320	Humor	Facilitating the patient to perceive, appreciate, and express what is funny, amusing, or ludicrous in order to establish relationships, relieve tension, release anger, facilitate learning, or cope with painful feelings
2120	Hyperglycemia Management	Preventing and treating above-normal blood glucose levels
4170	Hypervolemia Management	Reduction in extracellular and/or intracellular fluid volume and prevention of complications in a patient who is fluid overloaded
5920	Hypnosis	Assisting a patient to achieve a state of attentive, focused concentration with suspension of some peripheral awareness to create changes in sensation, thoughts, or behavior

Continued

NIC Intervention Label		Definition
2130	Hypoglycemia Management	Preventing and treating low blood glucose levels
3790	Hypothermia Induction Therapy	Attaining and maintaining core body temperature below 35° C and monitoring for side effects and/or prevention of complications
3800	Hypothermia Treatment	Rewarming and surveillance of a patient whose core body temperature is below 35° C
4180	Hypovolemia Management	Expansion of intravascular fluid volume in a patient who is volume depleted
6530	Immunization/Vaccination Management	Monitoring immunization status, facilitating access to immunizations, and providing immunizations to prevent communicable disease
4370	Impulse Control Training	Assisting the patient to mediate impulsive behavior through application of problem-solving strategies to social and interpersonal situations
7980	Incident Reporting	Written and verbal reporting of any event in the process of patient care that is inconsistent with desired patient outcomes or routine operations of the health care facility
3440	Incision Site Care	Cleansing, monitoring, and promotion of healing in a wound that is closed with sutures, clips, or staples
6820	Infant Care	Provision of developmentally appropriate family-centered care to the child under 1 year of age
6540	Infection Control	Minimizing the acquisition and transmission of infectious agents
6545	Infection Control: Intraoperative	Preventing nosocomial infection in the operating room
6550	Infection Protection	Prevention and early detection of infection in a patient at risk
7410	Insurance Authorization	Assisting the patient and provider to secure payment for health services or equipment from a third party
2590	Intracranial Pressure (ICP) Monitoring	Measurement and interpretation of patient data to regulate intracranial pressure
6830	Intrapartal Care	Monitoring and management of stages one and two of the birth process
6834	Intrapartal Care: High-Risk Delivery	Assisting with vaginal delivery of multiple or malpositioned fetuses
4190	Intravenous (IV) Insertion	Insertion of a needle into a peripheral vein for the purpose of administering fluids, blood, or medications
4200	Intravenous (IV) Therapy	Administration and monitoring of intravenous fluids and medications
4210	Invasive Hemodynamic Monitoring	Measurement and interpretation of invasive hemodynamic parameters to determine cardiovascular function and regulate therapy as appropriate
4740	Journaling	Promotion of writing as a means to provide opportunities to reflect upon and analyze past events, experiences, thoughts, and feelings
6840	Kangaroo Care	Promoting closeness between parent and physiologically stable preterm infant by preparing the parent and providing the environment for skin-to-skin contact
6850	Labor Induction	Initiation or augmentation of labor by mechanical or pharmacological methods
6860	Labor Suppression	Controlling uterine contractions prior to 37 weeks of gestation to prevent preterm birth

NIC Intervention Label | Definition

NIC Intervention Label		Definition
7690	Laboratory Data Interpretation	Critical analysis of patient laboratory data in order to assist with clinical decision-making
5244	Lactation Counseling	Use of an interactive helping process to assist in maintenance of successful breastfeeding
6870	Lactation Suppression	Facilitating the cessation of milk production and minimizing breast engorgement after giving birth
6560	Laser Precautions	Limiting the risk of laser-related injury to the patient
6570	Latex Precautions	Reducing the risk of systemic reaction to latex
5520	Learning Facilitation	Promoting the ability to process and comprehend information
5540	Learning Readiness Enhancement	Improving the ability and willingness to receive information
3460	Leech Therapy	Application of medicinal leeches to help drain replanted or transplanted tissue engorged with venous blood
4380	Limit Setting	Establishing the parameters of desirable and acceptable patient behavior
3480	Lower Extremity Monitoring	Collection, analysis, and use of patient data to categorize risk and prevent injury to the lower extremities
3840	Malignant Hyperthermia Precautions	Prevention or reduction of hypermetabolic response to pharmacological agents used during surgery
1480	Massage	Stimulation of the skin and underlying tissues with varying degrees of hand pressure to decrease pain, produce relaxation, and/or improve circulation
3300	Mechanical Ventilation Management: Invasive	Assisting the patient receiving artificial breathing support through a device inserted into the trachea
3302	Mechanical Ventilation Management: Noninvasive	Assisting the patient receiving artificial breathing support which does not necessitate a device inserted into the trachea
3310	Mechanical Ventilatory Weaning	Assisting the patient to breathe without the aid of a mechanical ventilator
2300	Medication Administration	Preparing, giving, and evaluating the effectiveness of prescription and nonprescription drugs
2308	Medication Administration: Ear	Preparing and instilling otic medications
2301	Medication Administration: Enteral	Delivering medications through a tube inserted into the gastrointestinal system
2310	Medication Administration: Eye	Preparing and instilling ophthalmic medications
2311	Medication Administration: Inhalation	Preparing and administering inhaled medications
2302	Medication Administration: Interpleural	Administration of medication through an interpleural catheter for reduction of pain
2312	Medication Administration: Intradermal	Preparing and giving medications via the intradermal route
2313	Medication Administration: Intramuscular (IM)	Preparing and giving medications via the intramuscular route
2303	Medication Administration: Intraosseous	Insertion of a needle through the bone cortex into the medullary cavity for the purpose of short-term, emergency administration of fluid, blood, or medication
2319	Medication Administration: Intraspinal	Administration and monitoring of medication via an established epidural or intrathecal route
2314	Medication Administration: Intravenous (IV)	Preparing and giving medications via the intravenous route

Continued

NIC Intervention Label

Definition

2320	Medication Administration: Nasal	Preparing and giving medications via nasal passages
2304	Medication Administration: Oral	Preparing and giving medications by mouth
2315	Medication Administration: Rectal	Preparing and inserting rectal suppositories
2316	Medication Administration: Skin	Preparing and applying medications to the skin
2317	Medication Administration: Subcutaneous	Preparing and giving medications via the subcutaneous route
2318	Medication Administration: Vaginal	Preparing and inserting vaginal medications
2307	Medication Administration: Ventricular Reservoir	Administration and monitoring of medication through an indwelling catheter into the lateral ventricle of the brain
2380	Medication Management	Facilitation of safe and effective use of prescription and over-the-counter drugs
2390	Medication Prescribing	Prescribing medication for a health problem
2395	Medication Reconciliation	Comparison of the patient's home medications with the admission, transfer, and/or discharge orders to ensure accuracy and patient safety
5960	Meditation Facilitation	Facilitating a person to alter his/her level of awareness by focusing specifically on an image or thought
4760	Memory Training	Facilitation of memory
4390	Milieu Therapy	Use of people, resources, and events in the patient's immediate environment to promote optimal psychosocial functioning
5330	Mood Management	Providing for safety, stabilization, recovery, and maintenance of a patient who is experiencing dysfunctionally depressed or elevated mood
8020	Multidisciplinary Care Conference	Planning and evaluating patient care with health professionals from other disciplines
4400	Music Therapy	Using music to help achieve a specific change in behavior, feeling, or physiology
4410	Mutual Goal Setting	Collaborating with patient to identify and prioritize care goals, then developing a plan for achieving those goals
1680	Nail Care	Promotion of clean, neat, attractive nails and prevention of skin lesions related to improper care of nails
1450	Nausea Management	Prevention and alleviation of nausea
2620	Neurologic Monitoring	Collection and analysis of patient data to prevent or minimize neurologic complications
6880	Newborn Care	Management of neonate during the transition to extrauterine life and subsequent period of stabilization
6890	Newborn Monitoring	Measurement and interpretation of physiologic status of the neonate for the first 24 hours after delivery
6900	Nonnutritive Sucking	Provision of sucking opportunities for the infant
7200	Normalization Promotion	Assisting parents and other family members of children with chronic illnesses or disabilities in providing normal life experiences for their children and families
1100	Nutrition Management	Assisting with or providing a balanced dietary intake of foods and fluids
1120	Nutrition Therapy	Administration of food and fluids to support metabolic processes of a patient who is malnourished or at high risk for becoming malnourished
5246	Nutritional Counseling	Use of an interactive helping process focusing on the need for diet modification

NIC Intervention Label

Definition

1160	Nutritional Monitoring	Collection and analysis of patient data to prevent or minimize malnourishment
1710	Oral Health Maintenance	Maintenance and promotion of oral hygiene and dental health for the patient at risk for developing oral or dental lesions
1720	Oral Health Promotion	Promotion of oral hygiene and dental care for a patient with normal oral and dental health
1730	Oral Health Restoration	Promotion of healing for a patient who has an oral mucosa or dental lesion
8060	Order Transcription	Transferring information from order sheets to the nursing patient care planning and documentation system
6260	Organ Procurement	Guiding families through the donation process to ensure timely retrieval of vital organs and tissue for transplant
0480	Ostomy Care	Maintenance of elimination through a stoma and care of surrounding tissue
3320	Oxygen Therapy	Administration of oxygen and monitoring of its effectiveness
4091	Pacemaker Management: Permanent	Care of the patient receiving permanent support of cardiac pumping through the insertion and use of a pacemaker
4092	Pacemaker Management: Temporary	Temporary support of cardiac pumping through the insertion and use of temporary pacemakers
1400	Pain Management	Alleviation of pain or a reduction in pain to a level of comfort that is acceptable to the patient
5562	Parent Education: Adolescent	Assisting parents to understand and help their adolescent children
5566	Parent Education: Childrearing Family	Assisting parents to understand and promote the physical, psychological, and social growth and development of their toddler, preschool, or school-aged child/children
5568	Parent Education: Infant	Instruction on nurturing and physical care needed during the first year of life
8300	Parenting Promotion	Providing parenting information, support, and coordination of comprehensive services to high-risk families
7440	Pass Facilitation	Arranging a leave for a patient from a health care facility
4420	Patient Contracting	Negotiating an agreement with an individual that reinforces a specific behavior change
2400	Patient-Controlled Analgesia (PCA) Assistance	Facilitating patient control of analgesic administration and regulation
7460	Patient Rights Protection	Protection of health care rights of a patient, especially a minor, incapacitated, or incompetent patient unable to make decisions
7700	Peer Review	Systematic evaluation of a peer's performance compared with professional standards of practice
0560	Pelvic Muscle Exercise	Strengthening and training the levator ani and urogenital muscles through voluntary, repetitive contraction to decrease stress, urge, or mixed types of urinary incontinence
1750	Perineal Care	Maintenance of perineal skin integrity and relief of perineal discomfort
2660	Peripheral Sensation Management	Prevention or minimization of injury or discomfort in the patient with altered sensation
4220	Peripherally Inserted Central (PIC) Catheter Care	Insertion and maintenance of a peripherally inserted catheter either midline or centrally located

Continued

PART IV - NIC

NIC Intervention Label		Definition
2150	Peritoneal Dialysis Therapy	Administration and monitoring of dialysis solution into and out of the peritoneal cavity
0630	Pessary Management	Placement and monitoring of a vaginal device for treating stress urinary incontinence, uterine retroversion, genital prolapse, or incompetent cervix
4232	Phlebotomy: Arterial Blood Sample	Obtaining a blood sample from an uncannulated artery to assess oxygen and carbon dioxide levels and acid-base balance
4234	Phlebotomy: Blood Unit Acquisition	Procuring blood and blood products from donors
4235	Phlebotomy: Cannulated Vessel	Aspirating a blood sample through an indwelling vascular catheter for laboratory tests
4238	Phlebotomy: Venous Blood Sample	Removal of a sample of venous blood from an uncannulated vein
6926	Phototherapy: Mood/Sleep Regulation	Administration of doses of bright light in order to elevate mood and/or normalize the body's internal clock
6924	Phototherapy: Neonate	Use of light therapy to reduce bilirubin levels in newborn infants
6580	Physical Restraint	Application, monitoring, and removal of mechanical restraining devices or manual restraints used to limit physical mobility of a patient
7710	Physician Support	Collaborating with physicians to provide quality patient care
6590	Pneumatic Tourniquet Precautions	Applying a pneumatic tourniquet, while minimizing the potential for patient injury from use of the device
0840	Positioning	Deliberative placement of the patient or a body part to promote physiological and/or psychological well-being
0842	Positioning: Intraoperative	Moving the patient or body part to promote surgical exposure while reducing the risk of discomfort and complications
0844	Positioning: Neurologic	Achievement of optimal, appropriate body alignment for the patient experiencing or at risk for spinal cord injury or vertebral irritability
0846	Positioning: Wheelchair	Placement of a patient in a properly selected wheelchair to enhance comfort, promote skin integrity, and foster independence
2870	Postanesthesia Care	Monitoring and management of the patient who has recently undergone general or regional anesthesia
1770	Postmortem Care	Providing physical care of the body of an expired patient and support for the family viewing the body
6930	Postpartal Care	Monitoring and management of the patient who has recently given birth
7722	Preceptor: Employee	Assisting and supporting a new or transferred employee through a planned orientation to a specific clinical area
7726	Preceptor: Student	Assisting and supporting learning experiences for a student
5247	Preconception Counseling	Screening and providing information and support to individuals of childbearing age before pregnancy to promote health and reduce risks

NIC Intervention Label / Definition

	NIC Intervention Label	Definition
6950	Pregnancy Termination Care	Management of the physical and psychological needs of the woman undergoing a spontaneous or elective abortion
1440	Premenstrual Syndrome (PMS) Management	Alleviation/attenuation of physical and/or behavioral symptoms occurring during the luteal phase of the menstrual cycle
6960	Prenatal Care	Monitoring and management of patient during pregnancy to prevent complications of pregnancy and promote a healthy outcome for both mother and infant
2880	Preoperative Coordination	Facilitating preadmission diagnostic testing and preparation of the surgical patient
5580	Preparatory Sensory Information	Describing in concrete and objective terms the typical sensory experiences and events associated with an upcoming stressful health care procedure/treatment
5340	Presence	Being with another, both physically and psychologically, during times of need
3500	Pressure Management	Minimizing pressure to body parts
3520	Pressure Ulcer Care	Facilitation of healing in pressure ulcers
3540	Pressure Ulcer Prevention	Prevention of pressure ulcers for an individual at high risk for developing them
7760	Product Evaluation	Determining the effectiveness of new products or equipment
8700	Program Development	Planning, implementing, and evaluating a coordinated set of activities designed to enhance wellness, or to prevent, reduce, or eliminate one or more health problems for a group or community
1460	Progressive Muscle Relaxation	Facilitating the tensing and releasing of successive muscle groups while attending to the resulting differences in sensation
0640	Prompted Voiding	Promotion of urinary continence through the use of timed verbal toileting reminders and positive social feedback for successful toileting
1780	Prosthesis Care	Care of a removable appliance worn by a patient and the prevention of complications associated with its use
3550	Pruritus Management	Preventing and treating itching
7800	Quality Monitoring	Systematic collection and analysis of an organization's quality indicators for the purpose of improving patient care
6600	Radiation Therapy Management	Assisting the patient to understand and minimize the side effects of radiation treatments
6300	Rape-Trauma Treatment	Provision of emotional and physical support immediately following a reported rape
4820	Reality Orientation	Promotion of patient's awareness of personal identity, time, and environment
5360	Recreation Therapy	Purposeful use of recreation to promote relaxation and enhancement of social skills
0490	Rectal Prolapse Management	Prevention and/or manual reduction of rectal prolapse
8100	Referral	Arrangement for services by another care provider or agency
6040	Relaxation Therapy	Use of techniques to encourage and elicit relaxation for the purpose of decreasing undesirable signs and symptoms such as pain, muscle tension, or anxiety

Continued

PART IV - NIC

NIC Intervention Label	Definition
5422 Religious Addiction Prevention	Prevention of a self-imposed controlling religious lifestyle
5424 Religious Ritual Enhancement	Facilitating participation in religious practices
5350 Relocation Stress Reduction	Assisting the individual to prepare for and cope with movement from one environment to another
4860 Reminiscence Therapy	Using the recall of past events, feelings, and thoughts to facilitate pleasure, quality of life, or adaptation to present circumstances
7886 Reproductive Technology Management	Assisting a patient through the steps of complex infertility treatment
8120 Research Data Collection	Collecting research data
8340 Resiliency Promotion	Assisting individuals, families, and communities in development, use, and strengthening of protective factors to be used in coping with environmental and societal stressors
3350 Respiratory Monitoring	Collection and analysis of patient data to ensure airway patency and adequate gas exchange
7260 Respite Care	Provision of short-term care to provide relief for family caregiver
6320 Resuscitation	Administering emergency measures to sustain life
6972 Resuscitation: Fetus	Administering emergency measures to improve placental perfusion or correct fetal acid-base status
6974 Resuscitation: Neonate	Administering emergency measures to support newborn adaptation to extrauterine life
6610 Risk Identification	Analysis of potential risk factors, determination of health risks, and prioritization of risk reduction strategies for an individual or group
6612 Risk Identification: Childbearing Family	Identification of an individual or family likely to experience difficulties in parenting, and prioritization of strategies to prevent parenting problems
6614 Risk Identification: Genetic	Identification and analysis of potential genetic risk factors in an individual, family, or group
5370 Role Enhancement	Assisting a patient, significant other, and/or family to improve relationships by clarifying and supplementing specific role behaviors
6630 Seclusion	Solitary containment in a fully protective environment with close surveillance by nursing staff for purposes of safety or behavior management
5380 Security Enhancement	Intensifying a patient's sense of physical and psychological safety
2260 Sedation Management	Administration of sedatives, monitoring of the patient's response, and provision of necessary physiological support during a diagnostic or therapeutic procedure
2680 Seizure Management	Care of a patient during a seizure and the postictal state
2690 Seizure Precautions	Prevention or minimization of potential injuries sustained by a patient with a known seizure disorder
5390 Self-Awareness Enhancement	Assisting a patient to explore and understand his/her thoughts, feelings, motivations, and behaviors
1800 Self-Care Assistance	Assisting another to perform activities of daily living
1801 Self-Care Assistance: Bathing/Hygiene	Assisting patient to perform personal hygiene

NIC Intervention Label

Definition

1802	Self-Care Assistance: Dressing/Grooming	Assisting patient with clothes and appearance
1803	Self-Care Assistance: Feeding	Assisting a person to eat
1805	Self-Care Assistance: IADL	Assisting and instructing a person to perform instrumental activities of daily living (IADL) needed to function in the home or community
1804	Self-Care Assistance: Toileting	Assisting another with elimination
1806	Self-Care Assistance: Transfer	Assisting a patient with limitation of independent movement to learn to change body location
5395	Self-Efficacy Enhancement	Strengthening an individual's confidence in his/her ability to perform a health behavior
5400	Self-Esteem Enhancement	Assisting a patient to increase his/her personal judgment of self-worth
5922	Self-Hypnosis Facilitation	Teaching and monitoring the use of a self-initiated hypnotic state for therapeutic benefit
4470	Self-Modification Assistance	Reinforcement of self-directed change initiated by the patient to achieve personally important goals
4480	Self-Responsibility Facilitation	Encouraging a patient to assume more responsibility for own behavior
5248	Sexual Counseling	Use of an interactive helping process focusing on the need to make adjustments in sexual practice or to enhance coping with a sexual event/disorder
8140	Shift Report	Exchanging essential patient care information with other nursing staff at change of shift
4250	Shock Management	Facilitation of the delivery of oxygen and nutrients to systemic tissue with removal of cellular waste products in a patient with severely altered tissue perfusion
4254	Shock Management: Cardiac	Promotion of adequate tissue perfusion for a patient with severely compromised pumping function of the heart
4256	Shock Management: Vasogenic	Promotion of adequate tissue perfusion for a patient with severe loss of vascular tone
4258	Shock Management: Volume	Promotion of adequate tissue perfusion for a patient with severely compromised intravascular volume
4260	Shock Prevention	Detecting and treating a patient at risk for impending shock
7280	Sibling Support	Assisting a sibling to cope with a brother or sister's illness/chronic condition/disability
3582	Skin Care: Donor Site	Prevention of wound complications and promotion of healing at the donor site
3583	Skin Care: Graft Site	Prevention of wound complications and promotion of graft site healing
3584	Skin Care: Topical Treatments	Application of topical substances or manipulation of devices to promote skin integrity and minimize skin breakdown
3590	Skin Surveillance	Collection and analysis of patient data to maintain skin and mucous membrane integrity
1850	Sleep Enhancement	Facilitation of regular sleep/wake cycles
4490	Smoking Cessation Assistance	Helping another to stop smoking
8750	Social Marketing	Use of marketing principles to influence the health beliefs, attitudes, and behaviors to benefit a target population

Continued

PART IV - NIC

NIC Intervention Label		Definition
5100	Socialization Enhancement	Facilitation of another person's ability to interact with others
7820	Specimen Management	Obtaining, preparing, and preserving a specimen for a laboratory test
5426	Spiritual Growth Facilitation	Facilitation of growth in patients capacity to identify, connect with, and call upon the source of meaning, purpose, comfort, strength, and hope in their lives
5420	Spiritual Support	Assisting the patient to feel balance and connection with a greater power
0910	Splinting	Stabilization, immobilization, and/or protection of an injured body part with a supportive appliance
6648	Sports-Injury Prevention: Youth	Reduce the risk of sports-related injury in young athletes
7850	Staff Development	Developing, maintaining, and monitoring competence of staff
7830	Staff Supervision	Facilitating the delivery of high-quality patient care by others
2720	Subarachnoid Hemorrhage Precautions	Reduction of internal and external stimuli or stressors to minimize risk of rebleeding prior to surgery or endovascular procedure to secure ruptured aneurysm
4500	Substance Use Prevention	Prevention of an alcoholic or drug use lifestyle
4510	Substance Use Treatment	Supportive care of patient/family members with physical and psychosocial problems associated with the use of alcohol or drugs
4512	Substance Use Treatment: Alcohol Withdrawal	Care of the patient experiencing sudden cessation of alcohol consumption
4514	Substance Use Treatment: Drug Withdrawal	Care of a patient experiencing drug detoxification
4516	Substance Use Treatment: Overdose	Monitoring, treatment, and emotional support of a patient who has ingested prescription or over-the-counter drugs beyond the therapeutic range
6340	Suicide Prevention	Reducing risk of self-inflicted harm with intent to end life
7840	Supply Management	Ensuring acquisition and maintenance of appropriate items for providing patient care
5430	Support Group	Use of a group environment to provide emotional support and health-related information for members
5440	Support System Enhancement	Facilitation of support to patient by family, friends, and community
2900	Surgical Assistance	Assisting the surgeon/dentist with operative procedures and care of the surgical patient
2920	Surgical Precautions	Minimizing the potential for iatrogenic injury to the patient related to a surgical procedure
2930	Surgical Preparation	Providing care to a patient immediately prior to surgery and verifying required procedures/tests and documentation in the clinical record
6650	Surveillance	Purposeful and ongoing acquisition, interpretation, and synthesis of patient data for clinical decision making
6652	Surveillance: Community	Purposeful and ongoing acquisition, interpretation, and synthesis of data for decision making in the community
6656	Surveillance: Late Pregnancy	Purposeful and ongoing acquisition, interpretation, and synthesis of maternal-fetal data for treatment, observation, or admission

NIC Intervention Label | Definition

NIC Intervention Label	Definition
6658 Surveillance: Remote Electronic	Purposeful and ongoing acquisition of patient data via electronic modalities (telephone, video, conferencing, e-mail) from distant locations, as well as interpretation and synthesis of patient data for clinical decision making with individuals or populations
6654 Surveillance: Safety	Purposeful and ongoing collection and analysis of information about the patient and the environment for use in promoting and maintaining patient safety
7500 Sustenance Support	Helping an individual/family in need to locate food, clothing, or shelter
3620 Suturing	Approximating edges of a wound using sterile suture material and a needle
1860 Swallowing Therapy	Facilitating swallowing and preventing complications of impaired swallowing
5602 Teaching: Disease Process	Assisting the patient to understand information related to a specific disease process
5603 Teaching: Foot Care	Preparing a patient at risk and/or significant other to provide preventive foot care
5604 Teaching: Group	Development, implementation, and evaluation of a patient teaching program for a group of individuals experiencing the same health condition
5606 Teaching: Individual	Planning, implementation, and evaluation of a teaching program designed to address a patient's particular needs
5640 Teaching: Infant Nutrition 0-3 Months	Instruction on nutrition and feeding practices through the first three months of life
5641 Teaching: Infant Nutrition 4-6 Months	Instruction on nutrition and feeding practices from the fourth month through the sixth month of life
5642 Teaching: Infant Nutrition 7-9 Months	Instruction on nutrition and feeding practices from the seventh month through the ninth month of life
5643 Teaching: Infant Nutrition 10-12 Months	Instruction on nutrition and feeding practices from the tenth month through the twelfth month of life
5645 Teaching: Infant Safety 0-3 Months	Instruction on safety through the first three months of life
5646 Teaching: Infant Safety 4-6 Months	Instruction on safety from the fourth month through the sixth month of life
5647 Teaching: Infant Safety 7-9 Months	Instruction on safety from the seventh month through the ninth month of life
5648 Teaching: Infant Safety 10-12 Months	Instruction on safety from the tenth month through the twelfth month of life
5655 Teaching: Infant Stimulation 0-4 Months	Teaching parents and caregivers to provide developmentally appropriate sensory activities to promote development and movement through the first four months of life
5656 Teaching: Infant Stimulation 5-8 Months	Teaching parents and caregivers to provide developmentally appropriate sensory activities to promote development and movement from the fifth month through the eighth month of life
5657 Teaching: Infant Stimulation 9-12 Months	Teaching parents and caregivers to provide developmentally appropriate sensory activities to promote development and movement from the ninth month through the twelfth month of life

PART IV - NIC

Continued

NIC Intervention Label | Definition

NIC Intervention Label	Definition
5610 Teaching: Preoperative	Assisting a patient to understand and mentally prepare for surgery and the postoperative recovery period
5612 Teaching: Prescribed Activity/Exercise	Preparing a patient to achieve and/or maintain a prescribed level of activity
5614 Teaching: Prescribed Diet	Preparing a patient to correctly follow a prescribed diet
5616 Teaching: Prescribed Medication	Preparing a patient to safely take prescribed medications and monitor for their effects
5618 Teaching: Procedure/Treatment	Preparing a patient to understand and mentally prepare for a prescribed procedure or treatment
5620 Teaching: Psychomotor Skill	Preparing a patient to perform a psychomotor skill
5622 Teaching: Safe Sex	Providing instruction concerning sexual protection during sexual activity
5624 Teaching: Sexuality	Assisting individuals to understand physical and psychosocial dimensions of sexual growth and development
5660 Teaching: Toddler Nutrition 13-18 Months	Instruction on nutrition and feeding practices from the thirteenth month through the eighteenth month of life
5661 Teaching: Toddler Nutrition 19-24 Months	Instruction on nutrition and feeding practices from the nineteenth month through the twenty-fourth month of life
5662 Teaching: Toddler Nutrition 25-36 Months	Instruction on nutrition and feeding practices from the twenty-fifth month through the thirty-sixth month of life
5665 Teaching: Toddler Safety 13-18 Months	Instruction on safety from the thirteenth month through the eighteenth month of life
5666 Teaching: Toddler Safety 19-24 Months	Instruction on safety from the nineteenth month through the twenty-fourth month of life
5667 Teaching: Toddler Safety 25-36 Months	Instruction on safety from the twenty-fifth month through the thirty-sixth month of life
5634 Teaching: Toilet Training	Instruction on determining the child's readiness and strategies to assist the child to learn independent toileting skills
7880 Technology Management	Use of technical equipment and devices to monitor patient condition or sustain life
8180 Telephone Consultation	Eliciting patient's concerns, listening, and providing support, information, or teaching in response to patient's stated concerns, over the telephone
8190 Telephone Follow-up	Providing results of testing or evaluating patient's response and determining potential for problems as a result of previous treatment, examination, or testing, over the telephone
3900 Temperature Regulation	Attaining and/or maintaining body temperature within a normal range
3902 Temperature Regulation: Intraoperative	Attaining and/or maintaining desired intraoperative body temperature
4430 Therapeutic Play	Purposeful and directive use of toys and other materials to assist children in communicating their perception and knowledge of their world and to help in gaining mastery of their environment
5465 Therapeutic Touch	Attuning to the universal healing field, seeking to act as an instrument for healing influence, and using the natural sensitivity of the hands to gently focus and direct the intervention process

NIC Intervention Label / Definition

NIC Intervention Label		Definition
5450	Therapy Group	Application of psychotherapeutic techniques to a group, including the utilization of interactions between members of the group
4270	Thrombolytic Therapy Management	Collection and analysis of patient data to expedite safe, appropriate provision of an agent that dissolves a thrombus
1200	Total Parenteral Nutrition (TPN) Administration	Preparation and delivery of nutrients intravenously and monitoring of patient responsiveness
5460	Touch	Providing comfort and communication through purposeful tactile contact
0940	Traction/Immobilization Care	Management of a patient who has traction and/or a stabilizing device to immobilize and stabilize a body part
1540	Transcutaneous Electrical Nerve Stimulation (TENS)	Stimulation of skin and underlying tissues with controlled, low-voltage electrical vibration via electrodes
0970	Transfer	Moving a patient with limitation of independent movement
7890	Transport: Interfacility	Moving a patient from one facility to another
7892	Transport: Intrafacility	Moving a patient from one area of a facility to another
5410	Trauma Therapy: Child	Use of an interactive helping process to resolve a trauma experienced by a child
6362	Triage: Disaster	Establishing priorities of patient care for urgent treatment while allocating scarce resources
6364	Triage: Emergency Center	Establishing priorities and initiating treatment for patients in an emergency center
6366	Triage: Telephone	Determining the nature and urgency of a problem(s) and providing directions for the level of care required, over the telephone
5470	Truth Telling	Use of whole truth, partial truth, or decision delay to promote the patient's self-determination and well-being
1870	Tube Care	Management of a patient with an external drainage device exiting the body
1872	Tube Care: Chest	Management of a patient with an external water-seal drainage device exiting the chest cavity
1874	Tube Care: Gastrointestinal	Management of a patient with a gastrointestinal tube
1875	Tube Care: Umbilical Line	Management of a newborn with an umbilical catheter
1876	Tube Care: Urinary	Management of a patient with urinary drainage equipment
1878	Tube Care: Ventriculostomy/Lumbar Drain	Management of a patient with an external cerebrospinal fluid drainage system
6982	Ultrasonography: Limited Obstetric	Performance of ultrasound exams to determine ovarian, uterine, or fetal status
2760	Unilateral Neglect Management	Protecting and safely reintegrating the affected part of the body while helping the patient adapt to disturbed perceptual abilities
0570	Urinary Bladder Training	Improving bladder function for those with urge incontinence by increasing the bladder's ability to hold urine and the patient's ability to suppress urination
0580	Urinary Catheterization	Insertion of a catheter into the bladder for temporary or permanent drainage of urine
0582	Urinary Catheterization: Intermittent	Regular periodic use of a catheter to empty the bladder

Continued

PART IV - NIC

NIC Intervention Label		Definition
0590	Urinary Elimination Management	Maintenance of an optimum urinary elimination pattern
0600	Urinary Habit Training	Establishing a predictable pattern of bladder emptying to prevent incontinence for persons with limited cognitive ability who have urge, stress, or functional incontinence
0610	Urinary Incontinence Care	Assistance in promoting continence and maintaining perineal skin integrity
0612	Urinary Incontinence Care: Enuresis	Promotion of urinary continence in children
0620	Urinary Retention Care	Assistance in relieving bladder distention
6670	Validation Therapy	Use of a method of therapeutic communication used with elderly persons with dementia that focuses on emotional rather than factual content
5480	Values Clarification	Assisting another to clarify her/his own values in order to facilitate effective decision making
9050	Vehicle Safety Promotion	Assisting individuals, families, and communities to increase awareness of measures to reduce unintentional injuries in motorized and nonmotorized vehicle
2440	Venous Access Device (VAD) Maintenance	Management of the patient with prolonged venous access via tunneled and nontunneled (percutaneous) catheters, and implanted ports
3390	Ventilation Assistance	Promotion of an optimal spontaneous breathing pattern that maximizes oxygen and carbon dioxide exchange in the lungs
7560	Visitation Facilitation	Promoting beneficial visits by family and friends
6680	Vital Signs Monitoring	Collection and analysis of cardiovascular, respiratory, and body temperature data to determine and prevent complications
1570	Vomiting Management	Prevention and alleviation of vomiting
1240	Weight Gain Assistance	Facilitating gain of body weight
1260	Weight Management	Facilitating maintenance of optimal body weight and percent body fat
1280	Weight Reduction Assistance	Facilitating loss of weight and/or body fat
3660	Wound Care	Prevention of wound complications and promotion of wound healing
3661	Wound Care: Burns	Prevention of wound complications due to burns and facilitation of wound healing
3662	Wound Care: Closed Drainage	Maintenance of a pressure drainage system at the wound site
3680	Wound Irrigation	Flushing of an open wound to cleanse and remove debris and excessive drainage

Index